Heart Failure:
Pharmacologic Management

*Dedication to*
Susan, Emilykate, Elizabeth Willa

# Heart Failure: Pharmacologic Management

EDITED BY

**Arthur M. Feldman,** MD, PhD

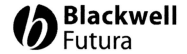

© 2006 by Blackwell Publishing
Blackwell Futura is an imprint of Blackwell Publishing

Blackwell Publishing, Inc., 350 Main Street, Malden, Massachusetts 02148-5020, USA
Blackwell Publishing Ltd, 9600 Garsington Road, Oxford OX4 2DQ, UK
Blackwell Science Asia Pty Ltd, 550 Swanston Street, Carlton, Victoria 3053, Australia

Library of Congress Cataloging-in-Publication Data

Heart failure : pharmacological management / edited by Arthur M.
   Feldman.
    p. ; cm.
   Includes bibliographical references.
   ISBN-13: 978-1-4051-0361-9
   ISBN-10: 1-4051-0361-2
   1. Congestive heart failure–Chemotherapy.   I. Feldman, Arthur
M. (Arthur Michael), 1949–.
   [DNLM: 1. Heart Failure, Congestive–drug therapy.   WG 370 H436535 2006]

RC685.C53H444 2006
616.1′29061–dc22

                                                    2005023990

ISBN-13: 978-1-4051-0361-9
ISBN-10: 1-4051-0361-2

A catalogue record for this title is available from the British Library

Commissioning Editor: Gina Almond
Development Editors: Vicki Donald and Beckie Brand

Set in 9.5/12 Minion by Newgen Imaging Systems (P) Ltd., Chennai, India
Printed and bound in Singapore by C.O.S. Printers Pte Ltd

For further information on Blackwell Publishing, visit our website:
www.blackwellcardiology.com

The publisher's policy is to use permanent paper from mills that operate a sustainable
forestry policy, and which has been manufactured from pulp processed using acid-free and
elementary chlorine-free practices. Furthermore, the publisher ensures that the text paper
and cover board used have met acceptable environmental accreditation standards.

**Notice:** The indications and dosages of all drugs in this book have been recommended in the medical
literature and conform to the practices of the general community. The medications
described do not necessarily have specific approval by the Food and Drug Administration for
use in the diseases and dosages for which they are recommended. The package insert for
each drug should be consulted for use and dosage as approved by the FDA. Because standards
for usage change, it is advisable to keep abreast of revised recommendations, particularly those
concerning new drugs.

# Contents

# Contributors

**Keith D. Aaronson, MD, MSc**
Associate Professor of Internal Medicine
Medical Director, Cardiac Transplant Program
University of Michigan Health System
Ann Arbor, MI, USA

**Abdul Al-Hesayen, MD, FRCPC**
Assistant Professor of Medicine
University of Toronto
Division of Cardiology
St. Michael's Hospital
Toronto, Ontario, Canada

**Bill Ayach, MSc**
FRWQ and Heart and Stroke Foundation Doctoral Fellow
Heart & Stroke/Richard Lewar Centre for Excellence
University of Toronto
Toronto, Ontario, Canada

**Biykem Bozkurt, MD, FACC**
Associate Professor of Medicine
Action Cheif, Section of Cardiology
Department of Medicine
Michael E. DeBakey Veterans Affairs
Medical Center & Winters Center for
   Heart Failure Research
Baylor College of Medicine
Houston, TX, USA

**Michael R. Bristow, MD, PhD**
Co-director, CU-CVI, Denver
Boulder and Aurora, Colorado
S. Gilbert Blount Professor of Medicine (Cardiology)
University of Colorado at Denver and Health Sciences Center
Denver, CO, USA

**Igino Contrafatto, MD**
Keck School of Medicine
University of Southern California
Los Angeles, CA, USA

**Deborah DeEugenio, Pharm D**
Jefferson Heart Institute
Philadelphia, PA, USA

**Anita Deswal, MD, MPH**
Assistant Professor of Medicine
Winters Center for Heart Failure Research
Baylor College of Medicine
Michael E. DeBakey Veterans Affairs Medical Center
Houston, TX, USA

**David H. Ellison, MD**
Head, Division of Nephrology & Hypertension
Professor of Medicine and Physiology & Pharmacology
Oregon Health & Science University
Portland, OR, USA

**Bonita Falkner, MD**
Professor of Medicine
Division of Nephrology
Jefferson Medical College
Philadelphia, PA, USA

**Arthur M. Feldman, MD, PhD**
Magee Professor and Chairman
Department of Medicine
Jefferson Medical College
Philadelphia, PA, USA

**Grace Chan**
Heart & Stroke/Richard Lewar Centre for Excellence
University of Toronto
Toronto, Ontario, Canada

**Koichi Fuse, MD, PhD**
CIHR/HSF TACTICS Research Fellow
Heart & Stroke/Richard Lewar Centre for Excellence
University of Toronto
Toronto, Ontario, Canada

**Olaf Hedrich, MD**
Division of Cardiology
Department of Medicine
Tufts-New England Medical Center
   and Tufts University School of Medicine
Boston, MA, USA

**Ray E. Hershberger,** MD
Professor of Medicine
Director, Heart Failure and Transplant Cardiology
Oregon Health & Science University
Portland, OR, USA

**Mariell Jessup,** MD
Professor of Medicine
University of Pennsylvania School of Medicine
Medical Director, Heart Failure/Transplant program
University of Pennsylvania Health System
Philadelphia, PA, USA

**Marvin A. Konstam,** MD, FACC
Chief of Cardiology
Professor of Medicine and Radiology
Tufts-New England Medical Center
Boston, MA, USA

**Marrick Kukin,** MD
Director, Heart Failure Program
St. Luke's Roosevelt Hospital
Professor of Clinical Medicine
Columbia University College of Physicians & Surgeons
New York, NY, USA

**Peter P. Liu,** MD
Heart and Stroke/Polo Chair Professor
   of Medicine and Physiology
Director, Heart and Stroke/Richard Lewar
Centre of Excellence in Cardiovascular Research
University of Toronto/Toronto General Hospital
Toronto, Ontario, Canada

**Donna M. Mancini,** MD
Professor of Medicine
College of Physicians and Surgeons
Columbia University Columbia
   Presbyterian Medical Center
New York, NY, USA

**Douglas L. Mann,** MD
Don W. Chapman Chair
Professor of Medicine, Molecular
   Physiology and Biophysics
Chief, Section of Cardiology
Baylor College of Medicine
Houston, TX, USA

**Paul J. Mather,** MD
Associate Professor of Medicine
Director, Advanced Heart Failure & Cardiac
   Transplant Center
Jefferson Heart Institute
Jefferson Medical College
Philadelphia, PA, USA

**Dennis M. McNamara,** MD, FACC
Associate Professor of Medicine
Director, Heart Failure/Transplantation Program
University of Pittsburgh Medical Center
Pittsburgh, PA, USA

**Geno J. Merli,** MD, FACP
Ludwig A. Kind Professor
Director, Division of Internal Medicine
Vice Chairman of Clinical Affairs
Department of Medicine
Jefferson Medical College
Philadelphia, PA, USA

**Srinivas Murali,** MD
Professor of Medicine
University of Pittsburgh School of Medicine
Associate Director, Clinical Services
Cardiovascular Institute Director, Heart Failure Network
Director, Pulmonary Hypertension Program
Pittsburgh, PA, USA

**Rimvida Obeleniene,** MD
St. Luke's Roosevelt Hospital
New York, NY, USA

**John D. Parker,** MD, FRCP(C), FACC
Pfizer Chair in Cardiovascular Research
Professor of Medicine and Pharmacology
University of Toronto
Head, Division of Cardiology
UHN and Mount Sinai Hospitals
Toronto, Ontario, Canada

**Theresa Pondok,** MD
Heart Failure Fellow
Jefferson Heart Institute
Thomas Jefferson University Hospital
Philadelphia, PA, USA

**Peter F. Robinson,** MD
Interventional Cardiology Fellow
University of Colorado at Denver
   and Health Sciences Center
Denver, CO, USA

**Alicia Ross,** MD
Fellow, Cardiovascular Medicine
Oregon Health & Science University
Portland, OR, USA

**Sharon Rubin,** MD
Associate Professor of Medicine
Jefferson Heart Institute
Thomas Jefferson University Hospital
Philadelphia, PA, USA

**Jonathan D. Sackner-Bernstein, MD**
Director of Clinical Research
Director of the Heart Failure Prevention Program
North Shore University Hospital
Long Island, NY, USA

**Leslie A. Saxon, MD**
Professor of Clinical Medicine
Director, Cardiac Electrophysiology
Keck School of Medicine
University of Southern California
Los Angeles, CA, USA

**Richard Sheppard, MD**
Assistant Professor of Medicine
McGill University
Division of Cardiology
Sir Mortimer B. Davis-Jewish General Hospital
Montreal, Quebec, Canada

**Hal Skopicki, MD, PhD**
Director of the Center for Cellular
    and Molecular Cardiology
North Shore-LIJ Research Institute
North Shore University Hospital
Long Island, NY, USA

**Rebecca Streeter, MD**
Clinical Cardiology Fellow
College of Physicians and Surgeons
Columbia University
Columbia Presbyterian Medical Center
New York, NY, USA

**Mei Sun, MD, PhD**
Heart and Stroke/ Richard Lewar Centre of Excellence
University of Toronto
Toronto, Ontario, Canada

**James Eric Udelson, MD, FACC**
Associate Chief, Division of Cardiology
Director, Nuclear Cardiology Laboratory
Department of Medicine/Division of Cardiology
Tufts-New England Medical Center
Associate Professor of Medicine and Radiology
Tufts University School of Medicine
Boston, MA, USA

**Howard H. Weitz, MD, FACC, FACP**
Professor of Medicine
Senior Vice Chairman for Academic Affairs
Department of Medicine
Co-Director, Jefferson Heart Institute
Jefferson Medical College
Philadelphia, PA, USA

# Introduction

Twenty years ago in the twenty-first edition of the *Principles and Practice of Medicine*, the authors described what was then the practice for the pharmacologic therapy of patients with heart failure, which included digoxin and a diuretic [1]. In addition, the authors noted that recent studies had supported the potential use of vasodilators in the treatment of this population of patients. Over the past two decades – a very short period of time in the evolution of science – enormous changes have occurred in our therapy for patients with this devastating disease. These changes have occurred in large part because of an explosion in our understanding of the basic biology of heart muscle disease, an increased level of sophistication in performing clinical research to evaluate the efficacy of new drugs and devices for the treatment of heart failure, and an improving understanding of how different genetic, racial, and gender backgrounds can influence a given patient's response to a given drug or device.

Epidemiologic studies have suggested that heart failure is a disease of epidemic proportions [2]. For example, it is estimated that over 550 000 new cases occur each year in the United States and that heart failure accounts for nearly 287 000 deaths (2002 Heart and stroke statistical update. Dallas: American Heart Association, 2001). Cross-sectional studies from large data sets have shown an increase in the point prevalence of heart failure in both the United States and Europe over the past three decades [3–5]. In addition, analyses of the National Health and Nutrition Examination Survey (NHANES) II showed similar trends and showed a prevalence estimate of 1.04% by subject self-report and 1.78% clinical evaluation in the US population [6]. More recently, McCullough and colleagues used administrative data sets from a large vertically integrated mixed model managed care organization

to assess the incidence of heart failure in a community setting [7]. They found that heart failure was a disease of epidemic proportion whose prevalence had increased over the previous decade. In addition, it has recently been demonstrated that the lifetime risk for developing heart failure is one in five for both men and women with risks being one in nine for men and one in six for women in the absence of a history of a myocardial infarction [8].

Despite the marked incidence of heart failure in the US population, recent epidemiologic studies suggest that 20 years of drug discovery has had an impact on the outcomes associated with this disease (and potentially on disease incidence by better control of risk factors). For example, the Framingham Heart Study demonstrated that over the past 50 years, the incidence of heart failure declined among women but not among men [9]. More importantly, survival after heart failure improved for both sexes with an overall improvement in the survival rate after the onset of heart failure of 12% per decade. Indeed, survival has improved to such an extent that clinicians have called for a reevaluation of the listing criteria for patients undergoing cardiac transplantation [10]. However, heart failure remains a progressive disease. Thus even patients with asymptomatic left ventricular dysfunction are at risk for symptomatic heart failure and death, even when only a mild impairment in ventricular function is present [11].

As will be described in the chapters of this text, a series of clinical trials have also demonstrated significant improvements in survivals as the baseline therapy for each of these trials changed. For example, the 2-year mortality rate in patients who had chronic heart failure, an ejection fraction of <45%, cardiac dilation, and reduced exercise tolerance and who were receiving digoxin and a diuretic in the Veterans Administration

Cooperative Study was 34% [12]. In the consensus trial, patients with severe heart failure symptoms who were receiving digoxin and a diuretic (and in some cases a vasodilator) had a 1-year moral— ity of 52% and a 6-month mortality of 44%. By contrast, patients with moderate to severe heart fail— ure symptoms receiving an angiotensin converting enzyme (ACE) inhibitor and a beta-blocker in the BEST trial had an annual mortality of 15% [13]. Furthermore, patients with moderate to severe heart failure symptoms receiving an ACE inhibitor, a beta-blocker, and an aldosterone antagonist in the recent COMPANION trial had a 1-year mortality of <10% [14]. Thus, while heart failure remains a dis— ease of epidemic proportions in the United States, our opportunity to improve both the length of life as well as the quality of the life of patients with this disease has improved remarkably over the past two decades.

An important concept that has received increas— ing attention is the finding that a large proportion of patients with the signs and symptoms of heart failure, that is, shortness of breath, edema, and fatigue actually have preserved left ventricular func— tion. Indeed, recent studies suggest that nearly half of all patients with symptoms of heart fail— ure have preserved left ventricular systolic function [15–17]. This finding is most commonly attrib— uted to patients who are older and are female [18]. Despite the fact that these patients have preserved function, their risk of readmission, disability, and symptoms subsequent to hospital discharge are comparable to that of heart failure patients with depressed systolic performance [19]. Indeed, in patients hospitalized with worsening heart failure, long-term prognosis was worse for patients with normal systolic function that for those with dimin— ished systolic performance despite a lower number of comorbidities [20]. Despite the increasing evid— ence of the importance of heart failure in patients with preserved systolic performance – and presum— ably diastolic dysfunction – there is little consensus regarding appropriate treatment strategies in these patients. Most studies that have been carried out to date are either small in size, nonrandomized or anecdotal. Thus, in this book we will focus largely on patients with heart failure secondary to systolic dysfunction, in whom seminal clinical trials have pointed the way in terms of treatment strategies.

However, where appropriate we will point out the potential role for pharmacologic agents in the ther— apy of patients with heart failure and preserved left ventricular function.

Despite the advances that have been made in the pharmacologic treatment of heart failure, the increasing armamentarium that is now in the hands of the practicing physician provides an interest— ing conundrum – how does one choose between the increasingly large number of treatment options, where does one start in a newly diagnosed patient, how does one monitor treatment once it is begun, and what are the side-effect profiles of these agents. Thus, the objective of this textbook is to act as an informative guide for the practicing physician in order that they be able to optimize their use of pharmacologic therapy in the treatment of patients with heart failure. In the chapters that follow, we have attempted to provide both the biologic and pathologic underpinning for the use of each pharmacologic agent currently recommended for the treatment of patients with heart failure, as well as provide an in depth presentation of the clinical investigations that have led to our under— standing of the risks and benefits associated with the use of these drugs. While the initial chapters focus on agents that have been well-characterized and are considered "standard care" for the patient with heart failure (i.e. diuretics, ACE inhibitors, angiotensin receptor antagonists, aldosterone ant— agonists, and beta-blockers), we have also included discussions of several agents that are currently under investigation (e.g. Vasopressin antagonists, erythropoietin) – but which we believe will have an important impact in the future. In addition, we have provided didactic discussion regarding the use of a group of agents about which there is some controversy, including inotropic agents, anti— arrhythmic drugs, and anticoagulants. We have also included a discussion on the emerging field of phar— macogenetics and how studies of the genetic profile of patients help us understand which patient pop— ulations are most likely to respond to a given class of drugs. Indeed, it is hoped that the emergence of pharmacogenetics will allow physicians to tailor design a pharmacologic regimen – avoiding those drugs (and their attendant risks) that will not add benefit and allowing the practitioner to optimize the dosing of those drugs that will add benefit based on a patients genotype. Finally, in the penultimate chapter of this book we have provided an algorithm for the physician that will help them utilize what has now become multidrug pharmacy for heart failure therapy.

This book could not have been completed without the commitment of each of the authors to provide a text that was informative and substantive and could provide the reader with up-to-date information that could allow them to understand the biologic and investigative basis for the rational use for heart failure drugs. In addition, the author thanks Marianne LaRussa for her technical and administrative assistance, editorial assistance and proof-reading.

## References

1 Harvey AM, Osler W. *The Principles and Practice of Medicine.* 21st edn. Conn.: Appleton-Century-Crofts, Norwalk, 1984.

2 Redfield MM. Heart failure – an epidemic of uncertain proportions. *N Engl J Med* 2002;**347**:1442–1444.

3 Hoes AW, Mosterd A, Grobbee DE. An epidemic of heart failure? Recent evidence from Europe. *Eur Heart J* 1998;**19**:L2–9.

4 Kannel WB, Ho K, Thom T. Changing epidemiological features of cardiac failure. *Br Heart J* 1994;**72**:S3–9.

5 Parameshwar J, Shackell MM, Richardson A, Poole-Wilson PA, Sutton GC. Prevalence of heart failure in three general practices in north west London. *Br J Gen Pract* 1992;**42**:287–289.

6 Schocken DD, Arrieta MI, Leaverton PE, Ross EA. Prevalence and mortality rate of congestive heart failure in the United States. *J Am Coll Cardiol* 1992;**20**:301–306.

7 McCullough PA, Philbin EF, Spertus JA, Kaatz S, Sandberg KR, Weaver WD. Confirmation of a heart failure epidemic: findings from the Resource Utilization Among Congestive Heart Failure (REACH) study. *J Am Coll Cardiol* 2002;**39**:60–69.

8 Lloyd-Jones DM, Larson MG, Leip EP *et al.* Lifetime risk for developing congestive heart failure: the Framingham Heart Study. *Circulation* 2002;**106**:3068–3072.

9 Levy D, Kenchaiah S, Larson MG *et al.* Long-term trends in the incidence of and survival with heart failure. *N Engl J Med* 2002;**347**:1397–1402.

10 Butler J, Khadim G, Paul KM *et al.* Selection of patients for heart transplantation in the current era of heart failure therapy. *J Am Coll Cardiol* 2004;**43**:787–793.

11 Wang TJ, Evans JC, Benjamin EJ, Levy D, LeRoy EC, Vasan RS. Natural history of asymptomatic left ventricular systolic dysfunction in the community. *Circulation* 2003;**108**:977–982.

12 Cohn JN, Archibald DG, Ziesche S *et al.* Effect of vasodilator therapy on mortality in chronic congestive heart failure. Results of a Veterans Administration Cooperative Study. *N Engl J Med* 1986;**314**:1547–1552.

13 A trial of the beta-blocker bucindolol in patients with advanced chronic heart failure. *N Engl J Med* 2001;**344**:1659–1667.

14 Bristow MR, Saxon LA, Boehmer J *et al.* Cardiac-resynchronization therapy with or without an implantable defibrillator in advanced chronic heart failure. *N Engl J Med* 2004;**350**:2140–2150.

15 Senni M, Tribouilloy CM, Rodeheffer RJ *et al.* Congestive heart failure in the community: a study of all incident cases in Olmsted County, Minnesota, in 1991. *Circulation* 1998;**98**:2282–2289.

16 Vasan RS, Larson MG, Benjamin EJ, Evans JC, Reiss CK, Levy D. Congestive heart failure in subjects with normal versus reduced left ventricular ejection fraction: prevalence and mortality in a population-based cohort. *J Am Coll Cardiol* 1999;**33**:1948–1955.

17 Kitzman DW, Gardin JM, Gottdiener JS *et al.* Importance of heart failure with preserved systolic function in patients ≥65 years of age. CHS Research Group. Cardiovascular Health Study. *Am J Cardiol* 2001;**87**:413–419.

18 Masoudi FA, Havranek EP, Smith G *et al.* Gender, age, and heart failure with preserved left ventricular systolic function. *J Am Coll Cardiol* 2003;**41**:217–223.

19 Smith GL, Masoudi FA, Vaccarino V, Radford MJ, Krumholz HM. Outcomes in heart failure patients with preserved ejection fraction: mortality, readmission, and functional decline. *J Am Coll Cardiol* 2003;**41**:1510–1518.

20 Varadarajan P, Pai RG. Prognosis of congestive heart failure in patients with normal versus reduced ejection fractions: results from a cohort of 2,258 hospitalized patients. *J Card Fail* 2003;**9**:107–112.

# CHAPTER 1

# Diuretics in congestive heart failure

*Alicia Ross,* MD, *Ray E. Hershberger,* MD *& David H. Ellison,* MD

## Introduction

Diuretics (see Table 1.1 for a physiological classification) remain an important part of the medical therapy for patients with congestive heart failure (CHF). They control fluid retention and rapidly relieve the congestive symptoms of heart failure (HF). The American College of Cardiology/American Heart Association assigned them a class I indication in patients with symptomatic heart failure who have evidence of fluid retention [1]. Indeed, diuretics are the only drugs used in the treatment of HF that control fluid retention and that rapidly produce symptomatic benefits in patients with pulmonary and/or peripheral edema. Because diuretics alone are unable to effect clinical stability in patients with HF, they should always be used in combination with an angiotensin converting enzyme (ACE) inhibitor and a $\beta$-blocker. Despite the widespread use of diuretics, there have yet to be large randomized clinical trials that evaluate their effects on mortality or morbidity (with the exception of aldosterone antagonists, which will be considered separately). Furthermore, care must be exercised in the use of diuretics as both hypovolemia secondary to over-diuresis and hypervolemia secondary to under-diuresis have profound effects on cardiac pathophysiology. Therefore, questions remain about appropriate diuretic use [2]. This chapter will explore the effects, pharmacokinetics, and clinical utility of diuretics in patients with congestive heart failure.

## Vascular effects of diuretics

Diuretics are believed to improve symptoms of congestion by several mechanisms. Loop diuretics induce hemodynamic changes that appear to be independent of their diuretic effect. They act as venodilators and, when giving intravenously, reduce right atrial and pulmonary capillary wedge pressure within minutes [3,4]. This initial improvement in hemodynamics may be secondary to the release of vasodilatory prostaglandins [5]. Studies in animals and humans have demonstrated that the loop diuretic furosemide directly dilates veins; this effect can be inhibited by indomethacin, suggesting that local prostaglandins may contribute to its vasodilatory properties [6]. In the setting of acute pulmonary edema from myocardial infarction, Dikshit *et al.* measured an increase in venous capacitance and decreasing pulmonary capillary wedge pressure within 15 min of furosemide infusion, while the peak diuretic effect was at 30 min [7]. Numerous other investigators have found similar results [8]. Other loop diuretics, such as bumetanide, have been reported to have differing effects [9]. There have also been reports of an arteriolar vasoconstrictor response to diuretics when given to patients with advanced heart failure [10]. A rise in plasma renin and norepinephrine levels leads to arteriolar vasoconstriction, resulting in reduction in cardiac output and increase in pulmonary capillary wedge pressure. These hemodynamic changes reverse over the next several hours, likely due to the diuresis. The vasoconstrictor response to loop

**Table 1.1** Physiological classification of diuretic drugs.

| Proximal diuretics | Loop diuretics | DCT diuretics | CD diuretics | Aquaretics |
|---|---|---|---|---|
| Carbonic anhydrase inhibitors | Na–K–2Cl (NKCC2) inhibitors | Na–Cl (NCCT) inhibitors | Na channel blockers (ENaC inhibitors) | Vasopressin receptor antagonists |
| Acetazolamide | Furosemide | Hydrochlorothiazide | Amiloride | Tolvaptan |
| | Bumetanide | Metolazone | Triamterene | Lixivaptan |
| | Torsemide | Chlorthalidone | Aldosterone antagonists | |
| | Ethacrynic acid | Indapamide* | Spironolactone | |
| | | Many others | Eplerenone | |

*Indapamide may have other actions as well.

DCT: Distal convoluted tubule. CD: Collecting duct. Aquaretics are pending approval for clinical use.

diuretic administration occurs more commonly in patients treated chronically with loop diuretics [10]. In this situation, chronic stimulation of the renal renin/angiotensin/aldosterone axis may prime the vascular system to vasoconstriction. It is likely that different diuretics have complex and multifactorial actions on the vascular system.

## Neurohormonal effects of diuretics

Diuretic drugs stimulate the renin–angiotensin–aldosterone (RAA) axis via several mechanisms. Loop diuretics stimulate renin secretion by inhibiting NaCl uptake into macula densa cells. Sodium/chloride uptake via the loop diuretic-sensitive $Na^+–K^+–2Cl^-$ cotransport system is a central component of the macula densa-mediated pathway for renin secretion [11]. Blocking $Na^+–K^+–2Cl^-$ uptake at the macula densa stimulates renin secretion directly, leading to a volume–independent increase in angiotensin II and aldosterone secretion. Loop diuretics also stimulate renal production of prostacyclin, which further enhances renin secretion. All diuretics can also increase renin secretion by contracting the extracellular fluid (ECF) volume, thereby stimulating the vascular mechanism of renin secretion. ECF volume contraction also inhibits the secretion of atrial natriuretic peptide. Among its other effects, atrial natriuretic peptide inhibits renin release. Interestingly, the combination of aggressive vasodilator therapy and diuresis to achieve improved hemodynamic parameters in turn led to diminished neurohormonal activation [12].

## Clinical use of diuretics in congestive heart failure

The mortality benefit of ACE inhibitors (or angiotensin receptor blockers) and $\beta$-adrenergic blockers in patients with systolic dysfunction is well documented (see Chapter 4). However, all recent heart failure mortality trials have included patients who were treated with diuretics as diuretics remain an important part of heart failure management. According to the SOLVD (Studies of Left Ventricular Dysfunction) registry, diuretics are the most commonly prescribed drugs for heart failure, used by 62% of patients [13].

When loop diuretics were introduced in the 1960s, they had a significant impact on heart failure treatment. They allowed the physician to aggressively treat fluid retention. However, few multicenter and randomized trials were carried out to assess the efficacy of diuretics and they rapidly became a standard part of the management of patients with this disease [14]. Indeed, it was not until the introduction of ACE inhibitors and elucidation of the neurohormonal pathophysiology of heart failure that regulatory mandates required that new drugs be evaluated with large randomized and placebo-controlled trials. By that time, it was clear to clinicians that diuretics dramatically improve the symptoms of congestion and they had become an inseparable part of the heart failure pharmacopeia.

Although diuretics have not been shown to improve survival in patients with heart failure (a trial that would now be considered unethical), investigators have attempted to gain a better understanding of the long-term benefits and risks of diuretic use from smaller clinical trials. For example, Odemuyiwa *et al.* [15] demonstrated that diuretic requirements did not decline after the addition of ACE inhibitors in patients with stable heart failures symptoms. Similarly, Grinstead *et al.* [16] evaluated 41 patients with stable, but symptomatic heart failure. After discontinuing diuretic therapy, patients were randomized to either lisinopril or placebo. Of this, 71% of patients restarted diuretic therapy because of worsening symptoms; however, there was no significant difference between the number of patients who restarted therapy in the placebo or lisinopril group. Interestingly, a baseline daily furosemide dose of >40 mg, a left ventricular ejection fraction <27%, and a history of systemic hypertension were independently predictive of the need for diuretic reinitiation.

It is tempting to think that ACE inhibitors would reduce extracellular fluid volume in the absence of other pharmacologic agents; however, in many cases they require the synergistic action of other drugs. The explanation for this paradox lies in the fact that, while diuretics shift the renal function curve to the left (Figure 1.1), permitting sodium excretion to increase at a constant mean arterial pressure and constant dietary salt intake, ACE inhibitors not only shift the renal function curve to the left but also reduce mean arterial pressure through peripheral vasodilation. Thus, in the absence of diuretics, ACE inhibitors are unable to effect a change in urinary sodium excretion because the shift in the renal function curve is offset by the reduction in blood pressure.

In another study that evaluated the effectiveness of diuretic therapy in patients with heart failure, Walma and colleagues evaluated the effects of diuretic withdrawal in a group of 202 elderly patients who were minimally symptomatic and who had not had a recent episode of worsening heart failure [17]. The subjects in this study were randomized to either continued therapy with a diuretic or discontinuation of their diuretic therapy. Diuretic reinstitution was required in 50 of 102 patients in the withdrawal group and 13 of 100 patients in the control arm. Heart failure was the most frequent cause of reinitiating diuretic therapy and 65% of patients who were originally prescribed diuretics for heart failure needed reinitiation of diuretic therapy during the trial. The authors concluded that

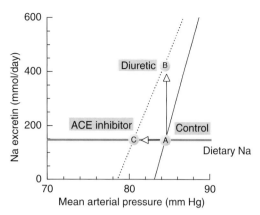

**Figure 1.1** Comparison of diuretic and ACE inhibitor effects on sodium (Na) excretion and mean arterial pressure. The figure shows two 'chronic renal function curves' relating dietary Na intake (grey line), urinary Na excretion (ordinate) and mean arterial pressure (abscissa). At baseline (point A), the urinary Na excretion equals dietary Na intake. Both diuretics and ACE inhibitors shift the renal function curve to the left (from the solid to the dotted line). Diuretics do not reduce arterial pressure directly, therefore urinary Na excretion rises (move from point A to point B). In contrast, ACE inhibitors reduce mean arterial pressure as well as shift the renal function curve, so urinary Na excretion is unchanged (move from point A to point C).

clinicians should be cautious while withdrawing diuretic therapy and when withdrawal is required it should be accompanied by assiduous monitoring, especially during the first 4 weeks after therapy is discontinued.

Important information regarding the use of diuretics also come from a number of large multicenter clinical trials that evaluated chronic therapy with diuretics in patients with hypertension, an important risk factor in the development of heart failure. In the Stop Hypertension in the Elderly Program (SHEP) [18], 4736 persons with isolated systolic hypertension were randomized to receive chlorthalidone, a thiazide-like diuretic, versus placebo, in a stepwise approach. The incidence of heart failure was reduced in the active group by 53% with 48 events being seen in the active treatment group and 102 events in the placebo group. Treatment with a diuretic compared to a calcium channel blocker or an ACE inhibitor was also evaluated in the Antihypertensive and Lipid-Lowering Treatment to Prevent Heart Attack Trial (ALLHAT) [19]. Chlorthalidone was superior to amlodipine in preventing the development of heart failure. The amlodipine group had a 38% ($p < 0.001$) higher risk of heart failure and a 6-year absolute risk difference of 2.5%. When all major long-term hypertension treatment trials were reviewed to evaluate the effects of diuretics on the development of heart failure, diuretics were found to decrease the risk of heart failure by 52% [20,21]. Thus, though indirect, the experience in hypertension supports the hypothesis that diuretics are beneficial in patients with heart failure as well as those at high risk of its development.

## Adverse effects associated with diuretic use

The adverse effects associated with the use of diuretics are reviewed in Table 1.2. However, the two most serious consequences of diuretic use are the development of arrhythmias and electrolyte abnormalities – the two being linked in many instances.

### Arrhythmias
Numerous studies have demonstrated an increased incidence of arrhythmias with the use of non-potassium-sparing diuretics [22]. Siscovick *et al.* demonstrated in a population-based case-control study that the presence and dose of thiazide diuretics was associated with an increased risk of primary cardiac arrest [23]. The SOLVD investigators similarly found that the baseline use of non-potassium-sparing diuretics was associated with an increased risk of arrhythmic death, while potassium-sparing diuretic use was not associated with an increased risk [24]. The presence or absence of ACE inhibitors or potassium supplementation did not affect this relationship and there was not a significant difference in potassium levels between patients who were receiving or not receiving an ACE inhibitor.

### Electrolyte abnormalities and other metabolic sequelae of diuretics
#### Hyponatremia
Hyponatremia develops in the setting of congestive heart failure because of the accumulation of excess free water within the vascular spaces. Free water retention occurs in the setting of increased tubular absorption of sodium and activation of the renin–angiotensin–aldosterone axis [2]. Water retention is caused at least in part by increased

Table 1.2 Complications of diuretics.

| Complications | Preventive measures |
| --- | --- |
| Electrolyte abnormalities | Periodic electrolyte monitoring when actively |
| Hypokalemia | diuresing or adjusting ACE inhibitor dose |
| Hyponatremia | |
| Hypomagnesemia | |
| | Caution with potassium-sparing diuretics |
| Arrhythmias | Keep serum K 4.0–5.0 |
| Extracellular fluid volume depletion | Daily weights |
| Metabolic alkalosis | Regular assessment by clinician |
| Azotemia | Regular assessment by clinician |
| | Medication review, that is, NSAIDs, etc. |
| Glucose intolerance | Regular assessment by clinician |
| Hyperlipidemia | |
| Hyperuricemia | |
| Erectile dysfunction | |
| Otoxicity | Limit rapid boluses, especially in uremia, use of aminoglycosides |
| | Limit rate of furosemide infusion to less than 240 mg/h |
| Progressive heart failure | Regular assessment by clinician |

levels of vasopressin and subsequent activation of vasopressin receptors in the kidney. Diuretics can contribute to the stimulation of vasopressin by reducing effective arterial volume [25,26]. Indeed, it has been recognized clinically that many patients enter the hospital with normal serum sodium, but develop hyponatremia after receiving aggressive diuresis with loop diuretics. Recent studies have demonstrated that even modest decreases in serum sodium (130 to 135 mEq/L) are associated with a worse outcome in patients hospitalized for worsening heart failure.

The management of hyponatremia includes efforts to improve cardiac function, decrease volume overload, and to restrict free water intake. Some patients may require intravenous inotropic support and/or low doses of dopamine to improve renal perfusion. Because hyponatremia is driven at least inpart by an impairment in effective arterial blood volume, the addition of an ACE inhibitor may lead to an improvement in the serum sodium level [27]. The recent development of vasopressin receptor antagonists (so-called aquaretic agents) shows promise in treating the water retention of heart failure and may become an important component of the treatment regimen for hyponatremic patients with heart failure [28,29]. The potential role for vasopressin antagonists will be discussed in Chapter 13.

## Disorders of potassium balance

Activation of the renin–angiotensin–aldosterone system leads to hypokalemia because of augmented exchange of sodium for potassium in the renal tubule [2]. Non-potassium-sparing diuretics potentiate this hypokalemia by presenting an increased sodium load to the distal tubule. This leads to urinary excretion of potassium, which has been associated with further activation of the renin–angiotensin–aldosterone axis [30]. As a result, many patients with chronic heart failure develop a reduction in whole-body potassium stores as potassium is released from intracellular storage pools in order to help balance the levels of potassium in the peripheral circulation. Aggressive diuresis in the setting of chronic hypokalemia can further reduce serum potassium levels. Hypokalemia is a significant risk factor for the development of malignant arrhythmias [4]. Although

not evaluated in a randomized, prospective trial, many experts believe that in patients with CHF, potassium concentrations should be maintained in the range of 4.5 to 5.0 mEq/L [2]. Historically, most heart failure patients who were receiving a loop diuretic were prescribed a potassium supplement. However, the incidence of hypokalemia in heart failure patients appears to be decreasing, with the wide utilization of ACE inhibitors/ARBs together with $\beta$-blockers and aldosterone antagonists. Indeed, a recent survey showed substantial increases in the rates of hospitalization for potentially harmful hyperkalemia as a result of increased utilization of aldosterone antagonists [31], an area that will be discussed in further detail in the chapter on the use of aldosterone antagonists. Preexisting serum potassium concentrations above 4 mM or even mild chronic kidney disease should prompt special caution in the use of potassium-sparing agents.

## Hypomagnesemia

Hypomagnesemia develops by similar mechanisms to hypokalemia; however, the importance of hypomagnesemia in heart failure is less well established. Hypomagnesemia has been associated with an increase in ectopy and mortality is some small trials; however, hypomagnesaemia was not associated with an increase in mortality in the large Prospective Randomized Milrinone Survival Evaluation (PROMISE) trial. Parenthetically, the presence of hypomagnesaemia is difficult to assess as there is poor correlation between serum and tissue magnesium concentrations [32]. Magnesium deficiency is less common in mild to moderate HF; however, there are several populations that are more susceptible including post cardiac transplant patients, patients in intensive care units, and patients with moderately severe to severe symptoms requiring hospitalization, high dose diuretic therapy, or patients who have coexisting hypokalemia [2]. Magnesium replacement should be strongly considered in these populations.

## Progressive heart failure

Because diuretic use is associated with activation of the renin–angiotensin–aldosterone system, there is reason to believe that its use may promote the progression of heart failure. In a retrospective analysis of the SOLVD trial, the risk of hospitalization for, or death from, worsening CHF was significantly increased in patients receiving non-potassium sparing diuretics (i.e. loop diuretics) compared to those patients not being treated with a diuretic or receiving a potassium sparing diuretic [13]. The investigators proposed that loop diuretics induce a loss of sodium that in turn activates the renin–angiotensin system and thereby contributes to disease progression. Thus, diuretics should always be used in conjunction with inhibitors of the renin–angiotensin system including ACE inhibitors, $\beta$-blockers, and an aldosterone inhibitor when appropriate.

## Practical considerations for the use of diuretics

### Diuretic choice and dosing

Most patients with a current evidence of volume overload or a history of fluid retention should be treated with a diuretic in combination with an ACE inhibitor and a $\beta$-blocker. In patients with new onset of fluid retention, a diuretic should be the first drug used as it will provide the most rapid improvement in symptoms. Some authors suggest that patients with mild symptoms should initially be treated with a thiazide diuretic [33]; however, there are no objective data to support this approach and many heart failure specialists believe that the thiazide diuretics have too little potency in a heart failure population. When patients have moderate to severe heart failure symptoms or renal insufficiency, a loop diuretic is required. Outpatient treatment should begin with low doses of diuretic with incremental increases in the dose until urine output increases and weight decreases ($\sim$1.0 kg/day). Some patients may develop hypotension or azotemia during diuretic therapy. While the rapidity of diuresis should be slowed in these patients therapy should be maintained at a lower level until euvolemia has been attained, as persistent volume overload may limit and/or compromise the effectiveness of other agents and persistently high filling pressures can enhance maladaptive cardiac remodeling.

A typical starting dose is 20 mg of furosemide in patients with normal renal function, although doses of 40–80 mg may be necessary. Further increases

in dose may be required to maintain urine output and weight loss. In patients with renal insufficiency, larger starting doses are often necessary, such as 40–80 mg of furosemide that may be increased up to 160 mg. Ceiling doses of loop diuretics in treating heart failure, single doses that appear to be maximally effective, have been described [33]. For furosemide, the maximal doses are 40–80 mg IV (160–240 mg PO). For torsemide, the maximal doses are 20–50 mg IV or PO. For bumetanide, the maximal doses are 2–3 mg IV or PO. Because of the steep dose-response curve for loop diuretics, an adequate dose is necessary that causes a clear diuretic response. Some experts recommend doubling the dose until this effect is demonstrated.

Although furosemide is the most commonly used loop diuretic, there are several limitations to its use. For example, its oral bioavailability is only approximately 50% and there is significant intra- and interpatient variability [34]. In patients with hepatic and bowel edema, the bioavailability of furosemide may be markedly decreased because of decreased gastric absorption. Therefore, some clinicians favor the use of bumetanide or torsemide because of their increased and more predictable bioavailability [35].

All of the commonly used loop diuretics are short acting. In CHF, the half-lives of these drugs are increased, but still less than 3 h [34]. After the period of diuresis, the diuretic concentration declines below its threshold and renal sodium reabsorption is no longer inhibited and "postdiuretic NaCl retention" begins [36]. If a patient is not restricting sodium intake, this retention can overtake the original diuresis. For this reason, loop diuretics usually need to be given at least twice daily and salt restriction is an important component of therapy. In addition, patients receiving diuretic therapy should monitor their weight on a daily basis.

### Diuretic resistance

An edematous patient may be deemed resistant to diuretic drugs when moderate doses of a loop diuretic do not achieve the desired reduction in ECF volume as noted by a change in weight, the amount of edema, the degree of liver enlargement, or the jugular venous pressure. Before labeling the patient as 'resistant' to diuretics and considering intensive diuretic therapy or combination therapy, it is important to exclude reversible causes. An inadequate ECF volume reduction does not necessarily indicate an inadequate natriuretic response (see Figure 1.1), Loop diuretics may induce natriuresis without contracting the ECF volume, if dietary NaCl intake is excessive. It should also be emphasized that the 'desired' ECF volume may not lead to an edema-free state; some patients may require a modest amount of peripheral edema to maintain adequate cardiac output: such patients may need to be counseled regarding local measures to reduce edema (support stockings, keeping the feet elevated) and the willingness to tolerate mild edema. When needed, however, intensive diuretic treatment is usually effective in reducing the ECF volume; each of the different approaches to intensive therapy is best employed under specific circumstances.

## Combination diuretic therapy

A common and useful method for treating the diuretic resistant patient is to administer two classes of diuretic drug simultaneously. For this discussion, it is assumed that the patient is already being given a loop diuretic at maximal or near maximal doses. Although some authors have advocated alternating two members of the same diuretic class together (such as ethacrynic acid and furosemide) controlled trials suggest little or no benefit from such an approach [37]. In contrast, adding a proximal tubule diuretic or a distal convoluted tubule diuretic (DCT) to a regimen of loop diuretics is often dramatically effective [38–40]. DCT diuretics (thiazides and the like) are the class of drugs most commonly added to loop diuretics and this combination has proven remarkably effective. The combination of loop and DCT diuretics has been shown to be synergistic (the combination is more effective than the sum of the effects of each drug alone) in formal permutation trials [41].

Adding a DCT diuretic to a regimen that includes loop diuretics may enhance NaCl excretion by several mechanisms, none of which is mutually exclusive. DCT diuretics do not appear to potentiate the effects of loop diuretics by altering their pharmacokinetics or bioavailability [42], but DCT diuretics do have longer half-lives than do loop diuretics. The first mechanism responsible for the efficacy of combination therapy is that DCT diuretics may prevent or attenuate postdiuretic NaCl retention. As shown in Figure 1.2, the natriuretic effects of a single dose of furosemide, bumetanide, and to a lesser extent torsemide, generally cease within 6 h. Before the next dose of diuretic is administered, intense renal NaCl retention frequently occurs (so called postdiuretic NaCl retention); this NaCl retention can be attenuated by DCT diuretics, which will continue to inhibit renal NaCl absorption after the loop diuretic has worn off. A second mechanism by which DCT diuretics potentiate the effects of loop diuretics is by inhibiting salt transport along the proximal tubule. When the kidney is strongly stimulated to retain NaCl, proximal NaCl reabsorption is enhanced. Most thiazide diuretics inhibit carbonic anhydrase, thereby reducing Na and fluid reabsorption along the proximal tubule. This leads to increase Na and fluid delivery to the loop of Henle [43], which leads to increases in delivery of $Na^+$ and $Cl^-$ into the collecting duct system. Because the loop diuretic drug is inhibiting loop segment solute reabsorption, the delivery of solute to the distal nephron will be greatly magnified. The importance of carbonic anhydrase inhibition in diuretic synergism is documented by the efficacy of carbonic anhydrase inhibitors (e.g. acetazolamide) when added to loop diuretics. Although carbonic anhydrase inhibitors are relatively weak diuretics when administered alone, they can be very potent when added to a regimen of a loop diuretic [44].

A third mechanism by which DCT diuretics may potentiate the effects of loop diuretics is by inhibiting NaCl transport along the distal convoluted tubule. Chronic loop diuretic administration leads to hypertrophy and hyperplasia of distal convoluted tubule cells, increasing their NaCl reabsorptive capacity by up to threefold [45–47]. Because DCT diuretics can inhibit thiazide-sensitive $Na^+/Cl^-$ cotransport completely even under these stimulated conditions [45], the effects of the DCT diuretics will be greatly magnified in the patient who has developed distal nephron hypertrophy from high doses of loop diuretics. Loon and colleagues [48] showed that the effect of chlorothiazide on urinary $Na^+$ excretion in humans is enhanced by one month's prior treatment with furosemide.

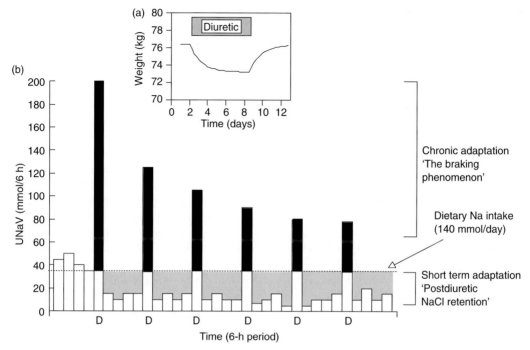

**Figure 1.2** Effects of diuretics on urinary Na excretion and ECF volume. (a) Effect of diuretic on body weight, taken as an index of ECF volume. Note that steady state is reached within 6–8 days despite continued diuretic administration. (b) Effects of loop diuretic on urinary Na excretion. Bars represent 6-h periods before (in Na balance) and after doses loop diuretic (D). The dotted line indicates dietary Na intake. The solid portion of the bars indicate the amount by which Na excretion exceeds intake during natriuresis. The hatched areas indicate the amount of positive Na balance after the diuretic effect has worn off. Net Na balance during 24 h is the difference between the hatched are (postdiuretic NaCl retention) and the solid area (diuretic-induced natriureisis). Chronic adaptation is indicated by progressively smaller peak natriuretic effects (The braking phenomenon) and is mirrored by a return to neutral balance [as indicated in (a)] where the solid and hatched areas are equal. As discussed in the text, chronic adaptation requires ECF volume depletion.

These data suggest that daily oral furosemide treatment, even in modest doses, may be sufficient to induce adaptive changes along the distal nephron, changes that may be treated with combination drug therapy.

The choice of drugs for combination diuretic therapy has been controversial [40,44,49–53]. In most cases, it is appropriate to add a DCT diuretic to a regimen of a loop diuretic. Alternative approaches, however, are appropriate in some circumstances and will be discussed later. In general, when a second class of diuretic is added, the dose of loop diuretic should not be altered. The shape of the dose-response curve to loop diuretics is not affected by the addition of other diuretics and the loop diuretic must be given in an effective or maximal safe dose. The choice of DCT diuretic that is to be added is arbitrary. Many clinicians choose metolazone

because its half-life, in the commonly employed formulation, is longer than that of some other DCT diuretics and because it has been reported to remain effective even when the glomerular filtration rate is low. Yet, direct comparisons between metolazone and several traditional thiazides have shown little difference in natriuretic potency when included in a regimen with loop diuretics in patients with congestive heart failure [51].

The DCT diuretics may be added in full doses (50–100 mg/day hydrochlorothiazide or 10 mg/day metolazone, see Table 1.3) when a rapid and robust response is needed, but such an approach is likely to lead to complications unless follow-up is assiduous. This approach should be reserved for hospitalized patients since fluid and electrolyte depletion may be excessive. Indeed, in one review of combination diuretic therapy, side effects were noted

**Table 1.3** Combination diuretic therapy.

| *To a maximal dose of a loop diuretic add* |
| --- |
| Distal convoluted tubule diuretics: |
|    metolazone 2.5–10 mg PO daily* |
|    hydrochlorothiazide (or equivalent) 25–100 mg PO daily |
|    chlorothiazide 500–1000 mg IV |
| Proximal tubule diuretics: |
|    acetazolamide 250–375 mg daily or up to 500 mg |
|      intravenously |
| Collecting duct diuretics: |
|    spironolactone 100–200 mg daily |
|    eplerenone 25–100 mg/day |
|    amiloride 5–10 mg daily |

*Metolazone is generally best given for a limited period of time (3–5 days) or should be reduced in frequency to three times per week once extracellular fluid volume has declined to the target level. Only in patients who remain volume expanded should full doses be continued indefinitely, based on the target weight. Be very cautious with higher doses of spironolactone or eplerenone in the setting of angiotensin converting enzyme inhibitors or angiotensin receptor blockers, hyperkalemia can occur [31].

to have occurred in about two-thirds of patients receiving therapy [39]. One rational approach to combination therapy is to achieve control of ECF volume by adding full doses of DCT diuretics on a daily basis initially and then to maintain control by reducing the dose of the DCT diuretic to three times weekly. However, many clinicians titrate the dose of the DCT diuretic in each patient and have found that in some patients only a single weekly dose is required to maintain an appropriate level of diuresis. A physiological rationale for such an approach is provided by the observation that chronic treatment with DCT diuretics down-regulates $Na^+/K^+$-ATPase activity [54] and transport capacity [55] along the distal convoluted tubule of rat. Thus, it may be speculated that adding a DCT diuretic to a regimen including a loop diuretic may decrease the structural and functional compensatory effects of loop diuretics.

Another approach to combination therapy is to use combination therapy for only a short fixed course. A comparison of different combination diuretic regimens suggested that a limited course of combination therapy may be as effective and perhaps safer than more prolonged courses [51]. Thus, for the outpatient, either a small dose of DCT diuretic, such as 2.5 mg/day metolazone or

a limited and fixed course of a higher dose (3 days of 10 mg/day metolazone) may be recommended as effective therapy that is less likely to lead to side effects. Because DCT diuretics are absorbed more slowly than loop diuretics, it may be reasonable to administer the DCT diuretic 1/2 to 1 h prior to the loop diuretic, although rigorous support for this contention is lacking.

Drugs that act along the collecting duct, such as amiloride and spironolactone, can be added to a regimen of loop diuretic drugs but their effects are generally less robust than those of DCT diuretics. For example, the combination of spironolactone and loop diuretics has not been shown to be synergistic but aldosterone antagonists can prolong life and help prevent hypokalemia [56]. Cortical collecting duct diuretics also reduce magnesium excretion, relative to other diuretics, making hypomagnesemia less likely than when loop diuretics are combined with DCT diuretics [57–60]. However, there is far less experience with these types of diuretics in heart failure patients.

One situation in which aggressive diuretic therapy is often indicated is for hospitalized patients, especially those in an intensive care unit who need urgent diuresis. While the causes of diuretic resistance delineated above may be present in these patients, many also receive obligate fluid and solute loads, some develop electrolyte complications, and many cannot take medications by mouth. Two IV drugs are available to supplement loop diuretics for combination therapy. Chlorothiazide (500–1000 mg once or twice daily) and acetazolamide (250–375 mg up to four times daily) are both available for IV administration: chlorothiazide has relatively potent carbonic anhydrase inhibiting capacity in the proximal tubule. It also blocks the 'thiazide-sensitive' Na–Cl cotransporter in the distal tubule; and chlorothiazide has a longer half-life than some other DCT diuretics. Both chlorothiazide and acetazolamide have been shown to act synergistically with loop diuretics when given acutely. Acetazolamide is especially useful when metabolic alkalosis and hypokalemia complicate the treatment of edema. Alkalosis may make it difficult to wean a patient from a ventilator and make it impossible to correct $K^+$ depletion. The use of acetazolamide can often correct these disorders [61] without the need to administer saline, which would otherwise be used to correct alkalosis in these patients. In other situations, combination diuretic therapy may be targeted at the underlying disease process. Low doses of dopamine are often employed to potentiate the action diuretics by improving renal perfusion. However, one study has suggested that dopamine is not effective as an adjunct to diuretic treatment unless it increases cardiac output [62].

A newer approach may include combining brain natriuretic peptide (nesiritide) with loop diuretic treatment. In animals, this combination was recently shown to result in enhanced natriuresis without stimulating aldosterone secretion [63]. This combination makes it attractive as an option for acutely ill patients, but awaits confirmatory studies in humans and will be discussed in detail in Chapter 11.

## High dose diuretic therapy

High doses of loop diuretics are frequently employed to treat severe volume overload, especially when treatment is urgent. Maximal effective doses of furosemide, bumetanide, and torsemide have been estimated (see "diuretic choice and dosing" discussed earlier), although some have used higher doses [64]. In diuretic sensitive patients, the most common complications of loop diuretics result directly from the diuresis and natriuresis. Hypokalemia, hyponatremia, and hypotension frequently result because of excessive fluid and electrolyte losses. For diuretic *resistant* patients, however, drug toxicity, most commonly ototoxicity, may also occur and is an important consideration during high dose or prolonged therapy. All loop diuretics have been reported to cause ototoxicity in experimental animals and clinical ototoxicity has been reported following ethacrynic acid, furosemide, and bumetanide administration [65,66]. Ototoxicity is usually reversible, but has been irreversible occasionally; its incidence may be increased in patients exposed to other ototoxic agents, such as the aminoglycosides. Ototoxicity may be especially common following ethacrynic acid administration. It appears to be related to the serum concentration of the drug. It has been suggested, and clinical experience seems to confirm, that ototoxicity of furosemide can be minimized by administering it no

faster than 15 mg/min [67]. Comparable data are not available for bumetanide and torsemide, but it seems reasonable to avoid rapid bolus administration of loop diuretics in general. Myalgias appear to be more common following high doses of bumetanide [68]. The avoidance of high peak levels and the concomitant toxicity is one reason that continuous infusion of diuretics (discussed later) has become popular as an alternative approach to treat diuretic resistant patients.

It has long been appreciated that many patients suffering from CHF experience symptomatic relief from IV boluses of loop diuretics before significant volume and NaCl losses have occurred. In some patients, loop diuretics reduce pulmonary capillary wedge pressure acutely [7]. Loop diuretics are also known to stimulate secretion of vasodilatory prostaglandins. Pretreatment of animals with indomethacin greatly attenuates furosemide-induced venodilation, suggesting that prostaglandin secretion contributes importantly to the effects of loop diuretics by altering vascular reactivity. Although venodilation and improvements in cardiac hemodynamics frequently result, other reports suggest that the hemodynamic response to IV loop diuretics may be more complex. In two series, 1–1.5 mg/kg furosemide boluses, administered to patients with chronic CHF, resulted in transient *deteriorations* in hemodyanamics during the first hour [10,69] and exacerbation of CHF symptoms. These changes were related to activation of both the sympathetic nervous system and the renin–angiotensin system by the diuretic. Although these data provide cautionary information concerning the use of loop diuretics in acute cardiogenic pulmonary edema, it should be emphasized that IV loop diuretics remain the most important and useful form of therapy for these patients because they rapidly ameliorate symptoms in most patients. Furthermore, they contribute to symptomatic improvement once natriuresis begins, an effect that should begin within 15 to 20 min of diuretic administration.

Another interesting complication of high dose furosemide treatment may be thiamine deficiency [70–74]. Studies in experimental animals have shown that chronic furosemide administration can lead to thiamine deficiency. In humans, several groups have reported thiamine deficiency in patients treated chronically with furosemide [74].

In one study, patients with CHF who received furosemide 80 mg daily for at least 3 months were randomized to receive IV thiamine or placebo. Intravenous thiamine led to improved hemodynamics and a natriuresis, compared with placebo, and to an improvement in the thiamine-pyrophosphate effect on erythrocyte transketolase activity [72].

**Continuous diuretic infusion**

For hospitalized patients who are resistant to diuretic therapy, another approach is to infuse diuretics continuously. Continuous diuretic infusions have several potential advantages over bolus diuretic administration. First, because it avoids troughs of diuretic concentration, continuous infusion prevents intermittent periods of positive NaCl balance (postdiuretic NaCl retention). When short-acting diuretics, such as the loop diuretics, are administered by bolus infusion or by mouth once or twice a day, a period of natriuresis and diuresis lasting about 6 h ensues. When diuretic serum concentrations decline, urine NaCl concentrations also decline to levels below basal. Because 24-h renal NaCl excretion is the sum of the natriuretic and antinatriuretic responses, negative salt balance may be limited, especially when dietary salt intake is high. Clearly, a constant infusion that leads to constant serum diuretic concentrations will minimize periods of sodium retention and might be expected to be more efficacious. Second, constant infusions appear to be more efficient than bolus therapy. In one study of patients with chronic renal failure, a continuous infusion of bumetanide was 32% more efficient than a bolus of the same drug when the amount of NaCl excreted per milligram of administered drug was compared [68]. In a crossover study of nine patients with NYHA class III–IV CHF (see Figure 1.2), 60–80 mg/day was more effective when given as a continuous infusion following a loading dose (30–40 mg) than when given as boluses three times daily (30–40 mg/dose) [75]. Third, some patients who are resistant to large doses of diuretics given by bolus have responded to continuous infusion [64]. Most studies of efficacy in diuretic resistant patients have not compared strictly equivalent doses or administered them is a randomized manner. Regardless, several studies do provide suggestive evidence that continuous infusion may elicit diuresis in some patients resistant to large boluses. Fourth, diuretic response can be titrated; in the intensive care unit where obligate solute and fluid administration must be balanced by solute and fluid excretion, control of NaCl and water excretion can be obtained by titration of diuretic dose. While this is important in every postoperative patient, it is especially important in patients who are hemodynamically compromised. Magovern reported successful diuresis of hemodynamically compromised patients after cardiac surgery by continuous furosemide infusion [76]. Because continuous infusion of loop diuretics may reduce the sympathetic discharge and activation of the renin–angiotensin system, continuous infusions may be the preferred mode of therapy for hemodynamically unstable patients in need of diuresis. Finally, drug toxicity from loop diuretics, such as ototoxicity (observed with all loop diuretics) and myopathies (with bumetanide), appear to be less common when the drugs are administered as continuous infusions. In fact, total daily furosemide doses exceeding 2 g have been tolerated well when administered over 24 h. Dosage regimens for continuous IV diuretic administration are shown in Table 1.4. Of note, although natriuretic efficacy may vary linearly with loop diuretic dose, high infusion rates (e.g. 2 g per day of furosemide) might lead to toxic serum concentrations if continued for prolonged periods. This is especially true in patients with renal failure, in whom larger doses are often required to initiate diuresis. Special care should be taken when administering large daily doses of loop diuretics over prolonged periods; in patients with renal failure, a drug such as torsemide that is cleared, in part, by hepatic metabolism, may be preferred when high or prolonged therapy is attempted.

**Ultrafiltration**

In contrast to loop diuretics, ultrafiltration has much more modest effects to stimulate the renin–angiotenin–aldosterone axis because it does not activate the macula densa mechanism [77]. Subsequent reports have corroborated that ultrafiltration is safe and can be an effective adjunct to diuretics, but controlled trials are still lacking [78].

**Table 1.4** Continuous infusion of loop diuretics.

| | Bolus (mg) | Infusion rate (mg/h) | | |
|---|---|---|---|---|
| | | <25 mL/min | 25–75 mL/min | >75 mL/min |
| Furosemide | 40 | 20 then 40 | 10 then 20 | 10 |
| Bumetanide | 1 | 1 then 2 | 0.5 then 1 | 0.5 |
| Torsemide | 20 | 10 then 20 | 5 then 10 | 5 |

At high continuous doses, toxicity may develop, especially during furosemide infusion in patients with impaired renal function. Doses derived from Brater [88].

**Table 1.5** Adequacy of diuresis.

*Adequacy of diuresis*

Jugular venous distension
Hepatojugular reflex
Hepatomegaly
Ascites, peripheral and sacral edema
Pulmonary rales
Cough, dyspnea on exertion
Orthopnea, paroxysmal nocturnal dyspnea
Documented elevated filling pressures by cardiovascular testing (i.e. cardiac catheterization, echo cardiography)

## Evaluation of adequacy of diuresis

Clinicians use various methods to determine the extent and adequacy of diuresis (Table 1.5). However, some of the more commonly used signs, such as resolution of pulmonary rales, are insensitive when determining adequacy of diuresis in patients with chronic heart failure. Many clinicians use measures of renal function as an indicator of over-diuresis; however, increased blood urea nitrogen (BUN)/serum creatinine ratio can be a marker for rapid diuresis rather than overdiuresis. Patients may be temporarily intravascularly depleted while evidence of increased total body fluid still remains. In patients with azotemia or hypotension but continued evidence of fluid retention, diuresis should continue, although at a slower rate. Overdiuresis that leads to hypotension may contribute to renal insufficiency in patients on vasodilators and ACE inhibitors. In this setting, hypotension can be managed by reducing the dose or frequency of diuretics. In some patients with advanced, chronic heart failure, elevated BUN and creatinine concentrations may be necessary to maintain control of congestive symptoms. Once patients are believed to be adequately diuresed, it is important to document this "dry weight" and have patients weigh themselves daily.

Natriuretic peptides are increasingly being used as both diagnostic and prognostic tools in CHF. Some investigators have encouraged their use to titrate therapy. Both b-type natriuretic peptide (BNP) and N-terminal-pro-BNP plasma concentrations have been demonstrated to improve with heart failure pharmacologic therapy [79–82]. In a study by Troughton *et al.* [82], patients with impaired systolic function and symptomatic heart failure were randomized to receive treatment guided by either N-BNP concentration (N-BNP < 200 pmol/L) or standardized clinical assessment. After a median of 9.5 months, there were fewer total cardiovascular events (death, hospital admission, or heart failure decompensation) in the BNP group compared to the clinical group (19 versus 54, $p = 0.02$). However, titration of heart failure therapy was accomplished by a predetermined protocol that first maximized ACE inhibitors and then increased the dose of the loop diuretics. Unfortunately, there have not been studies that investigate the role of natriuretic peptides in titration of diuretics in patients already maximized on ACE inhibitors and $\beta$-blockers.

## Monitoring the efficacy of diuretic therapy

Patients with CHF who are on diuretics should be monitored for complications of diuretics on a regular basis (Table 1.2). The interval for reassessment should be individualized based on severity of illness, recent medication changes, past history of electrolyte imbalances, or need for active diuresis.

The earliest indication of volume retention is usually a consistent or dramatic increase in weight. In some patients, they can be instructed to take an extra dose of their routinely prescribed loop diuretic. Metolazone or other long-acting thiazide diuretics also can be used to improve diuresis. A dose of 2.5 to 5.0 mg of metolazone in addition to routine loop diuretics can be used periodically. While the effectiveness of volume management by heart failure nurses and multidisciplinary heart failure clinics is well established [83–85], this commonly prescribed practice of patient-guided management of diuretics has not been adequately studied [86]. Some clinicians in cognitively intact and motivated patients have used this practice in order to prevent heart failure hospitalizations [87]; however, this practice could lead to over treatment with diuretics. Therefore, it should be reserved for those patients who are hemodynamically stable, well motivated, and consistently compliant. Routine use of extra diuretics should prompt reevaluation by a clinician.

## Summary

Diuretics are a mainstay of therapy in patients with heart failure. They rapidly produce an improvement in symptoms, can be effective in alleviating pulmonary and peripheral edema, and can adequately control fluid retention with chronic therapy. However, diuretics most be utilized with care. First and foremost, they must be used in combination with an ACE inhibitor and a $\beta$-blocker in order to optimize their effectiveness and decrease risk. Furthermore, care must be taken to avoid inappropriately high doses of diuretics and resultant volume contraction as well as to avoid underutilization and associated hypervolemia. Furthermore, care should be taken to avoid alterations in serum electrolyte levels that can accompany diuretic use. Although appropriate cautions are warranted, it should be recognized that an optimal use of diuretics serves as a cornerstone in the treatment of patients with heart failure.

## References

1 Hunt SA, Baker DW, Chin MH *et al.* ACC/AHA guidelines for the evaluation and management of chronic heart failure in the adult: executive summary. *J Heart Lung Transplant* 2002;**21**:189–203.

2 Leier CV, Dei Cas L, Metra M. Clinical relevance and management of the major electrolyte abnormalities in congestive heart failure: hyponatremia, hypokalemia, and hypomagnesemia. *Am Heart J* 1994;**128**:564–574.

3 Larsen FF. Haemodynamic effects of high or low doses of furosemide in acute myocardial infarction. *Eur Heart J* 1988;**9**:125–131.

4 Stampfer M, Epstein SE, Beiser GD, Braunwald E. Hemodynamic effects of diuresis at rest and during intense upright exercise in patients with impaired cardiac function. *Circulation* 1968;**37**:900–911.

5 Kramer BK, Schweda F, Kammerl M, Riegger GA. Diuretic therapy and diuretic resistance in cardiac failure. *Nephrol Dial Transplant* 1999;**14**:39–42.

6 Pickkers P, Dormans TP, Russel FG *et al.* Direct vascular effects of furosemide in humans. *Circulation* 1997;**96**:1847–1852.

7 Dikshit K, Vyden JK, Forrester JS, Chatterjee K, Prakash R, Swan HJC. Renal and extrarenal hemodynamic effects of furosemide in congestive heart failure after acute myocardial infarction. *N Engl J Med* 1973; **288**:1087–1090.

8 Raftery EB. Haemodynamic effects of diuretics in heart failure. *Br Heart J* 1994;**72**:44–47.

9 Kelly DT. Vascular effects of diuretics in heart failure. *Br Heart J* 1994;**72**:48–50.

10 Francis GS, Siegel RM, Goldsmith SR, Olivari MT, Levine B, Cohn JN. Acute vasoconstrictor response to intravenous furosemide in patients with chronic congestive heart failure. *Ann Intern Med* 1985;**103**:1–6.

11 Skott O, Briggs JP. Direct demonstration of macula densa-mediated renin secretion. *Science* 1987;**237**:1618–1620.

12 Johnson W, Omland T, Hall C *et al.* Neurohormonal activation rapidly decreases after intravenous therapy with diuretics and vasodilators for class IV heart failure. *J Am Coll Cardiol* 2002;**39**:1623–1629.

13 Domanski M, Norman J, Pitt B, Haigney M, Hanlon S, Peyster E. Diuretic use, progressive heart failure, and death in patients in the Studies Of Left Ventricular Dysfunction (SOLVD). *J Am Coll Cardiol* 2003;**42**:705–708.

14 Hampton JR. Results of clinical trials with diuretics in heart failure. *Br Heart J* 1994;**72**:68–72.

15 Odemuyiwa O, Gilmartin J, Kenny D, Hall RJ. Captopril and the diuretic requirements in moderate and severe chronic heart failure. *Eur Heart J* 1989;**10**:586–590.

16 Grinstead WC, Francis MJ, Marks GF, Tawa CB, Zoghbi WA, Young JB. Discontinuation of chronic diuretic therapy in stable congestive heart failure secondary to coronary artery disease or to idiopathic dilated cardiomyopathy. *Am J Cardiol* 1994;**73**:881–886.

17 Walma EP, Hoes AW, van Dooren C, Prins A, van der Does E. Withdrawal of long-term diuretic medication in elderly patients: a double blind randomised trial. *BMJ* 1997;**315**:464–468.

18  Kostis JB, Davis BR, Cutler J *et al.* Prevention of heart failure by antihypertensive drug treatment in older persons with isolated systolic hypertension. SHEP Cooperative Research Group. *JAMA* 1997;**278**:212–216.

19  ALLHAT Officers and Coordinators for the ALLHAT Collaborative Research Group. The Antihypertensive and Lipid-Lowering Treatment to Prevent Heart Attack Trial. Major outcomes in moderately hypercholesterolemic, hypertensive patients randomized to pravastatin vs usual care: The Antihypertensive and Lipid-Lowering Treatment to Prevent Heart Attack Trial (ALLHAT-LLT). *JAMA* 2002;**288**:2998–3007.

20  Moser M, Hebert PR. Prevention of disease progression, left ventricular hypertrophy and congestive heart failure in hypertension treatment trials. *J Am Coll Cardiol* 1996;**27**:1214–1218.

21  Moser M. Diuretics in the prevention and treatment of congestive heart failure. *Cardiovasc Drugs Ther* 1997;**11**:273–277.

22  Multiple risk factor intervention trial. Risk factor changes and mortality results. Multiple Risk Factor Intervention Trial Research Group. *JAMA* 1982;**248**:1465–1477.

23  Siscovick DS, Raghunathan TE, Psaty BM *et al.* Diuretic therapy for hypertension and the risk of primary cardiac arrest. *N Engl J Med* 1994;**330**:1852–1857.

24  Cooper HA, Dries DL, Davis CE, Shen YL, Domanski MJ. Diuretics and risk of arrhythmic death in patients with left ventricular dysfunction. *Circulation* 1999;**100**:1311–1315.

25  Schrier RW, Gurevich AK, Cadnapaphornchai MA. Pathogenesis and management of sodium and water retention in cardiac failure and cirrhosis. *Semin Nephrol* 2001;**21**:157–172.

26  Schrier RW, Ecder T. Gibbs memorial lecture. Unifying hypothesis of body fluid volume regulation: implications for cardiac failure and cirrhosis. *Mt Sinai J Med* 2001;**68**:350–361.

27  Dzau VJ, Hollenberg NK. Renal response to captoprol in severe heart failure: role of furosemide in natriuesis and reversal of hyponatremia. *Ann Intern Med* 1984;**100**:777–790.

28  Doggrell SA. Is vasopressin-receptor antagonism an advancement in the treatment of heart failure? *Expert Opin Pharmacother* 2004;**5**:2181–2184.

29  Gheorghiade M, Gattis WA, O'Connor CM *et al.* Effects of tolvaptan, a vasopressin antagonist, in patients hospitalized with worsening heart failure: a randomized controlled trial. *JAMA* 2004;**291**:1963–1971.

30  Bayliss J, Norell M, Canepa-Anson R, Sutton G, Poole-Wilson P. Untreated heart failure: clinical and neuroendocrine effects of introducing diuretics. *Br Heart J* 1987;**57**:17–22.

31  Juurlink DN, Mamdani MM, Lee DS *et al.* Rates of hyperkalemia after publication of the Randomized Aldactone Evaluation Study. *N Engl J Med* 2004;**351**:543–551.

32  Eichhorn EJ, Tandon PK, DiBianco R *et al.* Clinical and prognostic significance of serum magnesium concentration in patients with severe chronic congestive heart failure: the PROMISE Study. *J Am Coll Cardiol* 1993;**21**:634–640.

33  Brater DC. Diuretic therapy. *N Engl J Med* 1998;**339**:387–395.

34  Vargo DL, Kramer WG, Black PK, Smith WB, Serpas T, Brater DC. Bioavailability, pharmacokinetics, and pharmacodynamics of torsemide and furosemide in patients with congestive heart failure. *Clin Pharmacol Ther* 1995;**57**:601–609.

35  Murray MD, Deer MM, Ferguson JA *et al.* Open-label randomized trial of torsemide compared with furosemide therapy for patients with heart failure. *Am J Med* 2001;**111**:513–520.

36  Ellison DH. Diuretic therapy and resistance in congestive heart failure. *Cardiology* 2001;**96**:132–143.

37  Chemtob S, Doray J-L, Laudignon N, Papageorgiou A, Varma DR, Aranda JV. Alternating sequential dosing with furosemide and ethacrynic acid in drug tolerance in the newborn. *Am J Dis Child* 1989;**143**:850–854.

38  Epstein M, Lepp BA, Hoffman DS, Levinson R. Potentiation of furosemide by metolazone in refractory edema. *Curr Ther Res* 1977;**21**:656–667.

39  Oster JR, Epstein M, Smoler S. Combined therapy with thiazide-type and loop diuretic agents for resistant sodium retention. *Ann Intern Med* 1983;**99**:405–406.

40  Oimomi M, Takase S, Saeki S. Combination diuretic therapy for severe refractory nephrotic syndrome. *Lancet* 1990;**336**:1004–1005.

41  Ellison DH. The physiologic basis of diuretic synergism: Its role in treating diuretic resistance. *Ann Intern Med* 1991;**114**:886–894.

42  Marone C, Muggli F, Lahn W, Frey FJ. Pharmacokinetic and pharmacodynamic interaction between furosemide and metolazone in man. *Eur J Clin Invest* 1985;**15**:253–257.

43  Okusa MD, Erik A, Persson G, Wright FS. Chlorothiazide effect on feedback-mediated control of glomerular filtration rate. *Am J Physiol* 1989;**257**:F137–144.

44  Garin EH. A comparison of combinations of diuretics in nephrotic edema. *Am J Dis Child* 1987;**141**:769–771.

45  Ellison DH, Velázquez H, Wright FS. Adaptation of the distal convoluted tubule of the rat: Structural and functional effects of dietary salt intake and chronic diuretic infusion. *J Clin Invest* 1989;**83**:113–126.

46  Kaissling B, Stanton BA. Adaptation of distal tubule and collecting duct to increased sodium delivery. I. Ultrastructure. *Am J Physiol* 1988;**255**:F1256–1268.

47 Stanton BA, Kaissling B. Adaptation of distal tubule and collecting duct to increased sodium delivery. II. $Na^+$ and $K^+$ transport. *Am J Physiol* 1988;**255**:F1269–1275.

48 Loon NR, Wilcox CS, Unwin RJ. Mechanism of impaired natriuretic response to furosemide during prolonged therapy. *Kidney Int* 1989;**36**:682–689.

49 Brater DC, Pressley RH, Anderson SA. Mechanisms of the synergistic combination of metolazone and bumetanide. *J Pharmacol Exp Ther* 1985;**233**:70–73.

50 Kruck F. Acute and long term effects of loop diuretics in heart failure. *Drugs* 1991;**41**:60–68.

51 Channer KS, McLean KA, Lawson-Matthew P, Richardson M. Combination diuretic treatment in severe heart failure: A randomised controlled trial. *Br Heart J* 1994;**71**:146–150.

52 Frishman WH, Bryzinski BS, Coulson LR *et al.* A multifactorial trial design to assess combination therapy in hypertension: Treatment with bisoprolol and hydrochlorothiazide. *Arch Intern Med* 1994;**154**:1461–1468.

53 Ellison DH. Intensive diuretic therapy: High doses, combinations, and constant infusions. In DW Seldin, G Giebisch, eds. *Diuretic Agents: Clinical Physiology and Pharmacology.* Academic Press, San Diego, 1997:281–300.

54 Garg LC, Narang N. Effects of hydrochlorothiazide on Na-K-ATPase activity along the rat nephron. *Kidney Int* 1987;**31**:918–922.

55 Morsing P, Velázquez H, Wright FS, Ellison DH. Adaptation of distal convoluted tubule of rats: II. Effects of chronic thiazide infusion. *Am J Physiol* 1991; **261**:F137–143.

56 Pitt B, Zannad F, Remme WJ *et al.* The Effect of Spironolactone on Morbidity and Mortality in Patients with Severe Heart Failure. *N Engl J Med* 1999;**341**:709–717.

57 Devane J, Ryan MP. The effects of amiloride and triamterene on urinary magnesium excretion in conscious saline-loaded rats. *Br J Pharmacol* 1981;**72**:285–289.

58 Palmer L. Interactions of amiloride and other blocking cations with the apical Na channel in the toad urinary bladder. *J Membr Biol* 1985;**87**:191–199.

59 Dyckner T, Wester P-O, Widman L. Amiloride prevents thiazide-induced intracellular potassium and magnesium losses. *Acta Med Scand* 1988;**224**:25–30.

60 Ellison DH. Divalent cation transport by the distal nephron: insights from Bartter's and Gitelman's syndromes [In Process Citation]. *Am J Physiol Renal Physiol* 2000;**279**:F616–625.

61 Miller PD, Berns AS. Acute metabolic alkalosis perpetuating hypercarbia: a role for acetazolamide in chronic obstructive pulmonary disease. *JAMA* 1977; **238**:2400–2401.

62 Vargo DL, Brater DC, Rudy DW, Swan SK. Dopamine does not enhance furosemide-induced natriuresis in patients with congestive heart failure. *J Am Soc Nephrol* 1996;**7**:1032–1037.

63 Cataliotti A, Boerrigter G, Costello-Boerrigter LC *et al.* Brain natriuretic peptide enhances renal actions of furosemide and suppresses furosemide-induced aldosterone activation in experimental heart failure. *Circulation* 2004;**109**:1680–1685.

64 Gerlag PGG, van Meijel JJM. High-dose furosemide in the treatment of refractory congestive heart failure. *Arch Intern Med* 1988;**148**:286–291.

65 Brown RD, Feldman AM. Pharmacology of hearing and ototoxicity. *Ann Rev Pharmacol Toxicol* 1978; **18**:233–252.

66 Ryback LP. Ototoxicity of loop diuretics. *Otolaryngol Clin N America* 1993;**26**:829–844.

67 Nierenberg DW. Furosemide and ethacrynic acid in acute tubular necrosis. *West J Med* 1980;**133**:163–170.

68 Rudy DW, Voelker JR, Greene PK, Esparza FA, Brater DC. Loop diuretics for chronic renal insufficiency: a continuous infusion is more efficacious than bolus therapy. *Ann Intern Med* 1991;**115**:360–366.

69 Goldsmith SR, Francis G, Cohn JN. Attenuation of the pressor response to intravenous furosemide by angiotensin converting enzyme inhibition in congestive heart failure. *Am J Cardiol* 1989;**64**:1382–1385.

70 Leslie D, Gheorghiade M. Is there a role for thiamine supplementation in the management of heart failure? *Am Heart J* 1996;**131**:1248–1250.

71 Rieck J, Halkin H, Almog S *et al.* Urinary loss of thiamine is increased by low doses of furosemide in healthy volunteers. *J Lab Clin Med* 1999;**134**:238–243.

72 Shimon I, Almog S, Vered Z *et al.* Improved left ventricular function after thiamine supplementation in patients with congestive heart failure receiving long-term furosemide therapy. *Am J Med* 1995;**98**:485–490.

73 Suter PM, Haller J, Hany A, Vetter W. Diuretic use: a risk for subclinical thiamine deficiency in elderly patients. *J Nutr Health Aging* 2000;**4**:69–71.

74 Zenuk C, Healey J, Donnelly J, Vaillancourt R, Almalki Y, Smith S. Thiamine deficiency in congestive heart failure patients receiving long term furosemide therapy. *Can J Clin Pharmacol* 2003;**10**:184–188.

75 Lahav M, Regev A, Ra'anani P, Thodor E. Intermittent administration of furosemide vs continuous infusion preceded by a loading dose for congestive heart failure. *Chest* 1992;**102**:725–731.

76 Magovern JA, Magovern GJ Jr. Diuresis in hemodynamically compromised patients: Continuous furosemide infusion. *Ann Thorac Surg* 1990;**50**:482–484.

77 Agostoni P, Marenzi G, Lauri G *et al.* Sustained improvement in functional capacity after removal of body fluid with isolated ultrafiltration in chronic cardiac insufficiency: Failure of furosemide to provide the same result. *Am J Med* 1994;**96**:191–199.

78 Sheppard R, Panyon J, Pohwani AL *et al.* Intermittent outpatient ultrafiltration for the treatment of severe refractory congestive heart failure. *J Card Fail* 2004; **10**:380–383.

79 Latini R, Masson S, Anand I *et al.* Effects of valsartan on circulating brain natriuretic peptide and norepinephrine in symptomatic chronic heart failure: the Valsartan Heart Failure Trial (Val-HeFT). *Circulation* 2002; **106**:2454–2458.

80 Murdoch DR, McDonagh TA, Byrne J *et al.* Titration of vasodilator therapy in chronic heart failure according to plasma brain natriuretic peptide concentration: randomized comparison of the hemodynamic and neuroendocrine effects of tailored versus empirical therapy. *Am Heart J* 1999; **138**:1126–1132.

81 Stanek B, Frey B, Hulsmann M *et al.* Prognostic evaluation of neurohumoral plasma levels before and during beta-blocker therapy in advanced left ventricular dysfunction. *J Am Coll Cardiol* 2001; **38**:436–442.

82 Troughton RW, Frampton CM, Yandle TG, Espiner EA, Nicholls MG, Richards AM. Treatment of heart failure guided by plasma aminoterminal brain natriuretic peptide (N-BNP) concentrations. *Lancet* 2000; **355**:1126–1130.

83 Capomolla S, Febo O, Ceresa M *et al.* Cost/utility ratio in chronic heart failure: comparison between heart failure management program delivered by day-hospital and usual care. *J Am Coll Cardiol* 2002; **40**:1259–1266.

84 Fonarow GC, Stevenson LW, Walden JA *et al.* Impact of a comprehensive heart failure management program on hospital readmission and functional status of patients with advanced heart failure. *J Am Coll Cardiol* 1997; **30**:725–732.

85 Kasper EK, Gerstenblith G, Hefter G *et al.* A randomized trial of the efficacy of multidisciplinary care in heart failure outpatients at high risk of hospital readmission. *J Am Coll Cardiol* 2002; **39**:471–480.

86 Macfadyen RJ, Struthers AD. Diuretic use and abuse in systolic cardiac failure: a recipe for renal impairment? *Heart* 2000; **83**:468.

87 Broadley AJ, Marshall AJ. Self administration of metolzaone reduces readmissions with decompensated congestive cardiac failure. *Heart* 1999; **82**:397–398.

88 Brater DC. Diuretic pharmacokinetics and pharmacodynamics. In DW Seldin, G Giebisch, eds. *Diuretic Agents: Clinical Physiology and Pharmacology.* Academic Press, San Diego, 1997:189–208.

**CHAPTER 2**

# Use of digoxin in the treatment of heart failure

*Deborah DeEugenio,* PHARM D *& Paul J. Mather,* MD

After all, in spite of opinion, prejudice or error, Time will fix the real value upon this discovery (digitalis glycosides), and determine whether I have imposed upon myself and others, or contributed to the benefit of science and mankind.

*William Withering, 1785*

## Introduction

Digoxin is one of the oldest drugs used for the treatment of heart failure. Despite over 200 years of use, the role of digoxin and other cardiac glycosides in heart failure is still a subject of ongoing debate. Proponents for the use of digoxin assert that its mild positive inotropic effects when administered orally, help prevent worsening of heart failure and improve the symptoms of low cardiac index. Opponents maintain that exposure to the continuous positive inotropism of digoxin therapy actually hastens myocardial cell demise.

## History and pharmacology

Cardiac glycosides have been used for centuries as therapeutic agents. Chemical compounds containing the molecular structure common to these agents, a steroid nucleus containing an unsaturated lactone at the C17 position and one or more glycoside residues at C3, are found in many plants and several toad species, usually acting as venoms or toxins that protect against predators [2]. Digitalis glycosides are among the earliest agents documented to be used for the treatment of heart failure. The first comprehensive description of *Digitalis* glycosides in the treatment of congestive heart failure, and other ailments, was described in a monograph in 1785 by William Withering. The monograph also gives an account of the efficacy and toxicities of the leaves

of the common foxglove plant, *Digitalis purpurea* (Figure 2.1) [1]. Withering believed that *digitalis* had a diuretic effect in patients with a weak and irregular pulse and *dropsy,* an edematous condition usually believed to be caused by kidney or heart disease in the 1700s [1].

Other clinically relevant glycosides are derived from the leaves of the *Digitalis lanata,* from which (Figure 2.2) digitoxin and digoxin are derived. Digoxin is currently the most commonly prescribed cardiac glycoside due to its convenient pharmacokinetics, alternative routes of administration, and the widespread availability of techniques to measure serum concentrations [2].

## Mechanism of action

### Inhibition of Na$^+$, K$^+$–ATPase

All cardiac glycosides are potent and highly selective inhibitors of the active transport of Na$^+$ and K$^+$ across cell membranes, by binding to a specific site on the Na$^+$/K$^+$–ATPase, the enzymatic equivalent of the cellular "sodium pump" (Figure 2.3) [2]. The sodium pump is an integral membrane protein responsible for sodium and potassium ion translocation across cell membranes, which is coupled with hydrolysis of high-energy ATP phosphate [3,4]. The sodium pump contains $\alpha$, $\beta$, and $\gamma$ subunits, however, the $\alpha$ subunit contains the important binding site for digitalis glycosides [3,5]. Enzymatic activity of the sodium

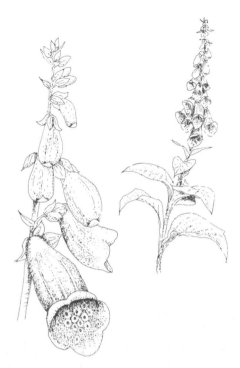

**Figure 2.1** Digitalis glycosides were originally derived from the common foxglove plant, digitalis purpurea. These plants are tall, perennial plants with numerous tubular flowers which bloom in the summer months.

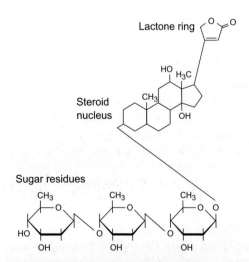

**Figure 2.2** The chemical structure of digoxin, the most commonly prescribed cardiac glycoside, contains a steroid nucleus with a lactone ring and sugar residues.

pump results in the exchange of three intracellular sodium ions for two extracellular potassium ions. Cardiac-glycoside induced inhibition of the sodium pump increases the intracellular sodium concentration or activity [5].

## Positive inotropic effect

It has been known for over 70 years that cardiac glycosides produce a positive inotropic effect. In the 1960s, Sonnenblick *et al.* showed that *Digitalis* increases the velocity of the shortening of the cardiac muscle, resulting in a shift upward and to the left of the left ventricular function (i.e. Frank–Starling curve), so that increased stroke work is generated for a given filling volume or pressure [2,6]. This effect is present in normal and failing myocardial tissue, in atrial and ventricular muscle, and it appears to be sustainable without desensitization or tachyphylaxis [2,7]. The increase in contractile force or positive inotropic effect is due to an increase in available cytosolic calcium primarily during systole, which interacts with contractile proteins to increase the velocity and extent of sarcomere shortenings [8]. Digoxin's positive inotropic action comes from an increase in cardiac myocyte intracellular calcium. This effect occurs due to digoxin's inhibition of cardiac sodium–potassium ATPase. Diminished outward sodium pumping leads to an increase in intracellular sodium that, in turn, increases intracellular calcium stores through enhanced calcium entry, reduced calcium efflux, or both – defects mediated via the sodium–calcium exchanger [3,8,9]. Diastolic calcium levels are minimally increased because of rapid sequestration of intracellular calcium by the sarcoplasmic reticulum; however, increased calcium is apparent during systole with the release of these stored ions [3,9,10].

Rahimtoola *et al.* summarized the hemodynamic benefits of *Digitalis* as decreased right atrial and wedge pressure and increased cardiac output at rest, and decreased right atrial and wedge pressure and increased cardiac output and left ventricular stroke-work index during exercise [11].

## Neurohumoral and autonomic effects

Traditionally heart failure was considered as a hemodynamic disorder. Hence original drug

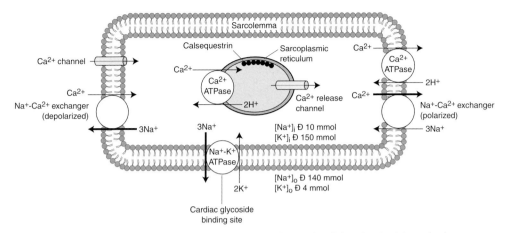

**Figure 2.3** Cardiac glycosides exert their therapeutic effects by binding to the alpha subunit of the $Na^+/K^+$–ATPase "sodium pump", thus increasing intracellular sodium content. These effects are beneficial in heart failure because they cause positive inotropic effects in cardiac tissues, and neurohumoral and autonomic changes in non-cardiac tissues.

treatment attempted to correct the hemodynamic abnormalities. It is now known that increased cardiac sympathetic activation plays an important role in the disease pathophysiology and neurohumoral modulation or inhibition plays an important role in heart failure treatment [12]. Digoxin was initially believed to be purely a positive inotropic agent and it is now known that positive hemodynamic effects may have deleterious effects on mortality [13–15]. Digoxin does not appear to increase mortality in heart failure patients [16], and this may be because it exerts sympathoinhibitory effects not seen with other inotropes like dobutamine [17]. It appears that digoxin may work in HF primarily by attenuating the activation of neurohormonal systems and not as a positive inotrope.

Digoxin exerts it's neurohormonal effects by inhibiting sodium–potassium ATPase in noncardiac tissues. Inhibition of sodium–potassium ATPase in vagal afferent fibers acts to sensitize cardiac baroreceptors [18]. Increased sympathetic nervous activity in heart failure is due, in part, to a reduction in the sensitivity of the arterial baroreflex response to blood pressure, resulting in a decline in tonic baroreflex suppression of CNS-directed sympathetic activity [19,20]. This desensitization of the normal baroreflex is thought to be responsible in part for sustained elevation of plasma norepinephrine, renin, and vasopressin levels in heart failure [2]. This increase in sympathetic activity in heart failure initially maintains cardiac

output and blood pressure, but eventually leads to increased cardiac dysfunction. Mason *et al.* initially showed that intravenous infusion of a cardiac glycoside, in patients with heart failure, led to decreased mean arterial pressure, decreased forearm vascular resistance, decreased venous tone, and decreased heart rate. These sympathoinhibitory effects are consistent with enhanced baroreceptor responsiveness [21]. In the kidney, digoxin inhibits sodium–potassium ATPase that reduces reabsorption of sodium thereby decreasing sodium delivery to the distal tubules and reducing renin secretion in the kidneys [18].

Acute administration of *Digitalis* preparations has been shown to decrease plasma concentrations of norepinephrine and plasma renin activity, which may be linked to improved baroreceptor sensitivity. This effect appears to be sustained with repeat dosing [19,20,22–25]. Digoxin has also been shown to prevent deterioration of heart rate variability [26], which indicates increased parasympathetic and baroreceptor sensitivity during therapy [27].

## Electrophysiologic effects
At therapeutic, nontoxic serum concentrations (1–2 ng/mL) digoxin decreases automaticity and increases maximal diastolic resting membrane potential in atrial and atrioventricular (AV) nodal tissues, due to an increase in vagal tone and a decrease in sympathetic activity. There is also a prolongation of the effective refractory period and

a decrease in conduction velocity in AV nodal tissue [2]. These actions are abolished by atropine and by cardiac denervation, as in cardiac transplantation [3]. In higher concentrations, digoxin may cause sinus bradycardia or arrest and/or prolongation of AV conduction or heart block [2]. Both systolic and diastolic calcium increase during *Digitalis*-induced arrhythmias, leading to the theory that intracellular calcium overload may cause *Digitalis*-induced arrhythmias. Spontaneous cycles of calcium release and reuptake result in after-polarizations and after-contractions [3].

## Dosing and monitoring

Patients should receive maintenance doses of 0.125 or 0.25 mg daily, with no loading dose, based on ideal body weight, age, and renal function. Patients with normal renal function should receive 0.25 mg daily. Patients with renal dysfunction, small stature, baseline conduction abnormalities, and the elderly should begin on 0.125 mg daily. Clinicians may consider checking a serum digoxin concentration in 1–3 weeks [28]. The level should be checked at least 6 h after an oral dose [28] to ensure appropriate drug distribution into tissues [27]. While some clinicians believe that it is not mandatory to check a serum digoxin concentration (SDC) in all patients, others would argue that there is little rationale for not obtaining what is relatively an inexpensive test [18]. By contrast, a serum digoxin level is strongly recommended in patients with a significant change in renal function or initiation of a concomitant interacting drug [27].

Although digoxin has been a mainstay of treatment for left ventricular dysfunction for over 200 years, no definitive data have been published to clarify the range of serum concentrations associated with clinical benefit. Many clinicians view the laboratory reference range of 0.8–2 ng/mL to be the desired serum concentration even though evidence from well-conducted clinical trials does not support this [29]. The ACC/AHA guidelines released in 2001, suggested that there may be little relationship between SDC and its therapeutic effects, and data suggest that large doses of digoxin may not be more effective than small doses in the treatment of HF [18]. It appears that higher concentrations may be necessary to

achieve maximal hemodynamic effects, however, beneficial neurohormonal effects tend to occur at lower serum concentrations seen with doses of 0.125–0.25 mg daily [27,29–33]. Digoxin may have increased adverse events at higher concentrations presumably due to arrhythmogenesis. Landmark clinical trials, which demonstrated digoxin's efficacy in patients with HF and normal sinus rhythm, used low concentrations of digoxin to achieve benefit. The average SDCs were 1.2, 1.2, and 0.8 ng/mL in the RADIANCE [34], PROVED [35], and DIG Trials [18], respectively. Adams *et al.* analyzed the PROVED and RADIANCE data and found digoxin's beneficial effects were consistent, regardless of SDC, when compared to placebo [30]. In an editorial, Gheorghiade and Pitt stated that "in the DIG Trial there was an association between serum digoxin concentration and mortality" and "this finding was significant even within the so-called therapeutic (laboratory reference) range" [36]. In a recent post hoc analysis of the DIG Trial data, higher SDC's were associated with higher crude all-cause mortality ($p = 0.006$ for trend), higher cardiovascular mortality ($p < 0.001$ for trend), but not increased mortality due to heart failure using Kaplan Meier survival curves. The authors recommend a therapeutic SDC of 0.5–0.8 ng/mL for patients with HF in sinus rhythm as these concentrations showed possible mortality benefit [37]. Indeed, we believe that a digoxin level of less than 1.0 ng/ml is advisable in patients with chronic heart failure.

## Clinical trials

### Historical clinical trials

Between 1969 and 1983, a number of uncontrolled trials of digoxin withdrawal were completed and have been summarized in several reviews [38–40]. These studies included heterogenous or undefined patient populations, such as patients with atrial fibrillation or normal sinus rhythm and diastolic or systolic dysfunction, and a wide variation in study design. Therefore, it is difficult to draw conclusions regarding its efficacy from these studies [38]. Jaeschke *et al.* completed a meta-analysis of seven randomized, double-blind placebo-controlled trials of digoxin published between the years of 1982 and 1989. They found a common odds ratio for HF deterioration, while receiving digoxin versus placebo of 0.28 (95%, CI 0.16–0.49) [41]. However, these results must be interpreted carefully due to the limitations of a meta-analysis. Demers *et al.* analyzed nine randomized, controlled trials comparing digoxin with angiotensin converting enzyme (ACE) inhibitors between 1987 and 1995. The author reported that these studies were not large enough to show differences in mortality or hospitalizations for heart failure. However, the overall data suggested digoxin was as effective as ACE inhibitors in improving exercise capacity and controlling signs and symptoms of HF. These studies had limitations including small size, a short treatment period, and the use of crossover and nonplacebo-controlled designs [42].

## Digoxin withdrawal trials: PROVED and RADIANCE

In the 1990s two well-designed trials helped digoxin to gain US FDA approval for the treatment of heart failure. PROVED [35] and RADIANCE [34] were companion trials designed to evaluate the effects of digoxin alone or in combination with ACE inhibitors. The trials had the same study design except that the use of ACE inhibitor was excluded in the PROVED trial, while its use was required for inclusion in the RADIANCE protocol. The studies were randomized, double-blinded, placebo-controlled trials of digoxin withdrawal in patients with mild to moderate heart failure (NYHA class II–III) and normal sinus rhythm who were clinically stable and receiving digoxin and diuretics. Patients were included if they had evidence of heart failure including; presence of dyspnea and/or fatigue on exertion, X-ray evidence of congestion, echocardiographic end-diastolic dimension ≥60 mm, diminished exercise capacity, and left ventricular dysfunction with a radionuclide ejection fraction <35% [39]. Patients were excluded if they had recent myocardial infarction (MI), unstable angina or stroke, primary, uncorrected valvular disease, hypertrophic cardiomyopathy, atrial or ventricular arrhythmia, uncontrolled hypertension or hypotension, significant hepatic, renal or pulmonary impairment, or use of concomitant $\beta$-blockers, antiarrhythmics or calcium channel blockers. Patients underwent an 8 week run-in

phase, in which all patients were stabilized on a digoxin dose maintaining levels between 0.9 and 2.0 ng/mL. Patients were then randomized to receive digoxin therapy (treatment group) or to withdrawal of digoxin (placebo group) for 12 weeks. The four primary endpoints were; incidence of treatment failure, time to treatment failure, maximum treadmill exercise time, and distance covered in the 6-min walk test.

The PROVED study enrolled 113 patients into the run-in phase and randomized 88 patients to the treatment phase. The PROVED trial was discontinued early because of difficulty with enrollment as many patients were receiving ACE inhibitors [39]. The PROVED data showed a significant improvement in the treatment group versus placebo in that patients in the treatment group demonstrated increased maximal exercise capacity ($p = 0.003$), decreased treatment failures ($p = 0.039$), and decreased time to treatment failure ($p = 0.037$). Patients who continued to receive digoxin also had lower body weight ($p = 0.044$), lower heart rate ($p = 0.003$), and higher left ventricular ejection fraction ($p = 0.016$) [42].

The RADIANCE trial, which required patients to be receiving concomitant ACE inhibitors, randomized 178 of 216 patients from the run-in phase [39]. Worsening heart failure necessitating withdrawal from the study occurred in 23 patients in the placebo group and only four patients continued to receive digoxin ($p < 0.001$). The relative risk of worsening heart failure in the placebo versus treatment group was 5.9 (95% CI 2.1–17.2). All measures of functional capacity showed deterioration in the placebo versus treatment groups ($p = 0.033$ for maximal exercise tolerance, $p = 0.01$ for submaximal exercise endurance, and $p = 0.019$ for NYHA class). Patients who had digoxin withdrawn also had lower quality of life scores ($p = 0.04$), decreased ejection fractions ($p = 0.001$), increased heart rates ($p = 0.001$), and increased body weights ($p < 0.001$) [34].

Some important limitations of these studies are noted. The run-in phase and withdrawal design of these studies produced selection bias in that patients were already tolerating and probably benefiting from digoxin therapy prior to enrollment [39]. It was also very short in duration and the results may have differed had the studies been carried out for a longer period of time. It was not powered to assess mortality differences. Finally, patients were not receiving what is currently considered optimal concomitant heart failure therapy, as $\beta$-blockers were contraindicated in both trials and ACE inhibitors were contraindicated in PROVED.

**Effects on mortality: the DIG trial**

The NIH designed a trial to attempt to address some of the limitations of the PROVED and RADIANCE trials: The *Digitalis* Investigation group [16]. This trial was a prospective, randomized, double-blind, placebo-controlled trial assessing the use of digoxin (3397 patients) versus placebo (3403 patients) in a study group that was receiving ACE inhibitors and diuretics. As 50% of patients were digoxin naïve, the study eliminated concerns regarding digoxin withdrawal. In addition, patients were assessed over a longer period of time than earlier studies and the trial was powered to assess digoxin's effects on mortality and hospitalizations. Eligible patients had heart failure with a left ventricular ejection fraction of $\leq$ 45% and normal sinus rhythm. The average dose of digoxin administered in the trial was 0.25 mg daily.

The primary endpoint was mortality and secondary endpoints included mortality from cardiovascular causes, death from worsening heart failure, hospitalization for worsening heart failure, and hospitalization for other causes. No statistically significant difference in mortality was noted between the two groups. There were 1181 deaths (34.8%) and 1194 deaths (35.1%) in the digoxin and placebo groups, (Figure 2.4a) respectively (risk ratio 0.99, 95% CI 0.91–1.07). There was a trend towards decreasing risk of death from heart failure in the digoxin group (risk ratio 0.88, 95% CI 0.77–1.01). This benefit was tempered by increased cardiovascular mortality in the digoxin group presumably due an increase in arrhythmias. There was however a statistically significant decrease in hospitalizations and need for cointerventions (defined as need for increasing doses of ACE inhibitors or diuretics or need to initiate new therapies due to worsening heart failure) in the digoxin group. There was an absolute 6% decrease in hospitalizations in the digoxin group and fewer patients were hospitalized

for worsening heart failure (26.8% versus 34.7%, risk ratio 0.72, 95% CI 0.66–0.79, $p < 0.001$). The authors reported that benefits were most pronounced in patients at higher risk including those with left ventricular ejection fractions <25%, enlarged hearts, and those in NYHA functional class III or IV. Benefits were also more pronounced in patients with nonischemic etiology [39]. However digoxin was still effective in patients with ejection fractions between 5% and 45%, ischemic etiology, smaller heart size, and NYHA class I and II symptoms, when considering the combined endpoint of death and hospitalizations [39]. Although digoxin did not improve mortality, these results are significant as previous trials with other inotropic agents have shown an excess of mortality [13–15].

In two post hoc analyses of the DIG trial, digoxin's effects on mortality were analyzed in women versus men and in patients with varying degrees of renal dysfunction. Rathore *et al.* [43] compared the effects of digoxin on mortality in men and women. In the study, women tended to be older, have more severe HF, and possess more significant comorbidities than men. In a multivariable analysis, digoxin was associated with a significantly higher risk of death among women (adjusted hazard ratio compared to placebo 1.23, 95% CI 1.02–1.47), but had no significant effect among men (adjusted hazard ratio 0.93, 95% CI 0.85–1.02). Shlipak *et al.* [44] showed that decreasing renal function, as evidenced by decreasing glomerular filtration rate (GFR) or increasing serum creatinine, significantly increase the risk of all-cause mortality in patients with HF. Patients with the highest creatinine levels were treated with the lowest doses of digoxin but had the highest serum digoxin concentrations. However, the effect of digoxin on all-cause mortality and the combined all-cause mortality plus hospitalization for worsening HF was comparable across all GFR groups.

**Digoxin use in clinical practice**

**Heart failure with left ventricular dysfunction**

Digoxin is recommended to be used for treatment of symptoms of heart failure unless contraindicated, class II, level B evidence [18].

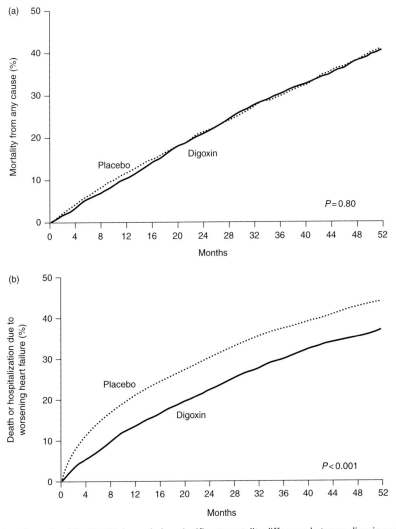

**Figure 2.4** Although results of the DIG Trial revealed no significant mortality difference between digoxin and placebo (a), digoxin did produce a significant decrease in the combined endpoint of death or hospitalization due to worsening heart failure due to a significant difference in hospitalizations for worsening heart failure in the digoxin group (b).

Conversely, there is no data to recommend the use of digoxin in patients with asymptomatic left ventricular dysfunction who are in sinus rhythm, thus it is a class III, level C recommendation. Data suggests that patients with left ventricular systolic dysfunction benefit from digoxin therapy despite only mild clinical evidence of HF [27], however, benefit may be more pronounced in patients with more severe disease. The results of the DIG trial suggest that digoxin may exert greater effects in higher-risk patients including those with

ejection fractions <25%, enlarged hearts, and NYHA class III and IV symptoms. However digoxin was effective in all patients with symptomatic left ventricular dysfunction [16].

Physicians may consider using digoxin to improve symptoms and the clinical status of patients with heart failure in conjunction with diuretics, ACE inhibitors, and β-blockers. Digoxin has been shown to decrease hospitalizations and emergency room visits, decrease the need for cointervention, and improve exercise capacity in patients with symptomatic HF and left ventricular dysfunction [27]. Digoxin may be used early on to reduce symptoms in patients who have initiated, but not yet responded to, ACE inhibitor and $\beta$-blocker therapy. Alternatively, clinicians may delay treatment with digoxin until the patient's response to ACE inhibitors and $\beta$-blockers has been defined and digoxin may be initiated in those patients who remain symptomatic. Digoxin's use should be avoided in patients with significant sinus or atrioventricular block, unless the patient has a permanent pacemaker. The drug should be used cautiously with other drugs that depress sinus or atrioventricular nodal function. Furthermore, it should be recognized that there is no role for digoxin "loading" and therefore it should not be used to stabilize patients with an acute exacerbation of heart failure.

## Diastolic dysfunction

Previously the major consensus has been that the use of *Digitalis* glycosides is inappropriate in patients with heart failure and normal left ventricular function [45]. However, the DIG trial investigators [16] included an ancillary trial that included patients with diastolic dysfunction or those with a left ventricular ejection fraction > 45%. The ancillary group, with diastolic dysfunction, had results consistent with the main trial with ejection fractions of 25–45% without evidence of excess arrhythmic or ischemic events. There was no significant difference in mortality with 23.4% mortality in both the digoxin and placebo groups (risk ratio 0.99, 95% CI 0.76–1.28). However, there was a trend towards a decrease in the combined outcome of death or hospitalization due to worsening heart failure (risk ratio 0.82, 95% CI 0.63–1.07).

It is unlikely that digoxin improves myocardial relaxation; however, it is possible that digoxin may produce a long-term improvement in LV compliance related to inhibition of left ventricular hypertrophy (LVH) and changes in the interstitium [45]. However, due to limited clinical evidence digoxin should not be routinely recommended for use in this patient population. Indeed, some clinicians would propose that digoxin is contraindicated in patients with heart failure and normal systolic function. However, the ACC/AHA Guidelines [18] recommend digoxin to minimize symptoms of heart failure in patients with diastolic dysfunction as a class IIB, level C recommendation due to limited evidence.

## Atrial fibrillation and heart failure

Digoxin is prescribed routinely in patients with HF and atrial fibrillation, but $\beta$-blockers may be more effective in controlling ventricular response especially during exercise [18,46–48]. Digoxin should generally not be used as monotherapy for rate control in patients with atrial fibrillation for two reasons (1) increased risk of toxicity with high doses and (2) decreased efficacy with exercise or increased sympathetic activity. The traditional practice of arbitrarily increasing the dose of digoxin to achieve adequate rate control leads to excessive toxicity. Therefore, digoxin should be dosed at typically recommended doses and other agents, that is, $\beta$-blockers, should be added to achieve adequate rate control. Digoxin slows ventricular response by increasing vagal tone. However, with exertion or increased sympathetic activity, vagal tone decreases and ventricular rate may increase. Therefore, a concomitant agent, that is, a $\beta$-blocker, should be used to control ventricular rate [27].

## Heart failure and myocardial infarction

The results of studies in animals indicate that digoxin might exacerbate arrhythmias and increase myocardial necrosis in the setting of experimental myocardial ischemia [49]. Canine models have shown digoxin may increase myocardial oxygen consumption [50] and increase the extent and severity of myocardial infarction [51–54]. In dogs it has been demonstrated that post-MI the ventricular myocardium may be more susceptible to digoxin toxicity, especially life-threatening ventricular arrhythmias [55]. Evaluation of the correlation between digoxin use and death after MI was assessed in several studies. These studies should be interpreted with caution as most of these studies were post hoc evaluations of completed clinical trials and digoxin use was not randomized, so digoxin-treated patients compared to placebo-treated patients, often possessed more comorbidities [49]. The study subjects in these post hoc analyses were also not generally receiving optimal therapy for heart failure including an ACE inhibitor and a $\beta$-blocker. In several of these early trials, digoxin appeared to increase the risk of death post-MI; however this risk decreased or was decreased or eliminated after adjusting for other comorbidities [56–60]. However, in several other studies, digoxin use remained an independent risk factor for increased mortality following MI [61–67]. It appears that increased mortality may be related to increased dose [49]; however, this theory has not been confirmed in well-designed trials. The evidence to support use of digoxin following MI is conflicting and a prospective randomized trial seems unlikely. Currently there are no defined guidelines for digoxin use in patients post-MI. The decision as to the use of digoxin in post-MI patients must be made by the clinician based on risk–benefit ratio while recognizing that the safety of digoxin in these patients has been questioned [49].

## Pharmacokinetics

The bioavailability of digoxin tablets, elixir, and intravenous formulations are 0.5–0.9 (generally 0.7–0.8), 0.8 and 1, respectively (Table 2.1). Most clinicians consider the oral tablets to have a bioavailability of 0.7 [28], thus conversion from oral to intravenous dosing would be in a ratio of 0.7 : 1. The average volume of distribution is approximately 7.3 L/kg [28]. This volume is decreased in patients with renal disease and hypothyroidism, necessitating a maintenance dose reduction in these patients [2,28]. The volume of distribution appears to be more closely related to ideal rather than actual body weight in obese patients [28]. Digoxin is distributed in the body in a two compartment model. It first distributes into a small initial volume of distribution, $V_i$, consisting of plasma and other rapidly equilibrating tissues, and then it slowly distributes into a larger, slowly equilibrating compartment, $V_t$. The myocardium behaves as though it were located in the larger, more slowly equilibrating compartment $V_t$. Therefore, plasma levels will not reflect pharmacologic effects on the myocardium for at least 4 h after an intravenous dose or 6 h after an oral dose of digoxin [28]. Plasma levels drawn early after a dose will be

**Table 2.1** Digoxin Pharmacokinetic Parameters

| | |
|---|---|
| Bioavailability (F) | IV $= 1$ |
| | Oral tablets $= 0.7$ |
| Salt form | S $= 1$ |
| Distribution | 2 Compartment Model |
| | $V_i =$ Initial |
| | $V_t =$ Larger, more slowly equilibrating (Myocardium) |
| Volume of distribution ($V_D$) | 7.3 L/Kg (IBW) |
| Clearance (Cl) | Cl $=$ Cl$_{metabolic} +$ Cl$_{renal}$ |
| Half-life ($T_{1/2}$) | NL renal function $\approx 2$ days |
| | ESRD $\approx 4$–6 days |

*Source*: Adapted from [28].

falsely elevated and will not be reflective of therapeutic or toxic effects of digoxin [28]. However, clinical effects of a dose can be seen much earlier than 4–6 h, as the distribution half-life of digoxin is 35 min [28]. Digoxin's clearance is the sum of it's metabolic and renal clearance. The renal clearance is equal to or slightly less than the creatinine clearance. The metabolic clearance may be decreased by one-half in patients with HF and the renal clearance may also be slightly reduced in these patients [28]. Digoxin's half-life is approximately 2 days, allowing once daily dosing in patients with normal or slightly impaired renal function [28]. In these patients, steady state serum digoxin concentrations can be estimated in four half-lives [2] or 7–14 days after drug initiation or dosage change [28]. The half-life in anephric patients may increase to 4–6 days, thus steady state in these patients may not be reached for 15–20 days in patients with end-stage renal disease [28]. Digoxin is not effectively removed by peritoneal or hemodialysis because of the drug's large volume of distribution, thus supplemental dosing after dialysis are unnecessary [2,28].

There are a large number of drugs that may interact with digoxin including clarithromycin, erythromycin, amiodarone, itraconazole, cyclosporine, verapamil, or quinidine, all of which can increase serum digoxin levels. Many of these drugs are commonly coadministered with digoxin for the treatment of heart failure and appropriate dosage adjustments must be made to avoid digoxin toxicities. Pharmacokinetic drug interactions with

**Table 2.2** Major pharmacokinetic drug–drug interactions [2, 28, 68, 69].

| Drug | Proposed mechanism(s) | Effect on digoxin blood levels |
|---|---|---|
| Amiodarone | Increased bioavailability and decreased renal and nonrenal clearance | Increase |
| Clarithromycin | Increased bioavailability | Increase |
| Erythromycin | (In 10–15% of patients due to change in enteric flora) | |
| Cyclosporine | Unknown, probably decreased renal clearance | Increase |
| Propafenone | Decreased volume of distribution and decreased clearance | Increase |
| Quinidine | Decreased volume of distribution and decreased renal and nonrenal clearance | Increase |
| Verapamil | Decreased nonrenal clearance | Increase |

digoxin occur when interacting medications cause changes in digoxin bioavailability, volume of distribution, metabolism, or clearance (see Table 2.2). Pharmacodynamic interactions may also occur making individuals more susceptible to digoxin's adverse effects.

## Digoxin toxicity

*Digitalis* intoxication, which was caused by taking high doses of the medication and generally resolved upon discontinuation, was first described by William Withering in 1785 [1]. The cardiac and extracardiac signs and symptoms of *Digitalis* intoxication are very nonspecific and unpredictable [70]. Digoxin toxicity has been correlated with increasing serum digoxin concentrations, especially above 2.0 ng/mL [70–72]. Other factors that increase sensitivity to *Digitalis* include electrolyte abnormalities, advanced age, cardiac disease, impaired renal function, pulmonary disease, hypoxemia, hypothyroidism, acid–base abnormalities, amyloidosis, and drug interactions [70].

Common extracardiac symptoms include fatigue, visual complaints, muscular weakness, nausea, anorexia, abdominal upset, psychiatric complaints, dizziness, and unusual dreams [73]. The cardiac arrhythmias associated with digoxin toxicity arise from two actions of the drug, atrioventricular block and enhanced automaticity, which may lead to arrhythmias and may generate lethal ventricular

tachyarrhythmias [74]. However, it is important to recognize that the cardiac effects of toxic levels of digoxin may precede rather than follow the gastrointestinal side effects in some patients. Thus, clinicians should be vigilant in measuring serum digoxin concentrations when there is any suspicion of toxicity. The first step in the treatment of *Digitalis* intoxication is to withhold its glycoside and to correct electrolyte abnormalities, acid–base disturbances, and/or hypoxemia [70]. Digoxin Immune Fab, specific antibodies for the reversal of digoxin toxicity, have been shown to be clinically efficacious and safe for use in humans with potentially life-threatening toxicity [70].

## Conclusions

Digoxin represents the first pharmacologic agent identified for the treatment of heart failure. More recently, with the advent of ACE inhibitors, $\beta$-blockers, aldosterone antagonists, and diuretics, the role of digoxin in the management of patients with heart failure becomes less clear. Certainly, in those with persistent symptoms despite optimal therapy digoxin may play a role. Digoxin may be added to the initial regimen in patients with severe symptoms, while treatment may be delayed until the effectiveness of ACE inhibitors and $\beta$-blockers has been assessed. The choice between whether to begin digoxin or an aldosterone inhibitor in a persistently symptomatic patient remains more complex. Regardless of when digoxin therapy is begun, care should be taken to ensure that the dose of digoxin is appropriate and the blood levels do not exceed 1.0 ng/mL. When the Writing Committee for the 2005 ACC/AHA Guidelines reviewed earlier data regarding the safety and efficacy of digoxin in the context of newer studies assessing the efficacy of new pharmacologic agents including aldosterone antagonists, they felt that *Digitalis* did not compare favorably with these agents. In particular, *Digitalis* afforded no mortality benefit with a relatively narrow risk–benefit ratio. Therefore, the Writing Committee decided to change the level of recommendation for *Digitalis* from class I to a class IIa: "*Digitalis* can be beneficial in patients with current or prior symptoms of heart failure and reduced left ventricular ejection fraction to decrease hospitalizations for heart failure (Level of Evidence: B) [15]."

## References

1 Kelly RA, Smith TW. Pharmacological treatment of heart failure. In: Louis S. Goodman, Alfred Gilman, Joel G. Hardman *et al.*, eds, *The pharmacological basis of therapeutics*. 9th edn. McGraw-Hill, New York, 1996: 809–838.

2 Withering W. An account of the Foxglove and some of its medicinal uses: with practical remarks in dropsy and other diseases. The Classics of Medicine Library, Birmingham, Alabama, 1978, 207p.

3 Dec GW. Digoxin remains useful in the management of chronic heart failure. *Med Clin N Am* 2003;**87**:317–337.

4 Shull GE, Greeb J, Lingrel JB. Molecular cloning of three distinct forms of the Na+, K+, ATPase alpha-subunit from the rat brain. *Biochem* 1986;**25**:8125–8132.

5 Hasenfuss G, Mulieri LA, Allen PD *et al.* Myocardial disease: Influence of isoproterenol and ouabain on excitation-contraction coupling, cross-bridge function, and energetics in failing human myocardium. *Circulation* 1996;**94**:3155–3160.

6 Sonnenblick EH, Williams JF, Glick G *et al.* Studies on digitalis. XV. Effects of cardiac glycosides on myocardial force-velocity relations in the nonfailing human heart. *Circulation* 1966;**34**:532–9.

7 Rasmussen HH, Okita GT, Hartzs RS *et al.* Inhibition of electrogenic Na$^+$ pumping in isolated atrial tissue from patients treated with digoxin. *J Pharmacol Exp Ther* 1990;**252**:60–4.

8 Marban E, Tsien RW. Enhancement of calcium current during digitalis inotropy in mammalian heart: Positive feedback regulation by intracellular calcium? *J Physiol* 1982;**329**:589–614.

9 Smith TW. Digitalis: Mechanisms of action and clinical use. *N Engl J Med* 1988;**318**:358–365.

10 McGarry SJ, Williams AJ. Digoxin activates sarcoplasmic reticulum Ca$^{++}$ release channels: a possible role in cardiac inotropy. *Br J Pharmacol* 1993;**108**:1043–1050.

11 Rahimtoola SH, Tak T. The use of digitalis in heart failure. *Curr Prob in Cardiol* 1996;**21**:781–853.

12 Veldhuisen DJ, deGraeff PA, Remme WJ *et al.* Value of digoxin in heart failure and sinus rhythm: New features of an old drug? *J Am Coll Cardiol* 1996;**28**:813–819.

13 Cohn JN. Inotropic therapy for heart failure: paradise postponed. *N Engl J Med* 1989;**320**:729–731.

14 Krell MJ, Kline EM, Bates ER *et al.* Intermittent, ambulatory dobutamine infusions in patients with severe congestive heart failure. *Am Heart J* 1986;**112**:787–91.

15 Packer M, Carver JR, Rodeheffer RJ *et al.* Effect of oral milrinone on mortality in severe chronic heart failure. *N Engl J Med* 1991;**325**:1468–75.

16 Rekka G, Gorlin R, Smith T, and the Digitalis Investigation Group. The effect of digoxin on mortality and morbidity in patients with heart failure. *N Engl J Med* 1997;**336**:525–533.

17 Schobel HP, Oren RM, Roach PJ *et al.* Contrasting effects of digitalis and dobutamine on baroreflex sympathetic control in normal humans. *Circulation* 1991;**84**:1118–1129.

18 Hunt SA, Abraham WT, Chin MH *et al.* ACC/AHA 2005 Update for the evaluation and management of chronic heart failure in the adult: A report of the American College of Cardiology/American Heart Association task force on practice guidelines (Committee to revise the 2001 Guidelines for the Evaluation and Management of Heart Failure). 2005. American College of Cardiology Website. Available at: http://www.acc.org/clinical/guidelines/ failure/ hf_index.htm. (Accessed 15 December, 2005.)

19 Williamson KM, Patterson JH. Is there an expanded role for digoxin in patients with heart failure and sinus rhythm? A protagonist viewpoint. *Ann Pharmacother* 1997;**31**:888–892.

20 Ferguson DW, Berg WJ, Sanders JS *et al.* Sympathoinhibitory responses to digitalis glycosides in heart failure patients: Direct evidence from sympathetic neural recordings. *Circulation* 1989;**80**:65–77.

21 Mason DT, Spann JF, Zelis R *et al.* Studies on digitalis X. Effects of ouabain on forearm vascular resistance and venous tone in normal subjects and in patients with heart failure. *J Clin Invest* 1964;**43**:532–543.

22 Covit AB, Schaer GL, Sealey JE *et al.* Suppression of the renin-angiotensin system by the intravenous digoxin in chronic congestive heart failure. *Am J Med* 1983;**75**:445–447.

23  Newton GE, Tong JH, Schofield M *et al.* Digoxin reduces cardiac sympathetic activity in severe congestive heart failure. *J Am Coll Cardiol* 1996;**28**:155–161.

24  Pistorello M, Cimolato M, Pedini F *et al.* Effect of digoxin on the in vitro secretion of renin and angiotensin II/III immunoreactivity by the human adrenal gland. *Acta Endo* 1992;**127**:210–214.

25  Ribner HS, Plucinski DA, Hsieh AM *et al.* Acute effects of digoxin on total systemic vascular resistance in congestive heart failure due to dilated cardiomyopathy: a hemodynamic-hormonal study. *Am J Cardiol* 1985;**56**:896–904.

26  Brouwer J, Veldhuisen DJ, Man in 't Veld AJ *et al.* Heart rate variability in patients with mild to moderate heart failure: effects of neurohormonal modulation by digoxin and ibopamine. The DIMT Study Group. *J Am Coll Cardiol* 1995;**26**:983–990.

27  Heart Failure Society of America Committee Members. Heart Failure Society of America Practice Guidelines: HFSA Guidelines for the management of patients with heart failure caused by left ventricular systolic dysfunction-pharmacological approaches. *J Card Fail* 1999;**5**:357–382.

28  Winter ME. *Basic Clinical Pharmacokinetics.* 4th edn. Lippincott Williams Wilkins, Philadelphia, 2004: 183–218.

29  Terra SG, Washam JB, Dunham GD *et al.* Therapeutic range of digoxin's efficacy in heart failure: What is the evidence? *Pharmacotherapy* 1999;**19**:1123–1126.

30  Adams KF, Gheorghiade M, Uretsky BF *et al.* Clinical benefits of low serum digoxin concentrations in heart failure. *J Am Coll Cardiol* 2002;**39**:946–953.

31  Gheorghiade M, Hall VB, Jacobsen G *et al.* Effects of increasing maintenance dose of digoxin on left ventricular function and neurohormones in patients with chronic heart failure treated with diuretics and angiotensin-converting enzyme inhibitors. *Circulation* 1995;**92**:1801–1807.

32  Rathore SS, Curtis JP, Wang Y *et al.* Association of serum digoxin concentration and outcomes in patients with heart failure. *J Am Med Assoc* 2003;**289**: 871–878.

33  Slatton ML, Irani WN, Hall SA *et al.* Does digoxin provide additional hemodynamic and autonomic benefit at higher doses in patients with mild to moderate heart failure and normal sinus rhythm?. *J Am Coll Cardiol* 1997;**29**:1206–1213.

34  Packer M, Gheorghiade M, Young JB *et al.* Withdrawal of digoxin from patients with chronic heart failure treated with angiotensin-converting enzyme inhibitors. *N Engl J Med* 1993;**329**:1–7.

35  Uretsky BF, Young JB, Shahidi FE *et al.* Randomized study assessing the effect of digoxin withdrawal in patients with

mild to moderate chronic congestive heart failure: Results of the PROVED Trial. *J Am Coll Cardiol* 1993;**22**:955–962.

36  Gheorghiade M, Pitt B. Digitalis Investigation Group trial: A stimulus for further research. *Am Heart J* 1997;**134**:3–12.

37  Rathore SS, Wang Y, Krumholz HM. Sex-based differences in the effect of digoxin for the treatment of heart failure. *N Engl J Med* 2002;**347**:1403–1411.

38  Gheorghiade M, Zarowitz BJ. Review of randomized trials of digoxin therapy in patients with chronic heart failure. *Am J Cardiol* 1992;**69**:48G–62G.

39  Riaz K, Forker AD. Digoxin use in congestive heart failure. Current status. *Drugs* 1998;**55**:747–758.

40  Tauke J, Goldstein S, Gheorghiade M. Digoxin for chronic heart failure: A review of the randomized controlled trials with special attention to the PROVEd and RADIANCE Trials. *Prog in Cardiovasc Dis* 1994;**37**:49–58.

41  Jaeschke R, Oxman A, Guyatt GH. To what extent do congestive heart failure patients in sinus rhythm benefit from digoxin therapy? A systematic overview and meta-analysis. *Am J Med* 1990;**88**:279–286.

42  Demers C, McKelvie RS, Yusuf S. The role of digitalis in the treatment of heart failure. *Coron Artery Dis* 1999;**10**:353–360.

43  Rathore SS, Wang Y, Krumholz HM. Sex-based differences in the effect of digoxin in the treatment of heart failure. *N Engl J Med* 2002;**347**:1403–1411.

44  Shlipak MG, Smith GL, Ratahore SS *et al.* Renal function, digoxin therapy, and heart failure outcomes: Evidence from the Digoxin Intervention Group. *J Am Soc Nephrol* 2004;**15**:2195–2203.

45  Massie BM, Abdalla I. Heart failure in patients with preserved left ventricular systolic function: Do digitalis glycosides have a role? *Prog in Cardiovasc Dis* 1998;**40**:357–369.

46  David D, Segni ED, Klein HO *et al.* Inefficacy of digitalis in the control of heart rate in patients with chronic atrial fibrillation: beneficial effect of an added beta adrenergic blocking agent. *Am J Cardiol* 1979;**44**:1378–1382.

47  Farshi R, Kistner D, Sarma JS *et al.* Ventricular rate control in chronic atrial fibrillation during daily activity and programmed exercise: a crossover, open–label study of five drug regimens. *J Am Coll Cardiol* 1999;**33**:304–310.

48  Matsuda M, Matsuda Y, Yamagishi T *et al.* Effects of digoxin, propranolol and verapamil on exercise in patients with chronic isolated atrial fibrillation. *Cardiovasc Res* 1991;**25**:453–457.

49  Leor J, Goldbourt U, Behar S. Is it safe to prescribe digoxin after acute myocardial infarction? Update on continued controversy. *Am Heart J* 1995; 130:1322–1326.

50  Gross GJ, Warltier DC, Hardman HFB *et al.* The effect of ouabain on nutritional circulation and regional myocardial blood flow. *Am Heart J* 1977;**93**:487–495.

51  Lynch JJ, Simpson PJ, Gallagher KP *et al.* Increase in experimental infarct size with digoxin in a canine model of myocardial ischemia-reperfusion injury. *Am Heart J* 1988;**115**:1171–1182.

52  Maroko PR, Kjekshus JK, Sobel BE. Factors influencing infarct size following experimental coronary artery occlusions. *Circulation* 1971;**43**:67–71.

53  Lynch JJ, Montgomery DG, Lucchesi BR. Facilitation of lethal ventricular arrhythmias by therapeutic digoxin in conscious post infarction dogs. *Am Heart J* 1986;**111**:883–890.

54  Lynch JJ, Lucchesi BR. Effect of digoxin on the extent of injury and the severity of arrhythmias during acute myocardial infarction in the dog. *J Cardiovasc Pharmacol* 1988;**11**:193–203.

55  Iesaka Y, Kazutaka A, Gosselin AJ. Susceptibility of infracted canine hearts to digitalis-toxic ventricular tachycardia. *J Am Coll Cardiol* 1983;**2**:45–51.

56  Bigger JT, Fleiss JL, Rlonitzky LM *et al.* Effect of digitalis treatment on survival after acute myocardial infarction. *Am J Cardiol* 1985;**55**:623–630.

57  Byington R, Goldstein S. Association of digitalis therapy with mortality in survivors of acute myocardial infarction: observations in the Beta-Blocker Heart Attack Trial. *J Am Coll Cardiol* 1985;**6**:976–982.

58  Moss AJ, Davis HT, Conrad DL *et al.* Digitalis-associated cardiac mortality after myocardial infarction. *Circulation* 1981;**64**:1150–1156.

59  Madsen EB, Gilpin E, Henning H *et al.* Prognostic importance of digitalis after acute myocardial infarction. *J Am Coll Cardiol* 1984;**3**:681–689.

60  Muller JE, Turi ZG, Stone PH *et al.* Digoxin therapy and mortality after myocardial infarction. Experience in the MILIS study. *N Engl J Med* 1986;**314**:265–271.

61  Akiyama T, Pawitan Y, Campbell WB *et al.* Effects of advancing age on the efficacy and side effects of antiarrhythmic drugs in post-myocardial infarction patients with ventricular arrhythmias. The CAST Investigators. *J Am Ger Soc* 1992;**40**:666–672.

62  Anonymous. The mortality risk associated with digitalis treatment after myocardial infarction. The Digitalis Subcommittee of the Multicenter Post-Infarction Research Group. *Card Drugs Ther* 1987;**1**:125–132.

63  Kober L, Torp-Pedersen C, Gadsboll N *et al.* Is digoxin and independent risk factor for long-term mortality after acute myocardial infarction? *Eur Heart J* 1994;**15**:382–388.

64  Molstad P, Abdelnoor M. Digitoxin-associated mortality in acute myocardial infarction. *Eur Heart J* 1991;**12**:65–69.

65  Zack PM, Chaitman BR, Davis KB *et al.* Survival patterns in clinical and angiographic subsets of medically treated patients with combined proximal left anterior descending and proximal left circumflex coronary artery disease (CASS). *Am Heart J* 1989;**118**:220–227.

66  Leor J, Goldbourt U, Rabinowitz B *et al.* Digoxin and increased mortality among patients recovering from acute myocardial infarction: importance of digoxin dose. The SPRINT Study Group. *Card Drug Ther* 1995;**9**:723–729.

67  Ryan TJ, Bailey KR, McCabe CH *et al.* The effects of digitalis on survival in high-risk patients with coronary artery disease. The Coronary ASrtery Surgery Study (CASS). *Circulation* 1983;**67**:735–741.

68  Tatro DS, ed. *Drug Interaction Facts.* Facts and Comparisons, St Louis, 2000. 431–475.

69  Rodin SM, Johnson BF. Pharmacokinetic interactions with digoxin. *Clin Pharmacol* 1988;**15**:227–244.

70  Allen NM, Dunham GD. Treatment of digitalis intoxication with emphasis on the clinical use of digoxin immune FAB. *Ann Pharmacother* 1990;**24**:991–998.

71  Williamson KM, Thrasher KA, Fulton KB *et al.* Digoxin toxicity: An evaluation in current clinical practice. *Arch Int Med* 1998;**158**:2444–2449.

72  Beller GA, Smith TW, Abelmann WH, et al. Digitalis intoxication: A prospective clinical study with serum level correlations. *N Engl J Med* 1971;**284**:989–997.

73  Lely AH, Van Enter CHJ. Large-scale digitoxin intoxication. *BMJ* 1970;**3**:737–740.

74  Moorman JR, Pritchett EL. The arrhythmias of digitalis intoxication. *Arch Intern Med* 1985;**145**:1289–1292.

**CHAPTER 3**

# Renin–angiotensin system and angiotensin converting enzyme inhibitors in chronic heart failure

*Rimvida Obeleniene,* MD *& Marrick Kukin,* MD

## Introduction

Hemodynamic alterations in heart failure (HF) activate neurohormonal pathways including the renin–angiotensin (RAS) system. The hormonal changes while initially compensatory to maintain blood pressure, often have long-term deleterious effects on the failing heart. Thus, the RAS system has served as a target for therapeutic intervention in patients with HF.

## The biology of angiotensin II and the RAS

The classic RAS system is viewed as an endocrine system [1]. Angiotensinogen, an alpha-1 globulin is produced primarily by the liver and released into the circulation. Renin, a large enzyme produced mostly in the kidney, acts on circulating angiotensinogen to produce angiotensin I, which is a decapeptide, in the plasma. Circulating angiotensin I is then converted by the plasma angiotensin converting enzyme (ACE) and by pulmonary endothelial ACE into angiotensin II, an octapeptide. The major determinant of the rate of angiotensin II production is the amount of renin released by the kidney [2].

Renin is synthesized, stored, and secreted into the renal arterial circulation by the granular juxtaglomerular cells that lie within the walls of the afferent arterioles as they enter the glomeruli. The half-life of circulating renin is approximately 15 min. The secretion of renin is controlled by a complex array of renal and CNS pathways. For example, an increase in sodium (Na) absorption in the macula densa of the kidney as well as increased expression of adenosine (through A1-adenosine receptor activation) inhibits renin release [3], while prostaglandins stimulate renin release [4]. The regulation of renin release in the macula densa also appears to be mediated through complex interactions between COX-2 (inducible cyclooxygenase) and nNOS (neuronal nitric oxide synthase [5–7]. Evidence for this comes from the finding that Na depletion upregulates nNOS and COX-2, increases nitric oxide and peroxynitrite biosynthesis in the macula densa, and activates prostaglandin receptors in the juxtaglomerular cells.

Renin release is also regulated by changes in renal perfusion pressure. Both increases and decreases in renal perfusion effect wall tension in the afferent arteriole with subsequent modulation of renin release through the baroreceptor pathway. In addition, activation of $\beta_1$-adrenergic receptor-mediated pathways in juxtaglomerular cells also enhances renin secretion. While angiotensinogen serves as the substrate for renin and is found in the kidney its major source of synthesis is the liver [8,9].

Angiotensin converting enzyme (kininase II) is a glycoprotein ectoenzyme. Circulating ACE represents membrane ACE that has undergone proteolysis [10]. ACE is nonspecific and cleaves dipeptide units from diverse amino acid sequences including those found in bradykinin. That ACE effects rapid conversion of angiotensin I to angiotensin II is demonstrated when angiotensin I is administered intravenously. This conversion has physiologic importance as angiotensin I is less than 1%

as potent a vasoconstrictor as angiotensin II. Angiotensin III is formed from angiotensin II or I by aminopeptidase or ACE, respectively but angiotensin III is only 25% as potent as angiotensin II in elevating blood pressure and 10% as effective in stimulating the adrenal medulla [2].

Several recent findings have added increased complexity to the area of ACE and ACE inhibition. One area of recent interest is angiotensin 1–7. Both, angiotensin I and II can be metabolized to angiotensin 1–7. In addition, ACE inhibitors increase tissue and plasma levels of angiotensin 1–7, largely as a result of an increase in the levels of angiotensin I. Angiotensin 1–7 releases vasopressin, stimulates prostaglandin biosynthesis, dilates some blood vessels, and inhibits proliferation of vascular smooth muscle cells [11].

Recent studies have also demonstrated the biologic importance of tissue-based ACE. Extrinsic local RAS is acting via ACE on the vascular endothelial cells producing angiotensin I and II primarily within or at the surfaces of the blood vessel wall [12–14]. Intrinsic local RAS exists in many tissues: brain, blood vessels, pituitary, heart, kidney [15–17]. Interestingly, angiotensin II production has non-ACE mediated mechanisms. Indeed, a variety of signaling molecules including cathepsin G, heart chymase, and tonin enzymes appear to be able to synthesize angiotensin I and II independent of ACE [17,18]. However, the role of these alternative pathways in the pathophysiology of HF is not fully understood.

The biological effects of angiotensin II are mediated through interactions with two angiotensin receptors, $AT_1$ and $AT_2$. These receptors are coupled to guanine-nucleotide regulatory proteins, which in turn activate a variety of down-stream signaling pathways including phospholipase, calcium, MAP kinase JAK/STAT pathways, NADP/NADPH oxidase, serine/threonin protein kinases, nonreceptor tyrosine kinases, GTP-binding proteins, and inducible transcription and translation factors [19–21]. Signal transduction mechanisms for the $AT_2$ receptor include activation of phosphatases, potassium channels, nitric oxide production and inhibition of calcium channels [22]. A summary of major effects of angiotensin II are presented in Table 3.1.

Activation of RAS has both acute and chronic effects on the vasculature and the myocardium. Short-term activation maintains vascular tone, renal function, and other neurohormonal pathways. Indeed, an immediate effect of angiotensin II production is enhanced cardiac output and reduced left ventricular filling pressures. By contrast, chronic overexpression of angiotensin II is deleterious to the heart as it results in maladaptive cardiac remodeling including fibrosis and cellular hypertrophy. It is the well-demonstrated effects of angiotensin II on pathologic remodeling that led investigators to hypothesize that inhibition of ACE and diminished levels of angiotensin II might prove beneficial in patients with HF [1,2] (Figure 3.1).

## Pharmacology of ACEIs

The primary pharmacologic effect of ACEIs is to inhibit the conversion of the angiotensin I to the active angiotensin II. However, ACEIs also interfere with the negative feedback in renin release by increasing renin release and the rate of angiotensin I formation. ACEIs also enhance the action of kinins and augment kinin-mediated prostaglandin synthesis, an action that might explain their enhanced

Table 3.1 Mechanisms of Angiotensin II effects.

| Altered peripheral resistance | Altered renal function | Altered cardiovascular structure |
|---|---|---|
| Direct vasoconstriction | Direct effect to increase sodium | Non hemodynamically mediated effects |
| Enhancement of peripheral | reabsorbtion in proximal tubule | Increased expression of proto-oncogenes |
| noradrenergic neurotransmission | Release of aldosterone | Production of growth factors |
| Increase sympathetic discharge | Altered renal hemodynamics | Synthesis of extracellular matrix proteins |
| Release of catecholamines from | | Hemodynamically mediated effects |
| medulla | | Increased afterload |
| | | Increased wall tension |

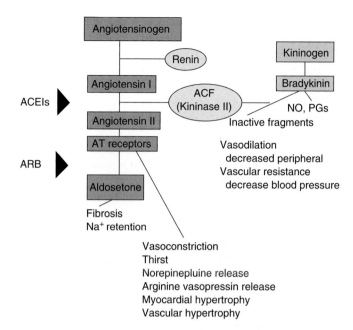

**Figure 3.1** Renin–angiotensin cascade and sites of action of ACEIs and angiotensin receptor blockers.

efficacy when compared with angiotensin receptor blockers in experimental systems. That non-ACE inhibition mechanisms also participate in the pharmacologic actions of ACEIs can be shown by the fact that administration of a kinin receptor blocker abrogates the advantage of ACE inhibition in experimental models [23].

Angiotensin converting enzyme inhibitors can be classified into three groups: sulfhydryl-containing (Captopril, Pivalopril, Zofenopril, Alacepril), dicarboxyl-containing (Enalapril, Lisinopril, Benazepril, Quinapril, Moexipril, Ramipril, Perindopril, Cilazapril), and phosphorus containing (Fosinopril) [1,2]. Currently available ACEIs are listed in Table 3.2. ACEIs differ markedly in tissue distribution and it is possible that this difference corresponds to local RAS, although clinical differences are not clearly established. ACEIs are predominantly cleared by the kidneys. Fosinopril has balanced elimination by the liver and kidneys [1].

## Clinical trials assessing the efficacy of ACEIs

A large number of seminal clinical trials have been performed over the past 20 years that demonstrate

**Table 3.2** FDA approved ACEIs and dosages.

| ACIEs | Dosage of Tablets (mg) |
| --- | --- |
| Benazepril (Lotensin) | 5, 10, 20, 40 mg tablets |
| Captopril (Capoten) | 12.5, 25, 50, 100 mg tablets |
| Enalapril (Vasotec) | 2.5, 5,10, 20 mg tablets |
| Enalaprilat | IV 1.25 mg/ml for injection |
| Fosinopril (Monopril) | 10, 20, 40 mg tablets |
| Lisinopril (Prinivil, Zestril) | 2.5, 5, 10, 20, 40 mg tablets |
| Moexipril (Univasc) | 7.5, 15 mg tablets |
| Perindopril (Aceon) | 2, 4, 8 mg tablets |
| Quinapril (Accupril) | 5, 10, 20, 40 mg tablets |
| Ramipril (Altace) | 1.25, 2.5, 5, 10 mg tablets |
| Trandolapril (Mavik) | 1, 2, 4 mg tablets |

the salutary benefits of ACEI in the therapy of HF. A review of these trials is relevant as it supports the current recommendations regarding the use of ACEI in HF therapy.

The first large randomized and placebo-controlled trial demonstrating the efficacy of ACEI in the therapy of HF was the Captopril multicenter trial (Captopril multicenter research group). This trial studied 92 patients with NYHA class II–III symptoms and EFs ≤40% despite treatment with diuretics and digoxin, who were randomized to captopril or placebo for a period of 3 months [24].

The dose of captopril was titrated from 25 mg tid to 100 mg tid over a period of 2 weeks. Patients randomized to captopril demonstrated increased exercise tolerance and improved symptoms when compared with placebo. In view of these salutary benefits of ACE inhibition, a second trial, the captopril–digoxin multicenter study was undertaken to compare the effects of captopril, digoxin, and placebo in patients with history of treatment with diuretics, an EF ≤40%, and NYHA class II symptoms [25]. The primary endpoints were exercise tolerance and symptoms. Captopril and digoxin were superior to placebo but interestingly indistinguishable from one another. Based on these studies, captopril was recommended as first-line therapy for patients with HF. However, important questions remained: were the benefits of captopril obvious with other ACEIs, could the use of ACEI's influence survival, and would inhibition of angiotensin II production benefit patients with either less severe or more severe disease. These important questions were addressed by a series of studies beginning in 1985.

Cooperative North Scandinavian Enalapril Study, CONSENSUS-I, was designed to determine the effect of ACEIs on survival [26]. The study included 257 patients with NYHA class IV HF, not responding to hospitalization and intensive therapy. Patients were randomized to enalapril (target dose 20 mg) twice daily, (mean total daily dose = 18 mg) or placebo. Enalapril reduced mortality from 44% to 26% at 6 months and from 52% to 36% at 12 months. CONSENSUS-I was a landmark study because it represented the first evidence that pharmacologic therapy could improve survival in patients with HF. However, its impact was superseded by the subsequent SOLVD trials that assessed the effects of enalapril in an even larger patient population. The SOLVD-treatment trial (studies on left ventricular dysfunction treatment trial), enrolled 2569 patients with NYHA class II and III HF symptoms and EFs ≤35% who were receiving diuretics and digoxin and randomized them to either enalapril (mean daily dose of 16.6 mg) or placebo [27]. In 41 month follow-up, the enalapril group demonstrated a 16% reduction in all-cause mortality and a 26% reduction in the combined endpoint of death or hospitalization for HF. Mortality reduction was attributed to a reduction

in the progression of HF as there was no discernible decrease in the incidence of sudden death. The results of SOLVD-treatment extended the benefits of ACEI in reducing mortality from the NYHA class IV patients as seen in CONSENSUS I to NYHA class II and III patients [28].

The SOLVD prevention trial studied asymptomatic patients (n = 4228) with an EF ≤35% and followed patients for up to 62 months [29]. Although enalapril did not effect a statistically significant reduction in mortality, it did effect a significant reduction (29%) in the prespecified combined endpoint of death or worsening HF. Thus, ACEIs reduced disease progression, and improved symptoms and prognosis in patients with preclinical disease. Importantly, the beneficial effects of enalapril therapy appear to be sustained over time as a recent 12-year follow-up of SOLVD demonstrated improved survival in patients enrolled in both the prevention arm (50.9% mortality enalapril versus 56.4% placebo) and the treatment arm (79.8% enalapril versus 80.8% placebo) despite a high rate of cross-over to ACEI therapy [30]. When data for the prevention and treatment trials were combined, the hazard ratio for death was 0.90 for the enalapril group compared with the placebo group. Indeed, enalapril extended median survival by 9.4 months in the combined trials. Similar results were found in the Munich mild heart failure trial [31]. This study enrolled 170 patients with NYHA class II symptoms and randomized them to either captopril or placebo with a median observation period of 2.7 years. Heart failure progressed to class IV in nine patients (10.8%) treated with captopril and in 23 patients (26.4%) treated with placebo and mean survival was 223 days longer in the captopril group. Thus, ACE inhibition early in the course of congestive HF slowed the progress disease.

The V-HeFT-II trial compared enalapril with the combination of hydralazine and isosorbide dinitrate in 804 patients with NYHA class II–III HF and EF of ≤45% [32]. The target dose of enalapril was 10 mg twice a day. Enalapril reduced mortality by 34% after 1 year and 28% after 2 years compared to the hydralazine–isordil combination, an improvement that was attributed to a decrease in sudden death. Since both ACEIs and hydralazine/isosorbide dinitrate have vasodilatory properties but only ACEIs blunt the neurohormonal axis, these results led investigators to suggest that the beneficial effects of ACE inhibition are due largely to their effects of angiotensin II – signaling. However, the recent trial demonstrating the benefits of the combination of hydralazine and isordil in African American patients with HF suggests that the mechanisms responsible for the beneficial effects of these agents might be far more complicated than was originally presumed (see Chapter 10).

That ACEIs benefit patients with HF was shown not just by the initial large seminal clinical trials but also by meta-analysis of a large number of studies using a variety of different ACEIs. For example, analysis of 32 studies utilizing 8 different ACEIs in a total of 7105 patients supported the benefits of ACEI use in this broad group of patients [33]. There was heterogeneity between the different drugs, supporting the class effect of ACEIs. Furthermore, ACEIs appeared to have a similar mortality benefit in patients 65 years of age or older who had an acute myocardial infarction [34]. These results came from a retrospective cohort study that used linked hospital discharge and prescription databases containing information on 18 453 patients 65 years of age or older who were admitted for an acute myocardial infarction [35].

## ACEIs, myocardial infarction, and heart failure

Heart failure is one of the major complications of myocardial infarction (MI) both acutely and chronically. The positive ACEI effect in established cases of HF encouraged further studies of these agents in patients following acute MI with or without HF. Four trials enrolled patients with left ventricular dysfunction following an acute MI: SAVE, AIRE, TRACE, and CONSENSUS II.

The SAVE (Survival and Ventricular Enlargement) trial was the first trial to evaluate ACEI in prevention of development of HF and mortality in patients within the post-MI period [36]. Within 3 to 16 days after MI, 2231 patients with EFs of $\leq 40\%$ without overt HF or symptoms of myocardial ischemia were randomly assigned to receive double-blind treatment with either placebo (1116 patients) or captopril 50 mg three times a day (1115 patients) and were followed for an average of

42 months. Mortality was significantly reduced by 19% as was the risk of recurrent MI in the ACEI group. In the AIRE (Acute Infarction Ramipril Efficacy Study) trial, the effect of ACE inhibition on the survival of patients with clinical HF after acute MI, was assessed [37] at an average follow-up time of 15 months. All-cause mortality was reduced from 22.6% (placebo group) to 16.9% (ramipril group) representing an absolute mortality reduction of 5.7% and a relative risk reduction of 27% in 2006 patients. In a long term follow-up study – AIRE Extension (AIREX) Study (Acute Infarction Ramipril Efficacy) – death from all causes occurred in 117 (38.9%) of 301 placebo and 83 (27.5%) of ramipril treated patients; a relative risk reduction of 36% and an absolute reduction in mortality of 11.4% (114 additional 5-year survivors per 1000 patients treated for an average of 12.4 months) [38]. Thus, there is evidence that administration of ramipril to patients with clinically defined HF after AMI results in a survival benefit that is not only large in magnitude, but also sustained over many years.

TRACE (Trandolapril Cardiac Evaluation Trial) [39] studied the effects of a third ACEI, trandolapril versus placebo in 1749 patients with a recent MI and left ventricular dysfunction (EF $\leq 35\%$). A total of 1749 patients were randomly assigned 3 to 7 days post-MI to receive oral trandolapril and patients were followed for 24 to 50 months. During the study period, 304 patients (34.7%) in the trandolapril group died, as compared with 369 (42.3%) in the placebo group. The relative risk of death in the trandolapril group, as compared with the placebo group, was 0.78. Trandolapril also reduced the risk of death from cardiovascular causes (relative risk, 0.75 and sudden death relative risk, 0.76). Progression to severe HF was less frequent in the trandolapril group (relative risk, 0.71). In contrast to SAVE, the risk of recurrent MI (fatal or nonfatal) was not significantly reduced (relative risk, 0.86). Similarly, SMILE (Survival of Myocardial Infarction Long-term Evaluation Study), randomized 1556 patients with a large anterior MI to the ACEI zofenopril or to placebo [40]. The overall prevalence of CHF was not reduced by zofenopril; however, the prevalence of severe HF (1.6% versus 2.6%, risk reduction 55.5%) and the combined occurrence of death or severe HF (4.8% versus 8.2%, risk reduction 59% were reduced at 6 weeks in the zofenopril group. In addition, the percentage of patients experiencing the development of severe HF after 1 year was significantly reduced with zofenopril (11.0% versus 24.3%). Thus, these results suggested that ACEIs should be considered for the prevention and treatment of CHF in patients with AMI [41].

By contrast with AIRE, SAVE and TRACE, CONSENSUS II assessed the use of intravenous enalaprilat early after a MI in 6090 patients [42]. All patients received subsequent oral enalapril unless the enalaprilat was not tolerated. This pharmacologic regimen had no effect on survival. Indeed, the CONSENSUS II trial was closed prematurely on the advice of the data and safety monitoring committee and the steering committee due to a 10% increase in risk in the enalapril treatment group. It was hypothesized that the increased incidence of hypotension from IV enalaprilat in the immediate post-MI period led to the lack of benefit for ACEI in this trial. This hypothesis was supported by Gruppo Italiano per lo Studio della Sopravvivenza nell'Infarto Miocardico (GISSI-3) [43] and the Fourth International Study of Infarct Survival (ISIS-4) [44] – both of which demonstrated a small benefit from early (within 24 h) short-term (4 to 6 weeks) treatment of patients with a MI who were not hypotensive. GISSI-3 randomized 19 394 patients to either lisinopril or control for 6 weeks and demonstrated a 12% decrease in mortality in the active treatment group while ISIS-4 demonstrated a 7% decrease in mortality in the active treatment group when 58 050 patients with an acute MI were randomized to either captopril or placebo, a finding that was substantiated by the Chinese cardiac study [45]. Thus, ACEIs have demonstrated consistent benefit in the post-MI patient with the greatest benefit being found in those patients with reduced EF.

Recently, investigators have sought to understand the mechanisms responsible for the salutary benefits of ACEIs in the post-MI population. For example, de Kam PJ *et al.* presented the results of meta-analysis of 845 patients form FAMIS, CAPTIN, and CATS studies, which evaluated the effect of ACE inhibition <9 h after MI on left ventricular (LV) dilation in patients receiving thrombolysis [45]. After 3 months, LV dilation was not significantly attenuated by very early treatment with an ACEI. However, subgroup analysis demonstrated that LV dilation was significantly attenuated by ACEI treatment only in patients in whom reperfusion was not successful. Furthermore, ACE inhibition prevented 6 deaths per 1000 treated and approximately 15 deaths due to HF per 1000 treated – benefits that were only seen with early administration of drug. Thus early administration and the avoidance of hypotension appear to be two important caveats in the use of ACE inhibition in the immediate post-MI period.

A second hypothesis regarding the use of ACE inhibition in the early post-MI period was that ACE inhibition effected salutary benefits through improvements in endothelial function. This hypothesis was evaluated by the TREND (Trial on Reversing ENdothelial Dysfunction) trial that assessed the effects of the ACEI quinapril in normotensive patients with coronary artery disease but without heart muscle dysfunction or major lipid abnormalities so that confounding variables that affect endothelial dysfunction could be minimized [47]. Using a double-blind, randomized, placebo-controlled design, TREND demonstrated that quinapril (40 mg daily) effected a beneficial effect on the constrictive responses to acetylcholine when compared with placebo at 6-months of therapy. That these salutary benefits on endothelial function were attributable to diminished bradykinin metabolism with subsequent release of endothelial nitric oxide is under active investigation.

## Clinical utility of ACEIs in patients with coronary artery disease and LV dysfunction

Despite the salutary benefits of ACE inhibition on morbidity and mortality in patients with symptomatic HF or with a recent MI, it should not be assumed that ACEIs provide salutary benefits in all forms of cardiovascular disease. For example, the QUITE trial (The Quinapril Ischemic Event Trial) was designed to test the hypothesis that quinapril 20 mg a day would reduce ischemic events (the occurrence of cardiac death, resuscitated cardiac arrest, nonfatal MI, coronary artery bypass grafting, coronary angioplasty, or hospitalization for angina pectoris) and the angiographic progression of coronary artery disease in patients without systolic LV dysfunction [48]. A total of 1750 patients were randomized to quinapril 20 mg a day or placebo and followed for a mean of 27 months. However, quinapril 20 mg did not significantly affect the overall frequency of clinical outcomes or the progression of coronary atherosclerosis [49]. Similarly, the QUASAR trial found that ACE inhibition had no effect on the incidence of transient ischemic events [50]. However, Flather *et al.* demonstrated in a meta-analysis of five long-term treatment trials consisting of a total of 12 763 patients who were randomized to either active treatment or placebo after an acute MI and followed for an average of 35 months [51] that ACEIs reduce the risk of death or readmission for HF in patients with lower EFs.

## Role of ACEIs in patients with coronary artery disease and preserved LV function

While treatment with ACEIs clearly reduces the rate of cardiovascular events among patients with LV dysfunction and those at high risk of such events, the role of ACEIs in preventing the development of HF was assessed in the HOPE trial. The HOPE study enrolled patients ($n = 9297$) with a high cardiovascular risk but excluded those with known impairment of systolic function as patients were required to have an EF >40%. In HOPE, the ACEI ramipril markedly reduced the combined endpoint of cardiovascular death, stroke, and MI. There was a highly significant 20% risk reduction in the rate of MI, a prospectively defined endpoint, over the average 4.5 year follow-up [52].

A group of European trials also assessed the same question, that is, can ACE inhibition benefit patients with coronary disease but with preserved ventricular function. The EUROPA trial (Efficacy of perindopril in reduction of cardiovascular events among patients with stable coronary artery disease), a randomized, double-blind, placebo-controlled, multicenter trial assessed whether the ACE inhibitor [53] perindopril reduced cardiovascular risk in a low-risk population with stable coronary heart disease and no apparent HF [54]. Patients had a cardiovascular history that included a previous MI (64%), angiographic evidence of coronary artery disease (61%), coronary revascularization (55%), or a positive stress test only (5%).

Nearly 13 000 patients were randomly assigned to perindopril 8 mg once daily ($n = 6110$) or to placebo ($n = 6108$). The mean follow-up was 4.2 years and the primary endpoint was a combination of cardiovascular death, MI, or cardiac arrest. The use of perindopril was associated with a 20% relative risk reduction – a benefit that was seen in all predefined subgroups. Perindopril demonstrated similar benefits in patients with diabetes who were receiving standard therapy including aspirin, statins, and beta-blockers [56]. The mechanisms responsible for the salutary benefits of ACE inhibition in this population will hopefully be clarified by the ongoing EUROPA-PERFECT substudy that is designed to test the hypothesis that the beneficial effects of ACE inhibition are mediated through alterations in sympathetic discharge and local vasodilating effects of enhanced nitric oxide and bradykinin release [57].

Thus, taken together with the retrospectively derived evidence from the HF trials there is now evidence supporting the hypothesis that the ACEIs can prevent MI and decrease overall cardiovascular risk as well as the risk of developing HF. However, whether the results of HOPE can be applied to other ACEIs remains to be determined. Furthermore, it is unclear as to whether these salutary benefits of ACEIs will also be seen with angiotensin receptor antagonists. The majority of patients with clinical HF have underlying ischemic heart disease. Prevention of MI and control of blood pressure are two key factors in the management of patients irrespective of systolic ventricular function.

## Dosing of ACEIs in HF

Despite the evidence for benefit of ACEIs, recent studies suggest that they are persistently used in lower doses in clinical practice than tested in the large-scale trials. This led investigators to designing the ATLAS (Assessment of Treatment with Lisinopril and Survival) trial, to compare high and low dose ACE inhibition. Patients (3164) with NYHA class II–IV HF symptoms were randomized to either high-dose (32.5–35.0 mg/day) or low-dose (2.5–5.0 mg/day) lisinopril. Patients in the high-dose lisinopril group had fewer hospitalizations (1.98 versus 2.22) and hospital days (18.28 versus 22.22) especially HF hospitalizations (0.64 versus 0.80) and fewer HF hospital days

(6.02 versus 7.45) compared with the low-dose group. Cost savings from fewer HF hospitalizations offset higher ACEI costs in the high-dose group. However, there was not a difference in mortality between the two groups [57]. Based on these findings and reports from other multicenter clinical trials, consensus panels have recommended that physicians make every effort to attain doses that are consistent with those used in successful multicenter trials.

## ACEI use in selected patient populations

There is a lack of information on the effects of ACEIs in the elderly. Pedone *et al.* [55] studied the frequency with which physicians wrote prescriptions for ACEIs in elderly patients with HF who were discharged from acute care hospitals and evaluated the effects of these drugs on 1-year mortality rates [58]. They used data from the GIFA. In the study, 818 patients (mean age of 79 years; range 65–101) were enrolled. One-fourth of the participants were aged 85 years or older. ACEIs were prescribed for only 550 patients (67.2%) at discharge. Older age and physical disability were negatively correlated with the use of ACEIs. However, elderly patients using ACEIs had a 40% reduction in mortality. Interestingly, the reduction in mortality was much stronger among individuals who were disabled. Thus, although not optimally utilized, ACEIs appear to have an equal benefit in the elderly.

Meta-analysis as well as post hoc analysis of large multicenter clinical trials have assessed the benefits of ACEIs according to gender, race, and the presence of diabetes [59,60]. When data was synthesized from six large trials of ACEIs that included a total of 10 213 men and 2373 women, beneficial reductions in all-cause mortality were seen in both black and white patients, men and women, and in patients with or without diabetes. Interestingly, while women with symptomatic LV systolic dysfunction benefited from ACEI use, women with asymptomatic LV systolic dysfunction did not demonstrate a reduction in mortality (pooled relative risk = 0.96; 95% confidence interval: 0.75 to 1.22). Thus, ACEIs appear to benefit a heterogenous group of patients. However, as will be discussed in Chapter 16 a patient's genotype may have a greater impact on their response to pharmacologic therapy than their phenotype.

## ACEIs and Arrhythmias

Patients with chronic heart failure (CHF) have an increased risk for sudden death. This increased risk has been associated with increased QT dispersion (QTd), a reflection of the heterogeneity in ventricular repolarization. Recently, ACEIs have been shown to decrease QTd, a marker for increased electrical instability [61]. Furthermore, experimental and clinical evidence suggests a preventive role for ACEIs on the development of atrial fibrillation. Augmented atrial apoptosis, increased angiotensin II expression, and activation of associated signaling pathways have been implicated in the experimental development of atrial fibrillation (AF), however, their clinical significance is poorly understood. For example, in a canine model of HF, atrial remodeling occurs through both angiotensin II-dependent and angiotensin II-independent pathways; however, ACE inhibition only partially prevents atrial structural remodeling [62]. In patients with HF and chronic AF, treatment with lisinopril effected a trend towards improvement in the maintenance of sinus rhythm after cardioversion although the difference was not statistically significant [63]. However, in a retrospective analysis of the SOLVD trial, the time to first hospitalization with atrial tachyarrhythmias or death was significantly lower in the enalapril group when compared with placebo. Furthermore, in a multivariate analysis adjusting for the presence of AF at study entry, enalapril treatment was associated with a reduction in the rate of hospitalization with atrial tachyarrhythmias or death (RR, 0.87). The incidence of hospitalization with atrial tachyarrhythmias was 7.9 hospitalizations per 1000 patient-years of follow-up in the enalapril group, compared with 12.4 per 1000 patient-years in the placebo group (RR, 0.64) [64]. Indeed, by Cox multivariate analysis, enalapril was the most powerful predictor for risk reduction of AF (hazard ratio, 0.22) [65]. In addition, in patients admitted for AF who required electrical cardioversion, the number of defibrillation attempts required for successful cardioversion was significantly less in patients receiving an ACEI [66]. Although the mechanisms by which ACE inhibition exerts protective effects against both atrial and ventricular tachyarrhythmias is undefined, these recent reports suggest that ACEIs may alter the electrical substrate of the heart.

## Effects of ACEIs on exercise tolerance

The effects of ACEIs on exercise tolerance remain controversial. In early clinical trials, ACE inhibitors increased the duration of treadmill exercise by 25%. Similarly, captopril and digoxin were superior to placebo in improving exercise tolerance in the captopril–digoxin multicenter study [24,25]. By contrast, when quinipril was evaluated in a double-blind placebo-controlled study in frail elderly HF patients with preserved systolic function, 6-min walk distance increased equally at 6 months in both the quinapril group and in the placebo group [67]. Similarly, in a substudy of the TRACE trial, 254 patients underwent exercise tolerance tests at 1, 3, and 12 months [68]. ACE inhibition use did not effect a significant improvement in exercise tolerance. Thus, while ACEIs improve morbidity and mortality in patients with HF, their effects on exercise performance remains unclear.

## ACEIs and the use of aspirin

A controversial issue in the use of ACEIs in patients with HF has been the effects of concomitant use of an ACEI and aspirin. In 1992, Hall et al. performed a double-blind, randomized, crossover study in 18 patients with EFs <40% using pulmonary artery catheters to measure changes in central hemodynamics in response to acutely administered enalapril when given before, concomitant to, or the day after a 350-mg dose of aspirin [69]. Prior or concomitant treatment with aspirin abolished the enalapril-induced decrease in left ventricular filling pressures, systemic and vascular resistance, and the increase in cardiac output [70].

In addition, in a substudy of only 10 patients with CHF, Nakamura et al. demonstrated that pretreatment with aspirin reduced the vasodilatory effect of intraarterial enalaprilat on forearm blood flow [71]. More recently, investigators have demonstrated that aspirin, but not ticlopidine, limited the hemodynamic response to an oral dose of enalapril [72].

Taken together, these acute studies raised concerns about the coadministration of these medications and led to the hypothesis that aspirin counteracted the beneficial hemodynamic effects of ACEIs, presumably by inhibiting prostaglandin synthesis [70]. Furthermore, in a retrospective analysis of 344 patients hospitalized for HF and were either receiving or not receiving aspirin, the combination of high-dose aspirin with an ACEI was independently associated with the risk of death (hazard ratio, 1.03) while the combination of low-dose aspirin with an ACEI was not (hazard ratio, 1.02) [74].

However, recent studies have not supported this hypothesis. In a randomized, double-blind, crossover design study of 13 patients with a mean LVEF of 21%, there was no significant difference in the hemodynamic effect of acute administration of captopril (25 mg) in the presence or absence of acute concomitant aspirin (236 mg), despite significant reductions with aspirin administration in circulating prostaglandin and thromboxane $B_2$ concentrations [75]. Furthermore, the role of aspirin in the treatment of HF was also evaluated by reviewing data from 22 060 patients from six long-term randomized trials of ACEIs that provided information regarding survival, MI, stroke, hospital admission for congestive HF, or revascularization [75]. Although baseline characteristics and prognosis in patients allocated to placebo differed strikingly between those who were or were not taking aspirin at baseline, the individual analyses of these trials with the exception of SOLVD did not suggest any significant differences between the proportional reductions in risk with ACEI therapy in the presence or absence of aspirin for the major clinical outcomes ($p = 0.15$), or in any of its individual components, except MI (interaction $p = 0.01$). Overall, ACEI therapy significantly reduced the risk a major clinical event by 22%, with clear reduction in risk both among those receiving aspirin at baseline and those who were not. Considering the totality of evidence on all major vascular outcomes in these trials, there was not strong evidence that aspirin reduced the benefit of ACEI therapy. However, equipoise still exists in the medical and research community and physicians should therefore weigh the risks and benefits of aspirin use in each patient receiving therapy for HF.

The effects of the coadministration of aspirin and ACEIs on renal function in patients with HF have also been studied. In a randomized trial of 40 patients, Riegger *et al.* demonstrated that aspirin reduced renal prostaglandin E$_2$ with a commensurate decrease in renal sodium excretion [76]. Furthermore, a retrospective analysis by Dietz *et al.* suggested that the administration of aspirin worsened the ACEI-induced decrease in glomerular filtration rate and reduced the improvement in renal plasma flow [77]. However, the small size and retrospective design of these two trials obviated their utility in making clinical decisions.

## Adverse effects of ACEIs

Although ACEIs are well tolerated in patients with HF, clinicians must be aware of a group of side effects that may limit their use in some patients. Perhaps the most common side effect of ACEIs, consistent with their vasodilatory properties, is hypotension. Because of this common side effect, treatment should be started with small doses as a steep fall in blood pressure may occur following the first dose. Many HF patients with systolic blood pressures of 80–90 mmHg do tolerate these drugs. Thus, hypotensive symptoms rather than blood pressure itself should be limiting factor [1,2]. ACEIs have also been associated with an increased incidence of hyperkalemia. This adverse effect is seen most commonly in patients with renal insufficiency, patients taking potassium sparing agents, beta-receptor blockers and nonsteroidal anti-inflammatory drugs. Hyperkalemia, defined as a serum potassium >5.5 mEq/L, is considered a contraindication for ACEIs use and serum potassium needs to be monitored regularly with ACEI usage. The recent increase in the use of aldosterone antagonists requires especially close monitoring of serum potassium levels – a subject that will be discussed in greater detail in the Chapter 6 on Aldosterone Inhibitors.

Perhaps the most common side effect of ACEIs is a dry cough that is reported to occur in approximately 5% of all patients. It is usually not dose related, is diagnosed more frequently in women, usually develops after 1 week to 6 months of therapy, and may require discontinuation of therapy in some patients. Although cough has been considered

to be a "class effect", anecdotal reports have noted improvement or amelioration of symptoms with a change in the ACEI. Cough is most likely provoked by accumulating bradykinins, prostaglandins in the lungs, due to ACE inhibition. ACE inhibition has also been associated with acute renal failure. This is most commonly seen in patients with prerenal azotemia, dehydration, or renal artery stenosis. Indeed, patients with renal artery stenosis should not receive an ACEI – and patients developing rapid compromise of their renal function should be carefully evaluated for its presence. There is no strict contraindication regarding the usage of ACEIs in patients with mild to moderate renal dysfunction; however, patients with a >3.0 mEq/dcL do not usually tolerate these agents and such patients should undergo close monitoring of potassium and renal function.

The most worrisome acute side effect of ACEI use is angioedema, which can occur in between 0.1% and 0.2% of patients. Patients present with acute swelling of the lips, tongue, glottis, throat, bowel, and bronchial tree. This side effect is dose independent and disappears within hours after ACEI cessation. In pregnant women, ACEIs have been shown to be teratogenic and can cause oligohydraminos, fetal calvarial hypoplasia, fetal pulmonary hypoplasia, growth retardation, fetal death, neonatal anuria, and neonatal death. Thus, ACEIs should be discontinued in patients who are planning a pregnancy. Furthermore, ACEIs are classified as group C pharmacologic agents and therefore must be discontinued if a pregnancy is diagnosed.

## Practical considerations in the use of ACEIs

Treatment with an ACEI should be initiated at low doses with gradual increments in dosing as lower doses are tolerated. The target dose should be those doses that have proven efficacious in multicenter clinical trials. Although some patients may show an improvement in symptoms within 48 h, the long-term benefits for patients with HF may not be seen for months or years. It may be necessary to reduce the dose of ACEI or even discontinue the agent in patients who demonstrate clinical instability; however, every effort should be made to restart the ACEI when patients regain stability. In addition, in up-titrating the dose of an ACEI, it should be recognized that a decline in blood pressure should not obviate the use of these agents unless patients develop worsening renal function, syncope, or frank symptoms of hypotension. Furthermore, titration of other vasoactive agents including diuretics and vasodilators may be helpful. Alternatively, reduction in the dose of the ACEI may facilitate improvement in renal function.

Generally, ACEIs may be preferred to angiotensin receptor blockers because of the greater experience with these agents and the large number of clinical trials supporting their safety and efficacy. Although some ACEIs have been touted for their ability to inhibit tissue ACE, no clinical evidence exists suggesting one ACEI is better than the other. However, preference should be given to those ACEIs that have been shown in large multicenter clinical trials to reduce morbidity and mortality since these studies have defined a dose that is effective.

Physicians should not delay the initiation of beta-blockers in order to attain target doses of ACEIs. Patients with a current or recent history of fluid retention should also be treated with a diuretic in order to maintain sodium balance and prevent the development of edema. Indeed, because both hypovolemia and hypervolemia can adversely affect the outcome in patients receiving ACEIs; therefore, fluid balance should be assiduously monitored in all patients as should electrolyte balance and renal function. Renal function and serum potassium should be assessed within 1 to 2 weeks of the start of therapy and then routinely thereafter. Patients should also be warned against the use of nonsteroidal anti-inflammatory drugs as these can block the favorable effects of ACE inhibition and can potentially enhance its adverse effects [78].

## Conclusions

The ACEIs have been shown to alleviate symptoms, improve clinical status, enhance quality of life, and reduce the risk of death or hospitalization. Therefore, based on extensive clinical evidence, ACEI should be used in all patients with any degree of symptomatic HF, asymptomatic patients with LV dysfunction, and in patients at risk of developing LV dysfunction. All efforts should be made to achieve dosages similar to those in the clinical trials. The prevailing evidence is that the benefits of ACEI are a class effect. While recognizing that drug therapy for HF is a complex multidrug regimen, ACEI should be included as an essential part of the polypharmacy for patients with this disease.

## References

1  BG Katzung *Basic and Clinical Pharmacology*, 9th edn. McGraw Hill, New York, USA, 2004:177–183.
2  Goodman and Gilman's *The Pharmacological Basis of Therapeutics*, 10th edn. McGraw Hill, New York, USA, 2001:809–820.
3  Jackson EK. Adenosine: a physiological brake on renin release. *Annu Rev Pharmacol Toxicol* 1991;**31**:1–35.
4  Jackson EK, Branch RA, Oates JA. Participation of prostaglandins in the control of renin release. *Adv Prostaglandin Thromboxane Leukot Res* 1982;**10**:255–276.
5  Harris RC, McKanna JA, Akai Y, Jacobson HR, Dubois RN, Breyer MD. Cyclooxygenase-2 is associated with the macula densa of rat kidney and increases with salt restriction. *J Clin Invest* 1994;**94**:2504–2510.
6  Traynor TR, Smart A, Briggs JP, Schnermann J. Inhibition of macula densa-stimulated renin secretion by pharmacological blockade of cyclooxygenase-2. *Am J Physiol* 1999;**277**:F706–F710.
7  Beierwaltes WH. Macula densa stimulation of renin is reversed by selective inhibition of neuronal nitric oxide synthase. *Am J Physiol* 1997;**272**:R1359–R1364.
8  Campbell DJ, Habener JF. Angiotensinogen gene is expressed and differentially regulated in multiple tissues of the rat. *J Clin Invest* 1986;**78**:31–39.
9  Cassis LA, Saye J, Peach MJ. Location and regulation of rat angiotensinogen messenger RNA. *Hypertension* 1988;**11**:591–596.
10  Beldent V, Michaud A, Bonnefoy C, Chauvet MT, Corvol P. Cell surface localization of proteolysis of human endothelial angiotensin I-converting enzyme. Effect of the amino-terminal domain in the solubilization process. *J Biol Chem* 1995;**270**:28962–28969.
11  Tallant EA, Lu X, Weiss RB, Chappell MC, Ferrario CM. Bovine aortic endothelial cells contain an angiotensin-(1–7) receptor. *Hypertension* 1997;**29**:388–393.
12  Kato H, Iwai N, Inui H, Kimoto K, Uchiyama Y, Inagami T. Regulation of vascular angiotensin release. *Hypertension* 1993;**21**:446–454.
13  Taddei S, Virdis A, Abdel-Haq B *et al.* Indirect evidence for vascular uptake of circulating renin in hypertensive patients. *Hypertension* 1993;**21**:852–860.
14  Danser AH, van Kats JP, Admiraal PJ *et al.* Cardiac renin and angiotensins. Uptake from plasma versus in situ synthesis. *Hypertension* 1994;**24**:37–48.

15  Philipp CS, Dilley A, Saidi P *et al*. Deletion polymorphism in the angiotensin-converting enzyme gene as a thrombophilic risk factor after hip arthroplasty. *Thromb Haemost* 1998;**80**:869–873.

16  Saavedra JM, Correa FM, Seltzer A, Pinto JE, Viglione P, Tsutsumi K. Enhanced angiotensin converting enzyme binding in arteries from spontaneously hypertensive rats. *J Hypertens* 1992;**10**:1353–1359.

17  Dzau VJ, Sasamura H, Hein L. Heterogeneity of angiotensin synthetic pathways and receptor subtypes: physiological and pharmacological implications. *J Hypertens* 1993;**11**:S13–S18.

18  Wolny A, Clozel JP, Rein J *et al*. Functional and biochemical analysis of angiotensin II-forming pathways in the human heart. *Circ Res* 1997;**80**:219–227.

19  Griendling KK, Ushio-Fukai M, Lassegue B, Alexander RW. Angiotensin II signaling in vascular smooth muscle. New concepts. *Hypertension* 1997;**29**:366–373.

20  Inagami T, Eguchi S, Numaguchi K *et al*. Cross-talk between angiotensin II receptors and the tyrosine kinases and phosphatases. *J Am Soc Nephrol* 1999;**10**:S57–S61.

21  Blume A, Herdegen T, Unger T. Angiotensin peptides and inducible transcription factors. *J Mol Med* 1999;**77**:339–357.

22  Horiuchi M, Lehtonen JY, Daviet L. Signaling mechanism of the AT2 angiotensin II receptor: crosstalk between AT1 and AT2 receptors in cell growth. *Trends Endocrinol Metab* 1999;**10**:391–396.

23  Kenneth M McDonald, James Mock, Antonio D'Aloia *et al*. Bradykinin antagonism inhibits the antigrowth effect of converting enzyme inhibition in the dog myocardium after discrete transmural myocardial necrosis. *Circulation* 1995;**91**:2043–2048.

24  Captopril Multicenter Trial (Captopril Multicenter Research Group). A placebo controlled trial: captopril in refractory chronic congestive heart failure. *J Am Coll Cardiol* 1983;**2**:755–763.

25  Captopril-Digoxin Multicenter Research Group. Comparative effects of therapy with captopril and digoxin in patients with mild to moderate heart failure. *JAMA* 1988;**259**:539–544.

26  CONSENSUS Trial Study Group. Effects of enalapril on mortality in severe congestive heart failure: results of the Cooperative North Scandinavian Enalapril Study. *N Engl J Med* 1987;**316**:1429–1435.

27  SOLVD Investigators. Effect of enalapril on survival in patients with reduced left ventricular ejection fractions and congestive heart failure. *N Engl J Med* 1991;**35**:283–302.

28  Yusuf S, Pepine CJ, Garces C *et al*. Effects of enalapril on myocardial infarction and unstable angina in patients with low ejection fractions. *Lancet* 1992;**340**:1173–1178.

29  The SOLVD Investigators. Effects of enalapril on mortality and development of heart failure in asymptomatic patients with reduced left ventricular ejection fractions. *N Engl J Med* 1992;**327**:685–691.

30  Jong P, Yusuf S, Rousseau MF, Ahn SA, Bangdiwala SI. Effect of enalapril on 12-year survival and life expectancy in patients with left ventricular systolic dysfunction: a follow-up study. *Lancet* 2003;**361**:1843–1848.

31  Kleber FX, Niemoller L, Doering W *et al*. Impact of converting enzyme inhibition on progression of chronic heart failure: results of the Munich Mild Heart Failure Trial. *Br Heart J* 1992;**67**:289–296.

32  Cohn JN, Johnson G, Ziesche S *et al*. A comparison of enalapril with hydralazine-isosorbid dinitrate in the treatment of chronic congestive heart failure. *N Engl J Med* 1991;**325**:303–310.

33  Garg R, Yusuf S. Overview of randomized trials of angiotensin-converting enzyme inhibitors on mortality and morbidity in patients with heart failure. *JAMA* 1995;**273**:1450–1456.

34  Pilote L, Abrahamowicz M, Rodrigues E, Eisenberg MJ, Rahme E. Mortality rates in elderly patients who take different angiotensin-converting enzyme inhibitors after acute myocardial infarction: a class effect? *Ann Intern Med* 2004;**141**:102–112.

35  Hennessy S, Kimmel SE. Is improved survival a class effect of angiotensin-converting enzyme inhibitors? *Ann Intern Med* 2004;**141**:157–158.

36  Pfeffer MA, Braunwald E, Moye LA *et al*. Effect of captopril on mortality and morbidity in patients with left ventricular dysfunction after myocardial infarction. Results of the survival and ventricular enlargement trial. The SAVE Investigators. *N Engl J Med* 1992;**327**:669–677.

37  The Acute Infarction Ramipril Efficacy (AIRE) Study Investigators. Effect of ramipril on mortality and morbidity of survivors of acute myocardial infarction with clinical evidence of heart failure. *Lancet* 1993;**342**:821–828.

38  Hall AS, Murray GD, Ball SG *et al*. Follow-up study of patients randomly allocated ramipril or placebo for heart failure after acute myocardial infarction: AIRE Extension (AIREX) Study (Acute Infarction Ramipril Efficacy). *ACP J Club* 1997;**127**:57.

39  Kober L, Torp-Pedersen C, Carlsen *et al*. A clinical trial of the angiotensin-converting-enzyme inhibitor trandolapril in patients with left ventricular dysfunction after myocardial infarction. Trandolapril Cardiac Evaluation (TRACE) Study Group. *N Engl J Med* 1995;**333**:1670–1676.

40  Ambrosioni E, Borghi C, Magnani B. The effect of the angiotensin-converting-enzyme inhibitor zofenopril on mortality and morbidity after anterior myocardial infarction. The Survival of Myocardial Infarction Long-Term Evaluation (SMILE) Study Investigators. *N Engl J Med* 1995;**332**:80–85.

41 Borghi C, Ambrosioni E, Magnani B. Effects of the early administration of zofenopril on onset and progression of congestive heart failure in patients with anterior wall acute myocardial infarction. The SMILE Study Investigators. Survival of Myocardial Infarction Long-term Evaluation. *Am J Cardiol* 1996;**78**:317–322.

42 Swedberg K, Held P, Kjekshus J, Rasmussen K, Ryden L, Wedel H. Effects of the early administration of enalapril on mortality in patients with acute myocardial infarction. Results of the Cooperative New Scandinavian Enalapril Survival Study II (CONSENSUS II). *N Engl J Med* 1992;**327**:678–684.

43 GISSI-3-Gruppo Italiano per lo Studio della Sopravvivenza nell'Infarto Miocardico. GISSI-3 study protocol on the effects of lisinopril, of nitrates, and of their association in patients with acute myocardial infarction. *Am J Cardiol* 19928;**70**:62C–69C.

44 Flather M, Pipilis A, Collins R *et al.* Randomized controlled trial of oral captopril, of oral isosorbide mononitrate and of intravenous magnesium sulphate started early in acute myocardial infarction: safety and haemodynamic effects. ISIS-4 (Fourth International Study of Infarct Survival) Pilot Study Investigators. *Eur Heart J* 1994;**15**:608–619.

45 Chinese Cardiac Study (CCS-1) Collaborative Group. Oral captopril versus placebo among 14 962 patients with suspected acute myocardial infarction: a multicenter, randomized, double-blind, placebo controlled clinical trial. *Chin Med J (Engl)* 1997;**110**:834–838.

46 de Kam PJ, Voors AA, van den Berg MP *et al.* Effect of very early angiotensin-converting enzyme inhibition on left ventricular dilation after myocardial infarction in patients receiving thrombolysis: results of a meta-analysis of 845 patients. FAMIS, CAPTIN and CATS Investigators. *J Am Coll Cardiol* 2000;**36**:2047–2053.

47 Mancini GB, Henry GC, Macaya C *et al.* Angiotensin-converting enzyme inhibition with quinapril improves endothelial vasomotor dysfunction in patients with coronary artery disease. The TREND (Trial on Reversing ENdothelial Dysfunction) Study. *Circulation* 1996;**94**:258–265.

48 Cashin-Hemphill L, Holmvang G, Chan RC, Pitt B, Dinsmore RE, Lees RS. Angiotensin-converting enzyme inhibition as antiatherosclerotic therapy: no answer yet. QUIET Investigators. QUinapril Ischemic Event Trial. *Am J Cardiol* 1999;**83**:43–47.

49 Pitt B, O'Neill B, Feldman R *et al.* The QUinapril Ischemic Event Trial (QUIET): evaluation of chronic ACE inhibitor therapy in patients with ischemic heart disease and preserved left ventricular function. *Am J Cardiol* 2001;**87**:1058–1063.

50 Pepine CJ Rouleau JL, Annis K *et al.* Effects of angiotensin-converting enzyme inhibition on transient ischemia: the Quinapril Anti-Ischemia and Symptoms of Angina Reduction (QUASAR) trial. *J Am Coll Cardiol* 2003;**42**:2049–2059.

51 Flather MD Yusuf S, Kober L *et al.* Long-term ACE-inhibitor therapy in patients with heart failure or left-ventricular dysfunction: a systematic overview of data from individual patients. ACE-Inhibitor Myocardial Infarction Collaborative Group. *Lancet* 2000;**355**: 1575–1581.

52 Yusuf S, Sleight P, Pogue J, Bosch J, Davies R, Dagenais G. Effects of an angiotensin-converting-enzyme inhibitor, ramipril, on cardiovascular events in high-risk patients. The Heart Outcomes Prevention Evaluation Study Investigators. *N Engl J Med* 2000;**342**:145–153.

53 Pitt B, Poole-Wilson P, Segal R *et al.* Effects of losartan versus captopril on mortality in patients with symptomatic heart failure: rationale, design, and baseline characteristics of patients in the Losartan Heart Failure Survival Study – ELITE II. *J Card Fail* 1999;**5**: 146–154.

54 Fox KM. EURopean trial On reduction of cardiac events with Perindopril in stable coronary Artery disease Investigators. Efficacy of perindopril in reduction of cardiovascular events among patients with stable coronary artery disease: randomised, double-blind, placebo-controlled, multicentre trial (the EUROPA study). *Lancet* 2003;**362**:782–788.

55 Bots ML, Remme WJ, Luscher TF, Grobbee DE; EUROPA-PERFECT Investigators. PERindopril-Function of the Endothelium in Coronary Artery Disease Trial: the PERFECT study–substudy of EUROPA: rationale and design. *Cardiovasc Drugs Ther* 2002;**16**:227–236.

56 Daly CA, Fox KM, Remme WJ, Bertrand ME, Ferrari R, Simoons ML; EUROPA Investigators. The effect of perindopril on cardiovascular morbidity and mortality in patients with diabetes in the EUROPA study: Results from the PERSUADE substudy. *Eur Heart J.* 2005;**26**(14):1369–78.

57 Schwartz JS, Wang YR, Cleland JG, Gao L, Weiner M, Poole-Wilson PA; ATLAS Study Group. High- versus low-dose angiotensin converting enzyme inhibitor therapy in the treatment of heart failure: an economic analysis of the Assessment of Treatment with Lisinopril and Survival (ATLAS) trial. *Am J Manag Care* 2003;**9**:417–424.

58 Pedone C, Pahor M, Carosella L, Bernabei R, Carbonin P. For The GIFA Investigators Use of Angiotensin-converting enzyme inhibitors in elderly people with heart failure: prevalence and outcomes. *J Gerontol A Biol Sci Med Sci* 2004;**59**:M716–M721.

59 Shekelle PG, Rich MW, Morton SC *et al.* Efficacy of angiotensin-converting enzyme inhibitors and beta-blockers in the management of left ventricular systolic dysfunction according to race, gender and diabetic status:

a meta-analysis of major clinical trials. *J Am Cell Cardiol* 2003;**41**:1529–1538.

60 Dries DL, Strong MH, Cooper RS, Drazner MH. Efficacy of angiotension converting enzyme inhibition in reducing progression from asymptomatic left ventricular dysfunction to symptomatic heart failure in black and white patients. *J Am Cell Cardiol* 2002;**40**:1019.

61 Ranade V, Molnar J, Khokher T, Agarwal A, Mosnaim A, Somberg JC. Effect of angiotensin-converting enzyme therapy on QT interval dispersion. *Am J Ther* 1999;**6**:257–261.

62 Cardin S, Li D, Thorin-Trescases N, Leung TK, Thorin E, Nattel S. Evolution of the atrial fibrillation substrate in experimental congestive heart failure: angiotensin-dependent and -independent pathways. *Cardiovasc Res* 2003;**60**:315–325.

63 Van Den Berg MP, Crijns HJ, Van Veldhuisen DJ, Griep N, De Kam PJ, Lie KI. Effects of lisinopril in patients with heart failure and chronic atrial fibrillation. *J Card Fail* 1995;**1**:355–363.

64 Alsheikh-Ali AA, Wang PJ, Rand W. *et al.* Enalapril treatment and hospitalization with atrial tachyarrhythmias in patients with left ventricular dysfunction. *Am Heart J* 2004;**147**:1061–1065.

65 Vermes E, Tardif JC, Bourassa MG, *et al.* Enalapril decreases the incidence of atrial fibrillation in patients with left ventricular dysfunction: insight from the Studies Of Left Ventricular Dysfunction (SOLVD) trials. *Circulation* 2003;**107**:2926–2931.

66 Zaman AG, Kearney MT, Schecter C, Worthley SG, Nolan J. Angiotensin-converting enzyme inhibitors as adjunctive therapy in patients with persistent atrial fibrillation. *Am Heart J* 2004;**147**:823–827.

67 Zi M, Carmichael N, Lye M. The effect of quinapril on functional status of elderly patients with diastolic heart failure. *Cardiovasc Drugs Ther* 2003;**17**:133–139.

68 Abdulla J, Burchardt H, Z Abildstrom S, Kober L, Torp-Pedersen C; TRACE Study Group. The angiotensin converting enzyme inhibitor trandolapril has neutral effect on exercise tolerance or functional class in patients with myocardial infarction and reduced left ventricular systolic function. *Eur Heart J* 2003;**24**:2116–2122.

69 Hall D, Zeitler H, Rudolph W. Counteraction of the vasodilator effects of enalapril by aspirin in severe heart failure. *J Am Coll Cardiol* 1992;**20**:1549–1555.

70 Teerlink JR, Massie BM. The interaction of ACE inhibitors and aspirin in heart failure: torn between two lovers. *Am Heart J* 1999;**138**:193–197.

71 Nakamura M, Funakoshi T, Arakawa N, Yoshida H, Makita S, Hiramori K. Effect of angiotensin-converting enzyme inhibitors on endothelium-dependent peripheral vasodilation in patients with chronic heart failure. *J Am Coll Cardiol* 1994;**24**:1321–1327.

72 Spaulding C, Charbonnier B, Cohen-Solal A, Juillière Y, Kromer EP, Benhamda K *et al.* Acute hemodynamic interaction of aspirin and ticlopidine with enalapril: results of a double-blind, randomized comparative trial. *Circulation* 1998;**98**:757–765.

73 van Wijngaarden J, Smit AJ, de Graeff PA *et al.* Effects of acetylsalicylic acid on peripheral hemodynamics in patients with chronic heart failure treated with angiotensin-converting enzyme inhibitors. *J Cardiovasc Pharmacol* 1994;**23**:240–245.

74 Guazzi M, Brambilla R, Reina G, Tumminello G, Guazzi MD. Aspirin-angiotensin-converting enzyme inhibitor coadministration and mortality in patients with heart failure: a dose-related adverse effect of aspirin. *Arch Intern Med* 2003;**163**:1574–1579.

75 Teo KK, Yusuf S, Pfeffer M *et al.* Effects of long-term treatment with angiotensin-converting-enzyme inhibitors in the presence or absence of aspirin: a systematic review. *Lancet* 2002;**360**:1037–1043.

76 Riegger GA, Kahles HW, Elsner D, Kromer EP, Kochsiek K. Effects of acetylsalicylic acid on renal function in patients with chronic heart failure. *Am J Med* 1991;**90**:571–575.

77 Dietz R, Nagel F, Osterziel KJ. Angiotensin-converting enzyme inhibitors and renal function in heart failure. *Am J Cardiol* 1992;**70**:119C–125C.

78 Packer M. Adaptive and maladaptive actions of angiotensin II in patients with sever congestive heart failure. *Am J Kidney Dis* 1987;**10**:66–73.

**CHAPTER 4**

# Angiotensin receptor blockers in the treatment of heart failure

*Anita Deswal,* MD, MPH *& Douglas L. Mann,* MD

## Introduction

Activation of the renin–angiotensin system (RAS) plays a critical role in the pathogenesis of heart failure. Therefore, strategies for the treatment of heart failure have focused on the use of agents that block the RAS. Angiotensin-converting-enzyme (ACE) inhibitors are established as a cornerstone of therapy for heart failure and the role of angiotensin receptor blockers (ARBs) in patients with heart failure has also recently been clarified. In this chapter, we will review the rationale for the use of ARBs and their role in the treatment of patients with heart failure based on evidence from clinical trials.

## Rationale for use of ARBs in heart Failure

The deleterious effects of activation of the RAS in heart failure are mediated primarily through increased circulating and tissue levels of the neurohormone angiotensin II. The actions of angiotensin II, predominantly through the angiotensin II type 1 ($AT_1$) receptor, aggravate the hemodynamic derangements, accentuate symptoms, and accelerate vascular and cardiac pathology in patients with heart failure leading to increased morbidity and mortality (Table 4.1) [1]. On the other hand, the physiological role of the other angiotensin II receptor, the angiotensin II type 2 ($AT_2$) receptor, is only partly understood (Table 4.1) [1]. Because of the functions of the $AT_2$ receptor that include inhibition of cell growth and promotion of cell differentiation and apoptosis, it has been suggested that $AT_2$ receptors may play an important role in counterbalancing some of the effects of angiotensin II that are mediated through the $AT_1$ receptors.

The RAS may be inhibited at various levels as shown in Figure 4.1. ACE inhibitors block the action of ACE, the enzyme responsible for the conversion of angiotensin I to angiotensin II, thus reducing the angiotensin II that is available to stimulate the $AT_1$ and $AT_2$ receptors. However, the use of ACE inhibitors does not lead to complete suppression of angiotensin II levels in patients with heart failure and levels of plasma angiotensin II gradually increase despite chronic high-dose ACE inhibitor therapy [2–5]. With ACE inhibitors, competitive inhibition of ACE results in increases in both

**Table 4.1** Effects of angiotensin II.

| Angiotensin type I ($AT_1$) receptor stimulation | Angiotensin type II ($AT_2$) receptor stimulation |
|---|---|
| Vasoconstriction | Antiproliferation |
| Stimulation of aldosterone secretion | Cell differentiation |
| Stimulation of vasopressin secretion | Tissue repair |
| Sodium and water retention | Apoptosis |
| Cell growth and proliferation | Vasodilation? |
| Myocyte and smooth muscle cell hypertrophy | Renal sodium excretion? |
| Vascular and myocardial fibrosis | |
| Activation of the sympathetic nervous system | |
| Increased endothelin secretion | |
| Stimulation of plasminogen activator inhibitor-1 | |
| Stimulation of superoxide formation | |

**Figure 4.1** Activation of the renin–angiotensin system. Angiotensinogen is converted to angiotensin I by renin. Angiotensin I can be converted to angiotensin II through ACE and non-ACE dependent pathways. Angiotensin II exerts its biological effects binding to a type I ($AT_1$) and type II ($AT_2$) angiotensin receptor. Only 30–40% of angiotensin I to angiotensin II conversion occurs via the ACE pathway. Up to 60–70% of angiotensin I to angiotensin II conversion occurs via the non-ACE pathways including chymase, tonin, cathepsin, and kallikrein with angiotensin II-generating chymase being the predominant mechanism in human vasculature and the human heart. (Modified with permission from Annual Reviews 44.)

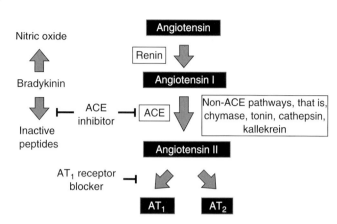

renin and angiotensin I, which then tend to overcome the blockade of this enzyme [6]. In addition, angiotensin II production also occurs through non-ACE pathways including other enzyme systems such as chymase, kallikrein, cathepsin G, and tonin that convert angiotensin I to angiotensin II [5,7,8]. For example, studies have shown that angiotensin II-generating chymase is the predominant pathway for the production of angiotensin II in the human vasculature with only 30–40% of angiotensin I to angiotensin II conversion occurring via the ACE pathway [9,10]. One study showed that only 13% of human heart angiotensin II production was blocked by ACE inhibitors with 87% of the angiotensin II being produced by non-ACE pathways [11]. Such observations provided the rationale for the development of angiotensin receptor antagonists that offer more complete protection against angiotensin II by directly blocking the $AT_1$ receptor. In addition, during chronic $AT_1$ receptor blockade, the increased levels of angoiotensin II that occur as a result of interruption of the normal negative feedback mechanism can stimulate the $AT_2$ receptors and therefore could theoretically be beneficial in patients with heart failure.

However, the beneficial effects of ACE inhibitors are also thought in part to be due to their augmentation of the effects of bradykinin (Figure 4.1). ACE inhibitors block the breakdown of bradykinin, mediated by kininase II, which is identical to ACE. Bradykinin has direct and indirect vasodilator activity through the release of nitric oxide and prostaglandin, as well as antimitotic and antithrombotic actions that could be of benefit in heart failure [12]. On the other hand, bradykinin is also likely to be responsible for the adverse reaction of cough with the use of ACE inhibitors [13] and it stimulates the release of catecholamines, which can be arrhythmogenic [14]. Compared to ACE inhibitors, ARBs do not appear to have similar effects on bradykinin. These differences in neurohormonal modulation and adverse effects between ACE inhibitors and ARBs suggest that the benefits and risks of these agents may differ in patients with heart failure and therefore warrant comparative evaluation of the two drug classes. Furthermore, the above observations also provide a rationale to evaluate a combination of the two classes of agents in patients with heart failure with a view towards combining the unique benefits of each class. Thus, the addition of an ARB to ACE inhibitor therapy may offer more complete $AT_1$ blockade of the RAS than could be achieved with ACE inhibition alone, while at the same time preserving the beneficial effects of bradykinin potentiation offered by ACE inhibitors.

Based on these theoretical considerations as well as promising results with preclinical and early clinical data, large-scale clinical trials have evaluated the beneficial effect of ARBs as alternatives to ACE inhibitors as well as the beneficial effect of the ACE inhibitor/ARB combination compared with

ACE inhibitors alone in patients with heart failure. Current available evidence for these strategies in patients with chronic heart failure as well as in high-risk patients with heart failure or depressed left ventricular ejection fraction post-acute myocardial infarction are reviewed in the following sections.

## ARBs in chronic heart failure

### ARBs as alternatives to ACE inhibitors in patients with chronic heart failure

With the proven efficacy of ACE inhibitors in heart failure with depressed systolic function, a number of trials have been performed to evaluate the efficacy of ARBs in comparison to ACE inhibitors. The Evaluation of Losartan In The Elderly I (ELITE I) trial was designed to compare the effects on renal function and tolerability of treatment with the ARB, losartan, to the ACE inhibitor, captopril, in patients with symptomatic heart failure [15]. Elderly patients with symptomatic heart failure secondary to left ventricular systolic dysfunction

were randomized to receive either captopril or losartan for 48 weeks (Table 4.2). There was no significant difference in the frequency of the primary endpoint of a persistent increase of $\geq 0.3$ mg/dL in serum creatinine between the losartan and captopril groups (10.5% in each group). Fewer patients in the losartan arm discontinued therapy for adverse events (12.2% versus 20.8% for captopril, $p = 0.002$). Death or hospital admission for heart failure tended to be lower in the losartan compared with the captopril group (9.4% versus 13.2%, $p = 0.075$), with the benefit being primarily driven by a 46% decrease in all-cause mortality. However, these apparent benefits of losartan were based on only a small number of events that did not constitute the primary endpoint of the study. Therefore, a second larger trial of 3152 patients, the Evaluation of Losartan In The Elderly II (ELITE II) compared the effects of captopril with losartan on mortality in heart failure patients similar to those enrolled in ELITE I [16]. However, ELITE II showed no significant difference in all-cause mortality (17.7%

**Table 4.2** Clinical trials of ARBs in heart failure.

| Trial | Study population | Target doses |
|---|---|---|
| Number of patients; average follow-up | | |
| ELITE I [15] | LVEF ≤40% | Captopril 50 mg three times daily versus |
| n = 722; 48 weeks | NYHA II–III | losartan 50 mg daily |
| | ≥65 years | |
| ELITE II [16] | LVEF ≤40% | Captopril 50 mg three times daily versus |
| n = 3152; 79 weeks | NYHA II–III | losartan 50 mg daily |
| | ≥60 years | |
| CHARM-alternative [19] | LVEF ≤40% | Candesartan 32 mg daily versus placebo |
| n = 2028; 34 months | NYHA II–IV | |
| | Intolerance to ACE inhibitors | |
| Val-HeFT [18] | LVEF <40% | Valsartan 160 mg twice daily versus placebo |
| n = 5010; 23 months | NYHA II–IV | |
| | 93% on ACE inhibitors | |
| CHARM-added [24] | LVEF ≤40% | Candesartan 32 mg daily versus placebo |
| n = 2458; 41 months | NYHA II–IV | |
| | All patients on ACE inhibitors | |
| CHARM-Preserved [28] | LVEF >40% | Candesartan 32 mg daily versus placebo |
| n = 3023; 37 months | NYHA II–IV | |
| OPTIMAAL [34] | Within 10 days post-acute MI with heart | Captopril 50 mg three times daily versus |
| n = 5477; 2.7 years | failure or Q-wave anterior infarction | losartan 50 mg daily |
| VALIANT [35] | Within 10 days post-acute MI with heart | Captopril 50 mg three times daily versus |
| n = 14 703; 24.7 months | failure or LVEF ≤35–40% | valsartan 160 mg twice daily versus captopril 50 mg three times daily + valsartan 80 mg twice daily |

versus 15.9% for losartan and captopril, respectively; hazard ratio 1.13, 95% CI 0.95–1.35, $p = 0.16$) or sudden death or resuscitated arrests (9.0 versus 7.3%, $p = 0.08$) between the two treatment groups [16]. Thus, in this study, blocking the $AT_1$ receptor was not superior to ACE inhibition; indeed, ACE inhibitors appeared to be marginally superior to ARBs. Though this finding may be interpreted as lending support to the possibility that the bradykinin effects of ACE inhibitors may indeed confer a practical benefit in patients with heart failure, it has also been suggested that the dose of losartan used in the ELITE trials (50 mg daily) may not fully block $AT_1$ receptors throughout the 24-h dosing interval and that higher doses may have been more effective[17]. Based on the ELITE II trial, ACE inhibitors continued to be the recommended agents of choice for patients with heart failure and depressed ejection fraction, but if patients were unable to tolerate ACE inhibitors for adverse events such as cough or angioedema, ARBs were offered as useful alternative agents to block the RAS. Further support for ARBs as an alternative strategy in patients with heart failure intolerant to ACE inhibitors was provided by results of the Valsartan in Heart failure Trial (Val-HeFT) in the small subgroup of patients not on an ACE inhibitors at baseline [18]. The results of this trial are discussed in detail in a later section of this chapter.

The definitive answer to whether ARBs are an effective alternative in patients with systolic heart failure who are intolerant to ACE inhibitors, was provided by the Candesartan in Heart failure: Assessment of Reduction in Mortality and Morbidity (CHARM)-alternative trial [19]. Patients with symptomatic heart failure with depressed ejection and history of intolerance to ACE inhibitors were randomized to either the ARB, candesartan, or to placebo (Table 4.2). The history of ACE inhibitor intolerance included cough in 72%, symptomatic hypotension in 13%, and renal dysfunction in 12% of patients. At baseline, 55% of patients were taking beta-blockers and 24% were taking spironolactone. The use of candesartan was associated with a significant 23% reduction in the primary composite outcome of cardiovascular mortality or heart failure hospitalization (hazard ratio 0.77, 95% CI 0.67–0.89; $p = 0.0004$). This benefit was noted individually on cardiovascular death and on heart failure hospitalization as well on other cardiovascular morbidity. The 23% reduction in cardiovascular mortality and heart failure hospitalizations is similar to the 26% reduction in these outcomes reported with the use of ACE inhibitors in the Studies of Left Ventricular Dysfunction (SOLVD) treatment trial and in an overview of large trials with ACE inhibitors in patients with left ventricular systolic dysfunction [20,21].

As expected, patients on candesartan in the CHARM alternative study were more likely to stop drug for renal dysfunction, hyperkalemia, and hypotension compared with placebo. In addition, patients in both groups who had previous ACE inhibitor intolerance because of renal dysfunction were likely to have the study drug discontinued because of increased serum creatinine. Furthermore, angioedema occurred in 3 of the 39 patients with a history of angioedema or anaphylaxis with ACE inhibitors. In two of the three cases, candesartan was restarted without recurrence and permanent discontinuation of drug occurred in only one case. The experience with these patients suggests that ARBs should be tried in patients with history of angioedema or anaphylaxis with ACE inhibitors, albeit with caution. Thus the results of the CHARM-alternative study, along with subgroup analysis in the Val-HeFT trial of 7% of patients who were not on ACE inhibitors, have shown that ARBs (specifically candesartan and valsartan) confer significant benefit on mortality and morbidity in patients with heart failure who are intolerant of ACE inhibitors and therefore constitute a good alternative strategy in these patients.

## ARBs in addition to ACE inhibitors in patients with chronic heart failure

Having demonstrated that ARBs offer a reasonable alternative to ACE inhibitors, and given the theoretical benefit of using a combination of ACE inhibitors and ARBs in patients with heart failure, the efficacy of ARBs as add-on therapy to ACE inhibitors in patients with left ventricular systolic dysfunction and symptomatic heart failure has been examined in several studies.

An early pilot study, the Randomized Evaluation Strategies for Left Ventricular Dysfunction (RESOLVD), investigated the favorable effects of a combination of the ARB, candesartan, and the ACE inhibitor, enalapril, compared with the effects of either agent alone on exercise tolerance, ventricular function, and quality of life in patients with chronic systolic heart failure [22]. In this study of 768 patients, no differences were noted in the effect of either drug alone compared with the combination in terms of quality of life or functional capacity. However, the combination of an ACE inhibitor and ARB appeared to have more beneficial effects on left ventricular remodeling than either agent alone.

Two large recent clinical trials, the Val-HeFT and the CHARM-added trial have since evaluated the benefit on morbidity and mortality of adding ARBs in patients with heart failure already on ACE inhibitors. Val-HeFT was designed to determine whether addition of the ARB, valsartan, could

reduce morbidity and mortality among patients with symptomatic systolic heart failure. At baseline, patients were already receiving standard therapy for heart failure, which included ACE inhibitors in 93% and beta-blockers in 35% of patients[18]. Patients with left ventricular systolic dysfunction and heart failure of NYHA class II–IV functional status were assigned to receive valsartan or placebo (Table 4.2). Valsartan was started at a dose of 40 mg twice daily, titrated up to 80 mg twice daily, and then to 160 mg twice daily. The two coprimary end points were all-cause mortality and the composite of mortality and morbidity. At follow-up, mortality was similar in the two groups (Table 4.3), but the combined mortality and morbidity end point was 13.2% lower with valsartan. The benefit was primarily because of a 24% reduction in the rate of hospitalizations for heart failure in patients in

**Table 4.3** Selected endpoints in the Val-HEFT [18] and CHARM-added [24] trials.

| Endpoint | Active drug number with event (%) | Placebo number with event (%) | Hazard ratio (95% CI) | p-value |
|---|---|---|---|---|
| *Val-HeFT* | *Valsartan (n = 2511)* | *Placebo (n = 2499)* | | |
| Death from any cause (co-primary end point) | 498 (19.7) | 484 (19.4) | 1.02 (0.88, 1.18*) | 0.80 |
| Combined endpoint (co-primary end point)** | 723 (28.8) | 801 (32.1) | 0.87 (0.77, 0.97*) | 0.01 |
| Death from any cause as first event | 356 (14.2) | 315 (12.6) | | |
| Hospitalization for HF | 346 (13.8) | 455 (18.2) | | |
| Cardiac arrest with resuscitation | 16 (0.6) | 26 (1.0) | | |
| Intravenous therapy | 5 (0.2) | 5 (0.2) | | |
| *CHARM* | *Candesartan (n = 1276)* | *Placebo (n = 1272)* | | |
| CV death or HF hospitalization (primary endpoint) | 483 (37.9) | 538 (42.3) | 0.85 (0.75, 0.96) | 0.01 |
| CV death | 302 (23.7) | 347 (27.3) | 0.84 (0.72, 0.98) | 0.03 |
| HF hospitalization | 309 (24.2) | 356 (28.0) | 0.83 (0.71, 0.96) | 0.01 |
| CV death, hospitalization for HF or MI | 495 (38.8) | 550 (43.2) | 0.85 (0.76, 0.96) | 0.01 |
| CV death, hospitalization for HF, MI, or stroke | 512 (40.1) | 559 (43.9) | 0.87 (0.77, 0.98) | 0.02 |
| CV death, hospitalization for HF, MI, stroke, or coronary revascularization | 548 (42.9) | 596 (46.9) | 0.87 (0.77, 0.97) | 0.02 |
| Death from any cause | 377 (30.0) | 412 (32) | 0.89 (0.77, 1.02) | 0.09 |

*97.5% CI.

**Combined endpoint of either hospitalization for heart failure, resuscitated sudden death, receipt of intravenous inotropic or vasodilator therapy for at least 4 h; CI = confidence intervals; HF = heart failure; CV = cardiovascular; MI = myocardial infarction.

**Table 4.4** Results of the heart failure morbidity endpoint in Val-HeFT based on baseline ACE inhibitor use.

|  | Without ACE inhibitor | | With ACE inhibitor | |
| --- | --- | --- | --- | --- |
|  | Placebo<br>(n = 181) | Valsartan<br>(n = 185) | Placebo<br>(n = 2318) | Valsartan<br>(n = 2326) |
| Events* (%) | 77 (42.5) | 46 (24.9) | 677 (31.2) | 724 (29.1) |
| Hazard ratio (95% CI) | 0.51 (0.35, 0.73) | | 0.92 (0.82, 1.02) | |
| p value | 0.0002 | | 0.0965 | |

*Combined endpoint of all-cause mortality, sudden death with resuscitation, hospitalization for heart failure, and the need for intravenous inotropic or vasodilatory drugs. (Data from [23].)

the valsartan arm (Table 4.3). Improvements were also seen with valsartan in several secondary end points including left ventricular ejection fraction, signs and symptoms of heart failure, and quality of life. The analyses of subgroups defined according to background therapy at baseline showed highly significant interactions. For instance, the small subgroup of 366 patients (7%) who were not receiving ACE inhibitors received maximal benefit with a 33% reduction in mortality and a 49% decrease in mortality and morbidity with valsartan compared to placebo, whereas the morbidity and mortality benefit of valsartan observed in the overall trial was no longer significant in patients already receiving background ACE inhibitor therapy (hazard ratio 0.92, p = 0.0965; Table 4.4). This modest favorable trend in the group receiving an ACE inhibitor was largely driven by the patients receiving less than the recommended dose of an ACE inhibitor [23]. Also, the larger subgroup of patients receiving both an ACE inhibitor and a beta-blocker at baseline had a statistically significant 42% increase in mortality with valsartan (p = 0.009) and a trend toward an increase in the mortality and morbidity composite (p = 0.10). To summarize, when added to standard therapy valsartan has no overall effect on mortality and produced a modest reduction in morbidity. However, this benefit was much larger in patients not receiving concomitant ACE inhibitor therapy and was not statistically significant in those who were already taking ACE inhibitors. A troublesome finding was the significant increase in mortality with valsartan in patients receiving both ACE inhibitor and beta-blocker therapy. Initially hypothesized to be due to possible deleterious effects of extensive inhibition of multiple neurohormonal systems in patients with heart

failure, this finding of harm with triple therapy of ACE inhibitors, ARBs, and beta-blockers has not been substantiated by subsequent trials with ARBs and was most likely a chance finding of multiple subgroup analyses.

More recently, the CHARM-added trial investigated whether combining the ARB, candesartan, with an ACE inhibitor improved clinical outcomes [24]. In this study, 2458 patients with symptomatic systolic heart failure already on treatment with an ACE inhibitor were randomized to receive either candesartan or placebo (Table 4.2). At baseline, therapy included beta-blockers in 55%, spironolactone in 17%, and diuretics in 90% of patients. Of note, about 73% of patients in this trial had NYHA class III functional class. After a median follow-up of 41 months, 38% of patients in the candesartan group and 42% of patients in the placebo group experienced the primary outcome of cardiovascular death or heart failure hospitalization (unadjusted hazard ratio 0.85; 95% CI 0.75–0.96; p = 0.01). This was the result of a significant reduction in cardiovascular mortality as well as heart failure hospitalizations in the candesartan group (Table 4.3). Candesartan also had a significant beneficial effect on other secondary cardiovascular outcomes (Table 4.3). In addition, the examination of subgroups revealed the benefit of candesartan on the primary outcome in all patients irrespective of baseline treatment with beta-blockers as well as in patients receiving recommended doses of ACE inhibitors. This subgroup analysis provided clarification on two important issues. First, the finding from Val-HeFT of increased mortality in patients receiving triple therapy with ACE inhibitors, ARBs, and beta-blockers was not substantiated in the CHARM study. Second, similar benefit with ARBs was noted even in patients already on target doses of ACE inhibitors.

Putting together the results of Val-HeFT and CHARM, there appears to be some morbidity benefit of adding an ARB to patients already on an ACE inhibitor, that is, a reduction in the hospitalization for heart failure. However, the benefit on cardiovascular mortality and a trend towards benefit on all-cause mortality was seen only in the CHARM study and not in Val-HeFT. The reasons for this difference are not clear. Therefore, at this point it may be prudent to recommend the use of ARBs in patients who appear to have continuing symptoms of progressive heart failure including heart failure hospitalizations or are hypertensive in spite of therapy with target doses of ACE inhibitors and beta-blockers, or in patients with heart failure who are on ACE inhibitors but unable to tolerate beta-blockers. Furthermore, in such patients with moderate to severe heart failure, there are no data to guide the decision of whether to first add an aldosterone receptor blocker (based on the beneficial effect seen in the Randomized Aldactone Evaluation Studies or RALES) or an ARB. In view of the fact that no major additive effect of the combined blockade with ACE inhibitors and ARBs has been demonstrated on the decrease in plasma aldosterone, especially in the long term [22] probably related to the non-angiotensin aldosterone activating pathways, it may be argued that the addition of an aldosterone receptor blocker may be more beneficial than addition of an ARB to ACE inhibitor therapy in patients with NYHA class III or IV functional status.

Irrespective of which strategy is chosen, the patients will need careful monitoring of renal function and serum potassium while initiating and up-titrating doses of ARBs, as demonstrated by the higher rate of discontinuation of the study drug for worsening renal function or hyperkalemia in patients on the ARB compared to those on placebo in the Val-HeFT and CHARM trials [18,24]. For example, in the CHARM study, discontinuation of study drug for increase in serum creatinine was 7.8% in the candesartan arm compared to 4.1% in the placebo group ($p = 0.0001$). Similarly, drug discontinuation for hyperkalemia was significantly higher in the candesartan arm (3.4%) compared to the placebo arm (0.7%, $p < 0.0001$).

## ARBs in patients with chronic heart failure and preserved ejection fraction

Large-scale clinical trial data evaluating treatment options is scant in patients with heart failure and preserved left ventricular ejection fraction. Because long-standing hypertension with left ventricular hypertrophy is thought to play a significant role in the development of heart failure in patients with preserved ejection fraction, a rationale exists for the evaluation of ARBs as well as ACE inhibitors in this patient population. ARBs as well as ACE inhibitors have been shown to slow the progression, or induce regression, of left ventricular hypertrophy through their effects on blood pressure as well as their effects on the myocardium [25]. In addition, angiotensin II has been shown to slow myocardial relaxation. A beneficial effect of RAS blockers in improving myocardial relaxation has been shown in patients with left ventricular hypertrophy as has an improvement in functional capacity and quality of life in patients with left ventricular hypertrophy, diastolic dysfunction, and exercise-induced hypertension [26,27].

Thus, the main objective of the CHARM-preserved trial was to assess whether the ARB, candesartan, would have a beneficial effect on the composite outcome of cardiovascular mortality or heart failure hospitalization in patients with heart failure and preserved ejection fraction. Patients with symptomatic heart failure, preserved left ventricular ejection fraction (>40%), and a history of a cardiovascular hospitalization, were randomized to either placebo or candesartan at a target dose of 32 mg daily (Table 4.2) [28]. At baseline, about 20% of patients were on ACE inhibitors and 56% were on beta-blockers. After a median follow-up of 37 months, the primary endpoint of cardiovascular death or heart failure hospitalization had occurred in 22% of patients in the candesartan group and 24% in the placebo group (hazard ratio 0.89, 95% CI 0.77–1.03; $p = 0.118$). Examining the components of the endpoint individually demonstrated no difference in cardiovascular death between the two arms (hazard ratio 0.99, 95% CI 0.80–1.22; $p = 0.92$), but a trend towards a reduction in heart failure hospitalizations with candesartan (hazard ratio 0.85, 95% CI 0.72, 1.01; $p = 0.072$). The number of patients who were admitted to the hospital for heart failure at least once during the trial was also significantly lower in the candesartan group ($n = 230$) than the placebo group ($n = 279$, $p = 0.017$) as was the total number of admissions for heart failure (402 in candesartan arm versus 566 in the placebo arm, $p = 0.014$). Thus, in patients with heart failure and preserved LVEF, use of ARBs was associated with only a modest reduction in morbidity, that is, heart failure hospitalizations and no benefit on mortality. However, it should be noted that the overall mortality in patients enrolled in this trial in the placebo group was significantly lower (approximately 5% annually) than reported for epidemiological studies of heart failure and preserved LVEF [29,30]. As would be expected, the blood pressure was lowered from baseline by 6.9 mmHg systolic and 2.9 mmHg diastolic more in the candesartan group compared with placebo ($p < 0.0001$), raising the question of how much better the blood pressure control with candesartan may have contributed to the reduction in heart failure hospitalizations. The ongoing I-PRESERVE trial is evaluating the ARB, irbesartan, in patients with heart failure and preserved ejection fraction and should provide further insight into the benefit of ARBs in this patient population.

## ARBs in high-risk patients post-myocardial infarction

ACE inhibitors have consistently been beneficial in improving morbidity and mortality in high-risk patients post-myocardial infarction [21,31–33]. Therefore, ARBs have been evaluated for benefit in high-risk patients post-myocardial infarction both as an alternative to ACE inhibitors and when added onto ACE inhibitor therapy.

In the Optimal Trial In Myocardial Infarction with the Angiotensin II Antagonist Losartan (OPTIMAAL), the ARB losartan (50 mg/day) was compared to the ACE inhibitor, captopril (150 mg/day), in high-risk patients post-acute myocardial infarction [34]. Patients who were within 10 days post-acute myocardial infarction with heart failure during the acute phase and/or Q-wave anterior infarction were enrolled (Table 4.2). The trial showed a strong but nonsignificant trend in favor of captopril over losartan in the primary endpoint of all-cause mortality (relative risk for losartan: captopril 1.13, 95% CI 0.99–1.28,

$p = 0.07$). A prespecified endpoint of cardiovascular mortality did reach significance in favor of captopril ($p = 0.03$) and first heart failure hospitalization trended in favor captopril (relative risk for losartan: captopril 1.16, 95% CI 0.98, 1.37, $p = 0.07$). The results for other secondary endpoints including reinfarction, all-cause hospitalizations, and need for revascularization were similar in the two groups. Thus, the OPTIMAAL trial raised important questions regarding the role of selective $AT_1$ receptor antagonism in high-risk patients following acute myocardial infarction.

However, the Valsartan in Acute Myocardial Infarction Trial (VALIANT) had better results with the ARB in a similar patient population. The VALIANT compared effects of the ARB, valsartan, the ACE inhibitor captopril, and the combination of valsartan and captopril in a high-risk patient population with clinical or radiological evidence of heart failure and/or evidence of left ventricular systolic dysfunction following acute myocardial infarction (Table 4.2) [35]. The primary endpoint of the study was all-cause mortality with a prespecified analysis that was designed to demonstrate the noninferiority, or equivalence, of valsartan to captopril in the event that valsartan was not clearly superior in the primary analysis. During a median follow-up of 24.7 months, mortality was 19.9 % in the valsartan group, 19.5 % in the captopril group, and 19.3% in the valsartan added to captopril group. The hazard ratio for valsartan versus captopril was 1.00 (97.5% CI, 0.90–1.11, $p = 0.98$) and for the valsartan-captopril combination versus captopril alone it was was 0.98 (97.5% CI 0.89–1.09, $p = 0.73$). Thus, the comparison of valsartan with captopril showed that these two agents were equivalent in terms of the overall mortality as well as the composite endpoint of fatal and nonfatal cardiovascular outcomes. Whereas patients receiving combined therapy experienced the most drug-related adverse events, adverse events were less common for monotherapy, with hypotension and renal dysfunction being more common in the valsartan group and cough, skin rash, and taste disturbance more common in the captopril group.

Taken together, the results suggest that valsartan (target dose 320 mg/day) is as effective as a dose of captopril (target dose 50 mg three times daily) that had been shown to be superior to placebo in reducing morbidity and mortality in high-risk patients with acute myocardial infarction [31–33,35].

However, there appears to be a discrepancy between the results of the VALIANT and the OPTIMAAL trials, both of which evaluated ARBs in high-risk post-myocardial infarction patients [36]. Apart from differences in pharmacokinetics between losartan and captopril, appropriate dosing may be important. That is, the dosing strategy of 50 mg/day of losartan versus 150 mg/day of captopril that favored captopril in the OPTIM-AAL trial [34] also favored the use of captopril over losartan in patients with moderate to severe heart failure in the ELITE II trial [16]. In contrast, in recently reported clinical trials of two high-risk patient populations with hypertensive left ventricular hypertrophy and with diabetic nephropathy, higher doses of losartan up to 100 mg/day were associated with a significant reduction in the incidence of heart failure [37,38], raising the question of whether higher doses of losartan may have been more effective in reducing cardiovascular outcomes in OPTIMAAL and ELITE II. VALIANT on the other hand tested a higher dose of valsartan (160 mg twice daily), a dose that is higher than its usual indicated dose in hypertension (160 mg daily). This may have contributed to its equivalent benefit compared to captopril in the trial. The fact that there were greater reductions in blood pressure and more frequent hypotension-related adverse effects with valsartan in VALIANT compared with losartan in OPTIMAAL relative to the captopril comparator, also supports this view.

Given that valsartan was as effective as captopril in reducing death and other adverse cardiovascular events, the question raised by the VALIANT trial is whether high-risk patients should receive an ACE inhibitor or an ARB following acute myocardial infarction. A number of factors may weigh in on the choice between these two agents including the cumulative clinical experience, tolerability, safety, convenience, and cost of the drugs. Given the much larger experience with ACE inhibitors in patients following acute myocardial infarction compared to the more limited clinical experience with ARBs, with comparable tolerability and safety of both agents, and given that the cost of using generic captopril is significantly lower than

that for valsartan, ACE inhibitors may at present be the first line of therapy for high-risk patients following acute myocardial infarction. However, in patients who cannot tolerate ACE inhibitors, valsartan appears to be a safe and equally effective alternative strategy [39].

Also VALIANT addressed the important issue of whether more complete blockade of the RAS using valsartan and captopril is more efficacious than captopril alone. In contrast to the two recently reported heart failure trials, wherein combined therapy with ACE inhibitors and ARBs was shown to be beneficial on cardiovascular morbidity (Val-HeFT) [18] and mortality (CHARM) [40], VALIANT showed that combined therapy resulted in an increase in adverse events without improving overall survival. A number of reasons have been offered for the discrepant results in the combination arm of VALIANT compared to those of the CHARM and Val-HeFT trials. First, the natural history of acute myocardial infarction (VALIANT) is different from chronic heart failure (CHARM and Val-HeFT). Heart failure hospitalizations tend to be a significant event for chronic heart failure patients, while myocardial infarction patients tend to have recurrent infarctions and early cardiac death. The main effects of drugs that block the RAS may be a reduction in heart failure events, as was the main effect shown with ARBs in the CHARM and Val-HeFT studies. Thus, it may be easier to show a benefit of combination therapy with an ACE inhibitor and an ARB in heart failure than in myocardial infarction patients. In addition, in the CHARM and Val-HeFT studies, the ARB was added on to treatment in patients who had already been taking ACE inhibitors long term, whereas in VALIANT both drugs were started concurrently. The RAS escape is seen in patients on chronic ACE inhibition therapy where significant angiotensin II is formed by non-ACE pathways. In that situation, a beneficial effect may be more likely to be seen if an ARB is added. But in the post-myocardial infarction state, if both the ACE inhibitors and ARB are started together, the escape mechanism may not be present leading to less benefit from an ARB. Furthermore, VALIANT is the only trial among the ARB trials in which the dose of the ACE inhibitor was titrated up to a maximum target. This resulted in a higher dose of ACE inhibitors in VALIANT (mean captopril dose 117 mg) than in CHARM (mean captopril dose of about 80 mg). This may have decreased the chances to observe the beneficial effect of addition of an ARB in VALIANT. Also, the VALIANT trial employed a high dose of valsartan (160 mg twice daily) in the monotherapy arm, but this dose was halved in the combination arm, raising the possibility that the dose may not have been high enough to show a benefit when added to full-dose ACE inhibition. This was in contrast to the CHARM and Val-HeFT, which used high-target ARB doses in all patients [41,42]. Taken together, the data does not support the routine addition of ARBs to standard therapy with target doses of ACE inhibitors and beta-blockers in high-risk patients post-acute myocardial infarction.

## ARBs in asymptomatic left ventricular systolic dysfunction

The ACE inhibitors are recommended for all patients with asymptomatic left ventricular systolic dysfunction to reduce progression to heart failure [43]. However, at present there is no data to support the combination of ACE inhibitors and ARBs in patients with asymptomatic left ventricular systolic dysfunction. Even though there is no data to confirm equivalence of ARBs to ACE inhibitors in this patient population, data from the post-MI patients and patients with symptomatic heart failure studies in the VALIANT and CHARM trials, allows us to extrapolate that the ARBs, valsartan, and candesartan should be used in patients with asymptomatic left ventricular systolic dysfunction who are intolerant to ACE inhibitors [19,41].

## Are all ARBs the same?

Although all ARBs as a group block the $AT_1$ receptor, they differ in pharmacokinetics including differences in binding characteristics. $AT_1$ receptor antagonism has been classified as surmountable and insurmountable based on the ability to shift the angiotensin-II concentration-response curve to the right [6]. Surmountable antagonism implies that the blockade by the antagonist can be overcome with increasing concentrations of agonist or angiotensin II, whereas with insurmountable antagonism, the blockade by the antagonist cannot be overcome with increasing concentrations of angiotensin II. Thus, insurmountable antagonism is associated with a reduction in maximal angiotensin II response whereas surmountable antagonism is not associated with a reduction in the maximal response to angiotensin II (Figure 4.2). With the use of ARBs, plasma angiotensin II concentrations increase as a result of interrupting the negative feedback in the RAS. This provides a theoretical rationale for more clinical benefit with use of an insurmountable $AT_1$ receptor blocker antagonist. An insurmountable, long-acting $AT_1$ receptor antagonist that displays tight binding characteristics is not likely to be overcome by the higher levels of circulating angiotensin II. Valsartan, irbesartan, candesartan, and an active metabolite of losartan, EXP3174, are insurmountable $AT_1$ receptor antagonists, while losartan is a surmountable antagonist [6]. Whether, this is a contributing factor to the better results seen in clinical trials using valsartan or candesartan in patients with heart failure compared to those with losartan is, however, not clear. Another important factor that

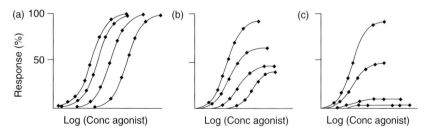

**Figure 4.2** Surmountable and insurmountable antagonism. (a) Surmountable antagonists produce parallel rightward shifts of the agonist concentration-response curves with no alteration of the agonist-maximal response. (b and c) Insurmountable antagonists produce parallel or nonparallel shifts of the agonist concentration-response curves with a depression of the maximal response to the agonist that cannot be overcome with increasing concentrations of the agonist. Conc = concentration. (Modified with permission from the American College of Pharmacology [6])

**Table 4.5** Selected ARBs evaluated in heart failure.

| Drug | Half-life (hours) | Recommended starting dose | Recommended target dose |
|---|---|---|---|
| Valsartan* | 9 | 40 mg twice daily | 160 mg twice daily |
| Candesartan* | 3.5–4 | 4 mg daily | 32 mg daily |
| Losartan (EXP 3174-active metabolite) | 2 (6–9) | 25 mg daily | 50 mg daily |

*Valsartan and candesartan are currently the ARBs of choice in patients with heart failure based on recent trials.

makes the interpretation of differences in benefits noted between different ARBs difficult is the issue of appropriate dosing as discussed earlier in the chapter. Choosing the appropriate dose of a therapeutic agent is perhaps equally as important as choosing the correct therapeutic agent.

Whether it is the differences in pharmacokinetics of the different ARBs or the inadequate dosing of losartan in the OPTIMAAL and ELITE trials, evidence from the CHARM and the VALIANT trials with candesartan and valsartan, respectively, suggest that valsartan and candesartan, at doses used in the clinical trials, may at present be the preferred ARBS in high-risk post-myocardial infarction patients as well as in patients with chronic heart failure. The recommended initial and target doses of these two agents are shown in Table 4.5.

Just as is the case with ACE inhibitors, renal function and serum potassium should be monitored closely after initiation and dose uptitration of ARBs, especially in patients with baseline renal insufficiency and serum creatinine greater than 2 mg/dL. If a significant increase in BUN and creatinine or orthostatic hypotension is noted after initiation or uptitration of ARBs, volume depletion requiring a decrease in diuretic dose should be considered before making a reduction in the dose of the ARB.

## Summary

Based on the clinical trial results discussed above, ARBs are a useful class of drugs in the treatment of patients with chronic heart failure and of high-risk patients post-MI. At present, based on a much larger experience and lower cost of ACE inhibitors compared to ARBs, ACE inhibitors continue to be first-line therapy for these patients. In patients intolerant of ACE inhibitors, the ARBs, valsartan and candesartan at target doses utilized in clinical trials, should be used as alternative agents. The routine addition of ARBs to ACE inhibitor therapy is not recommended in high-risk patients post-MI. However, in chronic heart failure, the addition of ARBs may be considered in patients who continue to be significantly symptomatic with heart failure or have uncontrolled hypertension, despite target doses of ACE inhibitors and beta-blockers. Even in this highly symptomatic patient population, it is at present unclear whether an aldosterone inhibitor or an ARB should be added first, and whether the combination of all three agents, that is, ACE inhibitors, ARBs, and aldosterone receptor antagonists, in addition to beta-blockers, is safe and efficacious.

## Acknowledgments

Dr. Deswal is supported by a VA cooperative studies program advanced clinical research career development award (# 712 A). This work is supported in part by grants from the Health Services Research and Development Service (# IIR 02-082-1) and the Clinical Science Research and Development Service of the Department of Veterans Affairs (to Dr Deswal) and by research funds from the Department of Veterans Affairs and the NIH (P50 HL-O6H and RO1 HL58081-01, RO1 HL61543-01, HL-42250-10/10, to Dr Mann).

## References

1 Burnier M, Brunner HR. Angiotensin II receptor antagonists. *Lancet* 2000; **355**:637–645.

2 Jorde UP, Ennezat PV, Lisker J *et al.* Maximally recommended doses of angiotensin-converting enzyme (ACE) inhibitors do not completely prevent ACE-mediated formation of angiotensin II in chronic heart failure. *Circulation* 2000; **101**:844–846.

3 Kawamura M, Imanashi M, Matsushima Y, Ito K, Hiramori K. Circulating angiotensin II levels under repeated administration of lisinopril in normal subjects. *Clin Exp Pharmacol Physiol* 1992; **19**:547–553.

4 de Gasparo M, Levens N. Does blockade of angiotensin II receptors offer clinical benefits over inhibition of angiotensin-converting enzyme? *Pharmacol Toxicol* 1998; **82**:257–271.

5 Wolny A, Clozel J-P, Rein J *et al.* Functional and biochemical analysis of angiotensin II-forming pathways in the human heart. *Circ Res* 1997; **80**:219–227.

6 McConnaughey MM, McConnaughey JS, Ingenito AJ. Practical considerations of the pharmacology of angiotensin receptor blockers. *J Clin Pharmacol* 1999; **39**:547–559.

7 Petrie MC, Padmanabhan N, McDonald JE, Hillier C, Connell JM, McMurray JJ. Angiotensin converting enzyme (ACE) and non-ACE dependent angiotensin II generation in resistance arteries from patients with heart failure and coronary heart disease. *J Am Coll Cardiol* 2001; **37**:1056–1061.

8 Dzau VJ. Multiple pathways of angiotensin production in the blood vessel wall: evidence, possibilities and hypotheses. *J Hypertens* 1989; **7**:933–936.

9 Okunishi H, Oka Y, Shiota N, Kawamoto T, Song K, Miyazaki M. Marked species-difference in the vascular angiotensin II-forming pathways: humans versus rodents. *Jpn J Pharmacol* 1993; **62**:207–210.

10 Liao Y, Husain A. The chymase-angiotensin system in humans: biochemistry, molecular biology and potential role in cardiovascular diseases. *Can J Cardiol* 1995; **11**:13F–19F.

11 Urata H, Healy B, Stewart RW, Bumpus FM, Husain A. Angiotensin II-forming pathways in normal and failing human hearts. *Circ Res* 1990; **66**:883–890.

12 Gavras I. Bradykinin-mediated effects of ACE inhibition. *Kidney Int* 1992; **42**:1020–1029.

13 Israili ZH, Hall WD. Cough and angioneurotic edema associated with angiotensin-converting enzyme inhibitor therapy. A review of the literature and pathophysiology. *Ann Intern Med* 1992; **117**:234–242.

14 Rump LC, Oberhauser V, Schwertfeger E, Schollmeyer P. Experimental evidence to support ELITE. *Lancet* 1998; **351**:644–645.

15 Pitt B, Segal R, Martinez FA *et al.* Randomized trial of losartan versus captopril in patients over 65 with heart failure (evaluation of losartan in the elderly study, ELITE). *Lancet* 1997; **349**:747–752.

16 Pitt B, Poole-Wilson PA, Segal R *et al.* Effect of losartan compared with captopril on mortality in patients with symptomatic heart failure: randomised trial–the Losartan Heart Failure Survival Study ELITE II. *Lancet* 2000; **355**:1582–1587.

17 Berlowitz MS, Latif F, Hankins SR *et al.* Dose-dependent blockade of the angiotensin II type 1 receptor with losartan in normal volunteers. *J Cardiovasc Pharmacol* 2001; **37**:692–696.

18 Cohn JN, Tognoni G. A randomized trial of the angiotensin-receptor blocker valsartan in chronic heart failure. *N Engl J Med* 2001; **345**:1667–1675.

19 Granger CB, McMurray JJ, Yusuf S *et al.* Effects of candesartan in patients with chronic heart failure and reduced left-ventricular systolic function intolerant to angiotensin-converting-enzyme inhibitors: the CHARM-Alternative trial. *Lancet* 2003; **362**:772–776.

20 The SOLVD Investigators. Effect of enalapril on survival in patients with reduced left ventricular ejection fractions and congestive heart failure. *N Engl J Med* 1991; **325**:293–302.

21 Flather MD, Yusuf S, Kober L *et al.* Long-term ACE-inhibitor therapy in patients with heart failure or left- ventricular dysfunction: a systematic overview of data from individual patients. ACE-Inhibitor Myocardial Infarction Collaborative Group. *Lancet* 2000; **355**:1575–1581.

22 McKelvie RS, Yusuf S, Pericak D *et al.* Comparison of Candesartan, Enalapril, and Their Combination in Congestive Heart Failure : Randomized Evaluation of Strategies for Left Ventricular Dysfunction (RESOLVD) Pilot Study: The RESOLVD Pilot Study Investigators. *Circulation* 1999; **100**:1056–1064.

23 Novartis:Diovan Prescribing Information. http://www.pharma.us.novartis.com / product / pi /pdf /diovan.pdf. Accessed 8–30–2004.

24 McMurray JJ, Ostergren J, Swedberg K *et al.* Effects of candesartan in patients with chronic heart failure and reduced left-ventricular systolic function taking angiotensin-converting-enzyme inhibitors: the CHARM-Added trial. *Lancet* 2003; **362**:767–771.

25 Dahlof B. Left ventricular hypertrophy and angiotensin II antagonists. *Am J Hypertens* 2001; **14**:174–182.

26 Kyriakidis M, Triposkiadis F, Dernellis J *et al.* Effects of cardiac versus circulatory angiotensin-converting enzyme inhibition on left ventricular diastolic function and coronary blood flow in hypertrophic obstructive cardiomyopathy. *Circulation* 1998; **97**:1342–1347.

27 Warner JG, Jr., Metzger DC, Kitzman DW, Wesley DJ, Little WC. Losartan improves exercise tolerance in

patients with diastolic dysfunction and a hypertensive response to exercise. *J Am Coll Cardiol* 1999; **33**: 1567–1572.

28 Yusuf S, Pfeffer MA, Swedberg K *et al.* Effects of candesartan in patients with chronic heart failure and preserved left-ventricular ejection fraction: the CHARM-Preserved Trial. *Lancet* 2003; **362**:777–781.

29 Senni M, Tribouilloy CM, Rodeheffer RJ *et al.* Congestive heart failure in the community: a study of all incident cases in Olmsted County, Minnesota, in 1991. *Circulation* 1998; **98**:2282–2289.

30 Gottdiener JS, McClelland RL, Marshall R *et al.* Outcome of congestive heart failure in elderly persons: influence of left ventricular systolic function. The Cardiovascular Health Study. *Ann Intern Med* 2002; **137**:631–639.

31 Pfeffer MA, Braunwald E, Moye LA *et al.* Effect of captopril on mortality and morbidity in patients with left ventricular dysfunction after myocardial infarction. Results of the survival and ventricular enlargement trial. The SAVE Investigators. *N Engl J Med* 1992; **327**: 669–677.

32 AIRE Study. Effect of ramipril on mortality and morbidity of survivors of acute myocardial infarction with clinical evidence of heart failure. *Lancet* 1993; **342**: 821–828.

33 Kober L, Torp-Pedersen C, Carlsen JE *et al.* A clinical trial of the angiotensin-converting-enzyme inhibitor trandolapril in patients with left ventricular dysfunction after myocardial infarction. *N Engl J Med* 1995; **333**:1670–1676.

34 Dickstein K, Kjekshus J. Effects of losartan and captopril on mortality and morbidity in high-risk patients after acute myocardial infarction: the OPTIMAAL randomised trial. Optimal Trial in Myocardial Infarction with Angiotensin II Antagonist Losartan. *Lancet* 2002; **360**:752–760.

35 Pfeffer MA, McMurray JJ, Velazquez EJ *et al.* Valsartan, captopril, or both in myocardial infarction complicated by heart failure, left ventricular dysfunction, or both. *N Engl J Med* 2003; **349**:1893–1906.

36 Mann DL, Deswal A. Angiotensin-receptor blockade in acute myocardial infarction–a matter of dose. *N Engl J Med* 2003; **349**:1963–1965.

37 Brenner BM, Cooper ME, de Zeeuw D *et al.* Effects of losartan on renal and cardiovascular outcomes in patients with type 2 diabetes and nephropathy. *N Engl J Med* 2001; **345**:861–869.

38 Dahlof B, Devereux RB, Kjeldsen SE *et al.* Cardiovascular morbidity and mortality in the Losartan Intervention For Endpoint reduction in hypertension study (LIFE): a randomised trial against atenolol. *Lancet* 2002; **359**:995–1003.

39 Mann DL, Deswal A. Angiotensin-Receptor Blockade in Acute Myocardial Infarction – A Matter of Dose. *N Engl J Med* 2003; **349**:1963–1965.

40 Pfeffer MA, Swedberg K, Granger CB *et al.* Effects of candesartan on mortality and morbidity in patients with chronic heart failure: the CHARM-Overall programme. *Lancet* 2003; **362**:759–766.

41 Pfeffer MA, McMurray JJ, Velazquez EJ *et al.* Valsartan, captopril, or both in myocardial infarction complicated by heart failure, left ventricular dysfunction, or both. *N Engl J Med* 2003; **349**:1893–1906.

42 VALIANT: Implications and explanations. Heart Wire News. 10 November 2003. http://www.theheart.org.

43 The SOLVD Investigators. Effect of enalapril on mortality and the development of heart failure in asymptomatic patients with reduced left ventricular ejection fraction. *N Engl J Med* 1992; **327**:685–691.

44 Mann DL, Deswal A, Bozkurt B, Torre-Amione G. New therapeutics for chronic heart failure. *Annu Rev Med* 2002; **53**:59–74.

**CHAPTER 5**

# Beta blockers

*Peter F. Robinson,* MD *& Michael R. Bristow,* MD, PHD

## Introduction

The medical treatment of chronic heart failure (CHF) has undergone a remarkable transition in the past 15 years. The approach has changed from a hemodynamic paradigm to a more long-term, reparative strategy that aims to favorably alter the biologic properties of the failing heart [1]. This is dramatically illustrated by the success in treating patients who suffer from mild to advanced CHF with $\beta$-adrenergic blocking agents. Initially it was thought that $\beta$-blocking was contraindicated in heart failure as increased adrenergic drive was thought to be critical for compensatory support of the failing heart. This belief was initially supported in the 1960s by evidence of a reduction of norepinephrine in myocardial tissue suggesting that adrenergic support was necessary but was deficient in heart failure, and early experiences that utilized standard doses of the first generation compound, propranolol, frequently led to worsening of heart failure signs and symptoms [2–4].

However, during the late 1970s and early 1980s, three separate lines of evidence contributed to a complete paradigm shift in the understanding of adrenergic mechanisms in heart failure. As recently summarized [5], these were: (1) the evidence that the failing human heart exhibited $\beta$-adrenergic receptor down-regulation and pathway desensitization, which are typical responses to excessive exposure to adrenergic drive, (2) the demonstration that coronary sinus norepinephrine levels were elevated in heart failure patients, reflecting an increase in interstitial levels despite the decrease in tissue stores, and (3) the apparently favorable clinical response to $\beta$-blocking agents when administered chronically to subjects with idiopathic dilated cardiomyopathy.

From a practical standpoint, two advances occurred during these years that allowed for the ultimate utilization of $\beta$-blocker therapy in this patient population. The first was the development of newer-generation compounds, initially $\beta_1$-selective compounds, or second generation agents, followed by the nonselective third-generation compounds that possessed vasodilatory properties. The second was simply the change in the way in which dosing with these compounds was initiated, utilizing low starting doses with a schedule of slow up-titration in an effort to allow the cardiovascular system to adapt slowly to the withdrawal of adrenergic stimuli. However, as recently discussed [6], new insights continue to modify existing antiadrenergic strategies. Consequently, it is likely that in the near future inhibition of the adrenergic nervous system will become much more effective than it is currently, where in terms of improving heart failure natural history it is the single most effective therapy available.

## The cardiovascular $\beta$-adrenergic system and the rationale for the use of $\beta$-blocker therapy

### Adrenergic signaling in the normal adult ventricle

There are three adrenergic receptors ($\beta_1$, $\beta_2$, and $\alpha_1$) in human cardiac myocytes that are coupled to positive inotropic, chronotropic, and growth responses [7–9]. In nonfailing human left and right ventricles, the relative $\beta_1 : \beta_2 : \alpha_1$ ratio is approximately $6 : 2 : 1$. Classically, $\beta$-adrenergic receptors are described as coupled to responses via the "stimulatory" G protein, $G_s$, to the effector enzyme adenylyl cyclase, which converts the substrate

MgATP to cAMP. CyclicAMP is a positively inotropic/lusitropic and chronotropic second messenger in addition to its strong growth promoting properties. In addition, there is increasing evidence that $\beta_1$-adrenergic receptors are coupled to important cell functions, many of them with pathologic potential, through cAMP-independent pathways involving intracellular effectors such as calcium/calmodulin activated kinase, calcineurin, and ERK1/2 MAP kinases [10–13].

In addition to their role as myocyte adrenergic receptors, $\beta_2$-receptors are also present on prejunctional adrenergic nerve terminals in the heart, where they facilitate norepinephrine release [14]. The $\beta_3$-receptor may also be present in the human heart as a counter-regulatory receptor coupled to the "inhibitory" G protein, $G_i$ [15], and there is also some evidence for a "$\beta_4$" receptor [16].

$\alpha_1$—Receptors are coupled via a different G protein, $G_q$, to the effector enzyme phospholipase C, which, through the second messenger diacyl glycerol, activates the growth-promoting protein kinase C family. Notably, the $\alpha_1$-receptor is not directly coupled to chronotropic activity and only very weakly coupled to the inotropic activity of the human myocyte.

## Adrenergic signaling in the chronically failing ventricle

In the resting state, there is no adrenergic support of the normally functioning human left ventricle [17]. However, the failing human heart is chronically adrenergically activated [17–19] under all conditions that helps to maintain cardiac performance over the short term by increasing both contractility and heart rate. Multiple lines of evidence [20–22] indicate that it is the increase in cardiac adrenergic drive rather than an increase in circulating norepinephrine that is both initially supportive and then ultimately damaging to the failing human heart. The neurotransmitter norepinephrine (NE) is the primary signaling molecule of cardiac adrenergic activity. NE is a powerful mediator of pathologic cardiac hypertrophy and myocardial damage [23]. In fact, it has been shown that transgenic animals incapable of synthesizing NE do not develop pathologic hypertrophy [24]. NE is also a powerful activator of apoptosis [25] and a promoter of ischemia [26]. When administered chronically at high levels

or when mimicked by transgenic $\beta_1$-receptor overexpression, NE can also directly cause contractile dysfunction [27]. In humans, pathologic hypertrophy and its molecular marker "fetal gene" induction, are $\beta_1$-receptor-mediated [28]. Apoptosis [25], tachycardia-exacerbated ischemia [29], and the majority of myocardial damage are also $\beta_1$-receptor mediated [30,31].

In the failing human ventricle, there is selective downregulation of the $\beta_1$-receptor, effectively increasing the relative abundances of the $\beta_2$- and $\alpha_1$-adrenergic receptors. Additionally, the absolute protein expression of the $\alpha_1$-receptor is increased in the failing heart. This combination of changes leads to a significant redistribution of adrenergic receptor subtypes from predominantly $\beta_1$ to a more mixed $2:1:1$ ratio of $\beta_1:\beta_2:\alpha_1$ receptors [9]. However, it is important to consider the relative affinity of NE for each receptor. Importantly, NE has a higher affinity for the human $\beta_1$-receptor than either the $\beta_2$-receptor or $\alpha_1$-receptor [32]. The relative potency of NE for $\beta_1:\beta_2:\alpha_1$-receptors is approximately $20:1:2$ [32–34]. This difference in affinity affects receptor occupancy. Given the approximate interstitial concentration of NE and epinephrine in patients with heart failure [35,36], this yields occupancies for $\beta_1:\beta_2:\alpha_1$ receptors of approximately $81:7:11\%$ and $88:6:6\%$ in respectively advanced and mild-moderate heart failure [32]. Thus the selectivity of NE for $\beta_1$-adrenergic receptors dictates that the vast majority of signaling traffic is carried by the $\beta_1$-receptor signal transduction pathways, in both nonfailing and failing human ventricular myocardium.

When expressed in transgenic animals at supraphysiologic levels, all three adrenergic signaling pathways appear to produce pathologic changes in the myocardium [37–43]. However, it requires approximately 10-fold greater expression of $\beta_2$-receptors to achieve the same degree of cardiomyopathy as with $\beta_1$-receptor expression [37,38,40]. Although overexpression of human $\alpha_{1b}$-receptors does produce a cardiomyopathy [41], expression of a constitutively active $\alpha_{1b}$-receptor produces only concentric hypertrophy without evidence of myopathy [42]. Additionally, in cultured cardiac myocytes exposed to norepinephrine, $\alpha_1$- [44] and $\beta_2$-receptor blockade [25] can produce an increase in apoptosis, indicating that there may be beneficial aspects to signaling through these pathways. In contrast, increased cardiac myocyte apoptosis appears to be exclusively mediated by the $\beta_1$-receptor subtype, both *in vitro* [25,45] and *in vivo* [46]. In total, these data from animal model systems confirm that chronic adrenergic signaling is a harmful compensatory mechanism in the failing human heart and that the majority of this damage is mediated via the $\beta_1$-receptor signaling pathway.

Finally, in the intact failing heart, reversal of remodeling associated with deinduction of the fetal gene program is mediated by $\beta_1$-receptor blockade, with no obvious contribution by either the $\beta_2$- or the $\alpha_1$-receptor pathways. That is, it has been shown that both immediate release metoprolol and carvedilol, delivered in equal $\beta_1$-receptor blocking doses, produce virtually identical effects on functional, structural, and molecular remodeling [28].

### Rationale for $\beta$-blocker therapy in CHF

In addition to changes in relative adrenergic receptor protein expression noted above, the failing human heart also undergoes desensitization of $\beta$-adrenergic signal transduction in response to ongoing adrenergic stimulation. In the end-stage failing heart, 50–60% of the total signal transducing potential is lost [9]. This occurs via modifications at multiple sites, including desensitization changes in the $\beta_1$ and $\beta_2$ receptors themselves, an upregulation in the inhibitory G protein ($G_i$), an increase in an enzyme responsible for modulating receptor activity by phosphorylation ($\beta$ARK), and in some cases a downregulation in the expression of adenylyl cyclase [9,47]. These and other data from model systems [48] suggest that the $\beta$-adrenergic receptor pathway desensitization changes present in the failing human heart are adaptive changes, and that a potentially effective therapeutic strategy would be to add to this endogenous antiadrenergic strategy by inhibiting receptor signal transduction [49–51]. However, as an adaptive change $\beta$-receptor desensitization is not particularly effective, as substantial signal transduction capacity remains, and the partial loss of a mechanism that has a beneficial component contributes to a reduction in myocardial reserve and a compromise of functional capacity. In addition, the cAMP-independent pathways coupled to pathologic effects such as apoptosis and fetal gene induction may be upregulated in the failing human heart [10–13]. This means that $\beta$-receptor desensitization results in a partial loss of the benefits of adrenergic stimulation, and an increase in pathologic processes mediated through residual signaling that is amplified through these upregulated cAMP-independent signal transduction mechanisms. Put in this light, the regulated changes in $\beta$-receptor signal transduction are decidedly maladaptive. This overall interpretation is emphasized in Figure 5.1.

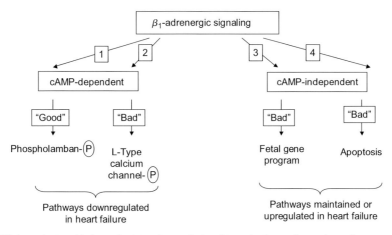

**Figure 5.1** cAMP dependent and independent $\beta_1$-adrenergic signal transduction pathways in cardiac myocytes in failing ventricles. Differential desensitization of cAMP dependent pathways and upregulation in cAMP independent signaling subserving pathologic processes such as fetal gene induction and apoptosis leads to a net upregulation in myopathic signal transduction.

In summary, the continuously increased adrenergic drive present in the failing human heart delivers adverse biologic signals to the cardiac myocyte and other myocardial cells via $\beta_1$- and to a lesser degree via $\beta_2$- and $\alpha_1$-adrenergic receptor signal transduction. This is the fundamental basis for the use of antiadrenergic agents in the treatment of CHF.

## Classes of $\beta$-blockers available

Table 5.1 lists various $\beta$-blockers that have at least some experience in heart failure therapy, by the generational classification [5] that is commonly used to categorize them. Table 5.2 gives additional pharmacological properties of heart failure $\beta$-blockers that may impact clinical efficacy.

### First generation compounds
Propranolol is the prototype "first generation" compound, introduced into clinical practice in 1968 as an antianginal agent. Propranolol and other first generation compounds, such as timolol, are nonselective agents with equal affinities for both $\beta_1$- and $\beta_2$-receptor subtypes and possessing no important pharmacologic properties other than $\beta$-blockade.

### Second generation compounds
In the 1970s, pharmaceutical companies developed "cardioselective" or second generation $\beta$-blockers that selectively antagonized $\beta_1$- compared to $\beta_2$-receptors. This was done in the mistaken belief that the human heart could be selectively $\beta$-blocked [7,8]. This belief arose from animal models in which only $\beta_1$-receptor-mediated responses were identified in the myocardium. At the time, it was hoped that a lack of $\beta_2$-receptor blockade would also reduce some of the unwanted systemic side effects of $\beta$-blockers, such as bronchial smooth muscle reactivity. However, this hypothesis has never been conclusively proven.

**Table 5.1** Generations of $\beta$-blocking agents developed for cardiovascular indications; representative compounds with experience in CHF populations.

| Compound generation | $K_H\beta_1$ (nM) | $K_L\beta_2$ (nM) | $\beta_1/\beta_2$ affinity | $K_i\alpha_1$ (nM) | $\beta_1/\alpha_1$ affinity |
|---|---|---|---|---|---|
| First propranolol | 4.1 | 8.5 | 2.1 | — | — |
| Second metoprolol | 50 | 3825 | 79 | — | — |
| Bisoprolol | 69 | 7135 | 102 | — | — |
| Third Carvedilol | 4.0 | 29 | 7.3 | 9.4 | 3.1 |
| Bucindolol | 3.6 | 5.0 | 1.4 | 249 (69) | 66 (19) |
| Nebivolol | 0.7 | 225 | 352 | 330 | 471 |
| Fourth??? | To be developed, for a heart failure indication exclusively | | | | |

**Table 5.2** Pharmacologic properties of $\beta$-blocking agents used to treat heart failure.

| Compound (Device) | Pharmacologic properties (0–4+) | | | | | |
|---|---|---|---|---|---|---|
| | $\beta_1$-AR blockade | $\beta_2$-AR blockade | $\alpha_1$-AR blockade | *ISA human | Inverse agonism | Sympatholysis |
| Metoprolol | ++++ | ++ | 0 | 0 | +++ | 0 |
| Bisoprolol | ++++ | ++ | 0 | 0 | +++ | 0 |
| Carvedilol | ++++ | +++ | ++++ | 0 | + | + |
| Bucindolol | ++++ | ++++ | + | 0 | 0 - + | +++ |
| Nebivolol | ++++ | + | 0 | 0 | ? | ? |

*Intrinsic sympathomimetic activity in functioning human heart.

The first selective $\beta_1$-blocking agent was practolol [52], which was sufficiently $\beta_1$-selective that it was used alongside propranolol to demonstrate the presence of a third subtype, the $\beta_3$ receptor. It was ultimately shown that these three distinct subtypes were the byproducts of distinct genes [53–56]. Practolol was the first $\beta$-blocking agent to be therapeutically administered to a patient with CHF [57]. Ultimately, immunologic side effects forced the removal of practolol from clinical practice and it was replaced by metoprolol in exploratory studies. Metoprolol is approximately 75-fold selective for human $\beta_1$- versus $\beta_2$-receptors (Table 5.1). In the 1980s, pharmaceutical companies developed even more $\beta_1$-selective compounds, including bisoprolol, which is 120-fold selective. Interestingly, this incrementally increased selectivity has not been associated with enhanced efficacy or reduced adverse events, as in heart failure clinical trials selective $\beta_1$-blockers and nonselective third-generation agents perform similarly, on average [58–64].

## Third-generation compounds

In the 1970s and 80s, another drug development effort aimed originally at improving the treatment of hypertension led to the creation of $\beta$-blockers with vasodilatory properties. The prototype agent of these "third generation" compounds is labetalol. Labetalol is a nonselective $\beta$-blocking agent with additional $\alpha$-blocking properties. In fact, labetalol has higher affinity for the $\alpha$-receptor than either the $\beta_1$- or $\beta_2$-receptor [60]. Although labetalol has never been systematically studied in heart failure populations, it has been shown to improve myocardial function in subjects with hypertensive cardiomyopathy [61]. However, carvedilol, bucindolol and nebivolol, three other $\beta$-blocking agents with vasodilating activity, have been extensively evaluated in the treatment of CHF [62–66].

As shown in Table 5.1, carvedilol is slightly (by seven-fold) $\beta_1$-selective at lower doses and in effect becomes nonselective at higher target doses [67,68]. It is also a potent $\alpha_1$-blocker with only a two- to three-fold selectivity for the $\beta_1$-receptor over the $\alpha_1$-receptor; this gives rise to its moderate vasodilator properties. In addition, carvedilol has been reported to possess multiple "ancillary properties", including antioxidant, antiendothelin,

antiapoptotic, and antiproliferative effects [69–71]. Although intriguing, the contribution of these ancillary properties to carvedilol's clinical benefits has yet to be established. In addition, carvedilol exhibits extremely slow offset kinetics from $\beta$-adrenergic receptors [72,73], and "tight binding" [74] that makes it difficult to be washed out of membranes or be displaced by competing ligands. These latter properties may contribute to the clinical efficacy of carvedilol. As discussed in the outcome trial section, there is now extensive experience with carvedilol in heart failure, and in the United States carvedilol is the only $\beta$-blocker with an indication for mortality reduction [62,63].

Bucindolol is a completely nonselective $\beta$-blocking agent with only mild vasodilator properties. Its vasodilator properties may be mediated through weak $\alpha_1$-blockade, where bucindolol's binding affinity is 60–70-fold less than for either the $\beta_1$- or the $\beta_2$-receptor [5,75–78] or through some other property, such as nitric oxide generation (Mason P, personal communication). Notably, as shown in Table 5.2, compared to other $\beta$-blocking agents used to treat CHF, bucindolol possess the lowest amount of "inverse agonism", or the ability of an antagonist to inactivate active-state receptors [79]. This likely explains its association with a low incidence of symptomatic bradycardia [79,80]. This same low-inverse-agonist profile may contribute to the apparent low amount of myocardial depression observed on acute administration of bucindolol [81]. In addition, the lack of significant $\alpha$-blockade in the presence of significant $\beta_2$-blockade at the prejunctional level gives bucindolol significant "sympatholytic" activity [82], which is unique among the $\beta$-blocker class of compounds (Table 5.2). Although bucindolol has a small amount of intrinsic sympathomimetic activity (ISA) in rodents and dogs, it is devoid of ISA in functioning human myocardium [80,83,84]. Bucindolol binds to $\beta_3$-receptors with high affinity [85] and $\beta_3$-agonism may contribute to its favorable metabolic effects [86].

Nebivolol is a third-generation compound with pronounced $\beta_1$-selectivity and vasodilatory properties related to nitric oxide (NO) generation [87–89]. Likely related to these properties, nebivolol has a unique hemodynamic profile among $\beta$-blocking agents; it reduces both preload and afterload (like carvedilol and bucindolol) but also improves arterial distensibility [89].

Because carvedilol and bucindolol block adrenergic receptors that are additional to $\beta_1$, and because all third-generation compounds possess vasodilatory properties, it has been argued that this class has a therapeutic advantage [75,80] compared to second- generation compounds. There are data to suggest that compared with second-generation compounds, third-generation compounds produce more beneficial effects on left ventricular function [75,90,91]. However, it is important to note that both second- and third-generation compounds improve intrinsic systolic function [88–90], prevent deterioration in function and progression in remodeling [90–94], and lead to reverse remodeling [94–99]. Most importantly and as discussed in the clinical trials section, in heart failure populations there is no evidence to suggest that third-generation $\beta$-blockers produce better clinical efficacy than second- generation compounds.

## Fourth generation compounds

The $\beta-$blockers used to treat CHF have all been initially developed for other cardiovascular indications, such as ischemic heart disease or hypertension. Despite their proven effectiveness, there has never been a $\beta$-blocker specifically developed for a heart failure indication. This situation will likely change in the near future, based on the degree of success of compounds that were secondarily directed to heart failure development. Possibilities for such a "fourth generation" $\beta$-blocker include compounds with both $\beta$-blocking and phosphodiesterase inhibitory activity, and compounds specifically targeted to $\beta$-receptor polymorphisms.

## $\beta$-blockers as therapy for CHF

### Therapeutic indications

Therapy with $\beta$-blockers is indicated for the treatment of patients who suffer from the clinical syndrome of CHF in the setting of left ventricular (LV) systolic dysfunction from either ischemic or nonischemic etiologies, in the absence of contraindications. Patients should be clinically compensated and on standard treatment, including diuretics and angiotensin-converting enzyme (ACE) inhibitors prior to initiation. However, the standard acceptance of initiating therapy with an ACE inhibitor prior to initiating a $\beta$-blocker has been put into question recently with the results of the Carvedilol ACE-Inhibitor Remodeling Mild CHF Evaluation (CARMEN) study, which showed that initiation with carvedilol concomitantly with enalapril was associated with a greater improvement in indices of LV function than either initiation with enalapril or carvedilol alone [100]. In general, if clinical compensation is achieved, $\beta$-blockade should likely be started as soon as possible and in the presence of ACE inhibitor therapy, and data has shown that initiation prior to discharge is associated with more frequent use of $\beta$-blockade at 60 days without a worsening of symptoms [101]. Therefore, this practice should be encouraged in an effort to increase the utilization of this important medication. However, more definitive outcome data may be necessary to make this a formal recommendation.

In the absence of symptoms, there are only limited data supporting the use of $\beta$-blocker agents in the setting of reduced LV systolic function [102,103]. Patients in the post-infarct time period should be treated with $\beta$-blocker therapy even with normal LV systolic function regardless of the presence of symptoms. See the clinical guidelines section for further details.

Recent data have shown $\beta$-blocker therapy to be beneficial not only for mild to moderate (NYHA class II–III symptoms) heart failure [58,59,65], but also for those with moderate to severe (NYHA class III–IV symptoms) heart failure [63,64]. Therapy needs to be initiated more cautiously in those at the more severe end of the spectrum, especially those with symptoms at rest. In these patients, therapy should likely be initiated under the supervision of a cardiologist.

When administered to heart failure patients, $\beta$-blockers should be uptitrated slowly to the maximal tolerated dose, typically limited either by significant bradycardia, hypotension, a decline in organ perfusion, or worsening of heart failure symptoms not amenable to increased diuretic dose or other alterations in the medical regimen [104]. Once heart failure subjects reach a maintenance dose of a $\beta$-blocker, treatment should be maintained indefinitely because of the risk of deterioration on withdrawal [105].

In the clinical utilization of $\beta$-blockers for CHF, there are situations where a patient treated chronically requires hospital admission due to a worsening in heart failure symptoms. There is at least a theoretical benefit to maintaining the patient on their dose of $\beta$-blocker if this is clinically possible. At times, however, a decrease in dose or even temporary discontinuation of the $\beta$-blocker may be necessary. Other clinical scenarios may necessitate the utilization of intravenous (IV) inotropic support. The presence of residual $\beta$-blockade may lead to an abrogation in the favorable hemodynamic effects typically seen if dobutamine (a $\beta_1$- and $\beta_2$-agonist) is used as the inotropic agent [106,107]. However, it has been shown that the hemodynamic effects of an IV form of a type III phosphodiesterase inhibitor, milrinone, is not adversely compromised [106,107]. Therefore, if a patient on a $\beta$-blocker for treatment of CHF requires IV inotropic support, a type III phosphodiesterase inhibitor (milrinone, enoximone, or levosimendan) is more beneficial in the acute setting than dobutamine.

## Effects on initiation of therapy

Because the failing heart is dependent on adrenergic support [2–4,14,17], the administration of any $\beta$-blocking agent to a subject with symptomatic heart failure from systolic dysfunction will cause some degree of myocardial depression that will clinically manifest to varying degrees. Acute administration of first-generation compounds, such as propranolol, causes a significant decrease in contractility [17] to a point where the intolerance rate is prohibitive [108]. This, coupled with a concomitant increase in systemic vascular resistance [4,80,109], leads to a marked reduction in cardiac output [17,34,80], resulting in a drug intolerance rate of >20% [108].

However, second-generation compounds can be administered in low starting doses to subjects even with severe left ventricular dysfunction [104] if done so in the appropriate clinical setting. The reason these compounds are effective is that selective $\beta_1$-receptor blockade leaves the $\beta_2$-receptor unblocked and capable of supporting myocardial function, either directly or through increased norepinephrine release mediated by presynaptic $\beta_2$-receptors [14]. Additionally, there is less reflex peripheral vasoconstriction because unblocked peripheral vascular $\beta_2$-receptors can mediate vasodilation [110]. The overall effect is that cardiac output and organ perfusion are reduced to a lesser extent than with first-generation compounds [104]. Consistent with the above, the drug tolerability rates for second-generation compound metoprolol range from 79–100%, starting at doses of 5 or 6.25 mg twice daily [80].

The third-generation compounds carvedilol, bucindolol, and nebivolol have the advantage of afterload reduction to counteract the negative inotropic properties of adrenergic withdrawal [80,81,111]. As a result, in grouped data, bucindolol does not lower cardiac output [34,80,81,111] and carvedilol is either neutral or may even increase it slightly [80,111]. However, the vasodilator properties do lead to an increased incidence of orthostatic hypotension upon initiation or uptitration of therapy, most of which are self-limiting or can be managed with a decrease in the dose of diuretic [104]. The balance of the above effects leads to a tolerability to carvedilol in approximately 92% of subjects with mild to moderate heart failure utilizing doses of 3.125 or 6.25 mg twice daily. Bucindolol is tolerated by the large majority (approximately 98%) of mild to moderate heart failure subjects challenged with 6.25 to 12.5 mg twice daily, owing to its more mild vasodilator effects [34,80,81]. Nebivolol appeared to be reasonably well-tolerated in the SENIORS Trial, which was a mixture of mild-moderate LV dysfunction and preserved LV function in elderly heart failure patients. However, 27% of patients withdrew from nebivolol study medication in SENIORS (21 months mean follow-up) [112], compared to 23% for bucindolol (24 months mean follow-up) in BEST [64] and 16% for carvedilol (10.4 months mean follow-up) in COPERNICUS [63].

In an attempt to safely initiate $\beta$-blocker therapy in those patients with the most severe symptoms, an approach of coupling the initiation of $\beta$-blockade with the temporary utilization of an oral inotropic agent, enoximone, has been studied with intriguing results [113,114]. Unfortunately, preliminary results suggest that this way was not successful in the overall study population in the ESSENTIAL trials but might have benefitted a subgroup of that population (unpublished results).

In summary, the vasodilatory properties of third-generation agents allows compounds with a nonselective profile, such as carvedilol and bucindolol, to be administered with an acceptable tolerability rate, allowing for administration of agents with a more comprehensive antiadrenergic profile [34,80]. Vasodilation also provides an additional mechanism of potential long-term benefit, although for carvedilol this property may not be durable [115,116] or may be overshadowed by the improvement in LV function [115]. Therefore, any outcome benefit demonstrated by third-generation compounds would not be readily explained solely by this feature. There may be other subtle differences between compounds that would require a properly designed, large study population to demonstrate differential clinical efficacy.

## Diastolic dysfunction

The vast majority of trials have been performed in patients with LV systolic function as a cause of heart failure symptoms. $\beta$-blocker therapy for patients who suffer from the clinical syndrome of heart failure with normal LV systolic function has not been well-studied. The one exception is the Study of the Effects of Nevibolol Intervention on Outcomes and Rehospitalisation in Seniors with Heart Failure (SENIORS) Trial, the results of which were published in early 2005 [112]. This trial utilized nebivolol for the treatment of heart failure regardless of the presence of LV systolic function and showed a significant reduction in the primary endpoint, although there were a relatively limited number of patients with preserved systolic function. Despite a lack of data, there are consensus-generated clinical guidelines for the management of patients with isolated diastolic dysfunction [33]. It is evident that $\beta$-blocker therapy plays a role in many of these areas, including treatment of hypertension, treatment of supraventricular arrhythmias, and management of ischemic symptoms.

## Pharmacokinetic issues

As stated previously, the strategy for administering all $\beta$-blocking agents in the setting of CHF is to start with extremely low doses [104] and increase the dose gradually, usually at weekly or biweekly intervals. Using this strategy, doses that can substantially reduce exercise heart rate (by 10–20 bpm) can be achieved within 4–6 weeks of drug initiation under close observation. Parenthetically, the reduction in exercise heart rate is considered the gold standard for evaluation of systemic $\beta_1$-blocking effect and reduction in resting heart rate is not a particularly accurate gauge of the degree of $\beta$-blockade. The pharmacologic half-lives of metoprolol tartrate (immediate release), carvedilol, and bucindolol dictate twice-daily dosing. However, clinical trial experience has suggested that metoprolol tartrate may require tid dosing in order to achieve comparable $\beta$-blockade over a 24-h period. Bisoprolol, metoprolol succinate CR/XL and nebivolol can be given once daily. Carvedilol, metoprolol, bucindolol, and nebivolol are all highly lipophilic compounds that are extensively metabolized and cleared by the liver; bisoprolol is less lipophilic and exhibits mixed hepatic/renal clearance [117]. The effects of lipophilicity on central nervous system access have not been extensively studied. First-pass metabolism occurs with all of these agents, so the bioavailability is relatively low, on the order of 20–50%. However, in the presence of liver congestion in advanced heart failure, the bioavailability increases and doses of lipophilic compounds produce relatively greater degrees of $\beta$-blockade. However, this may be tempered by increased intestinal congestion that may limit bioavailability and counteract these effects. Therefore in the setting of advanced heart failure, it is prudent to closely monitor the $\beta$-blockade achieved with each individual clinical scenario.

Pharmacokinetic interaction with other heart failure medications, including warfarin, does not typically occur with the $\beta$-blocking agents used in heart failure. Carvedilol does increase the oral bioavailability of digoxin, but the increase in plasma digoxin levels is relatively small, typically by 10–15% [118].

Essentially all of the lipophilic $\beta$-blocking agents used in heart failure management are hepatically metabolized by cytochrome P450 2D6 (CYP2D6) oxidation. In subjects with polymorphic variants of CYP2D6 responsible for the debrisoquin phenotype (the "poor metabolizer" present in 2–10%

of the US population), the elimination half-life may be prolonged, and plasma levels and the degree of $\beta$-blockade may be increased [119], but this does typically lead to serious adverse effects or altered clinical responses because of the large therapeutic index of $\beta$-blocking agents and target doses of $\beta$-blockers are already at high levels of receptor occupancy. Additionally, stereoselective metabolism by CYP2D6 occurs for some lipophilic $\beta$-blockers, including carvedilol and metoprolol. Carvedilol undergoes stereoselective metabolism of its $S$ isomer upon oral administration, which leads to plasma concentrations of the $R$ isomer that are two- to three-fold higher than the $S$ isomer [67,120]. It has been shown that the $S$ isomer has specificity for binding to $\beta$- and not to $\alpha$-adrenergic receptors [121]. Therefore, after oral administration, the $R$-isomer-predominant $\alpha$-blocking effects have been observed to about the same degree as the $\beta$-blocking effects, an effect not observed with IV administration [111,121,122]. In the poor metabolizer phenotype, the clearance of the $R$ isomer is further reduced relative to the $S$ isomer [123], which may lead to an even greater relative $\alpha$-blocking effect. However, it is unclear if this has any clinical relevance.

Metoprolol undergoes stereoselective metabolism by CYP2D6 but in favor of its $R$ isomer [124]. This results in only a small difference in relative $S/R$ plasma levels, typically 1.35-fold. However, this is reduced to <1 in poor metabolizers [124]. As the $S$ isomer of metoprolol has a relatively greater $\beta$-blocking effect than the $R$ isomer, this lowered ratio results in less $\beta$-blockade relative to total plasma levels [125], which tends to cancel out the effect of increased total plasma levels resulting from the lower oxidation rate. The end result, then, is that there is unlikely to be any clinically relevant importance related to this differential metabolism with metoprolol.

## Effects of long-term treatment on myocardial function, chamber characteristics, and other properties of the failing heart

The myocardial effects of long-term treatment with $\beta$-blocking agents have been reviewed in detail [1,34,75,80,126]. The marked generalization

about the long-term effects of $\beta$-blockade for the treatment of heart failure are that they are diametrically opposed to those seen with acute administration [1]. Put another way, every placebo-controlled trial that has been conducted for at least 3 months has shown an improvement in systolic function compared with the short-term negative inotropic effects previously characterized [1]. Later, between 4 and 12 months of therapy, a regression in myocardial mass and a normalization in ventricular size and shape, a phenomena referred to as reverse remodeling [1,34,75,80,96], is consistently observed on the average in heart failure populations with dilated cardiomyopathy phenotypes. These time-dependent effects of $\beta$-blocker therapy appear to be $\beta$-blocker overall class effects, as they have been observed with both second- and third-generation compounds. Importantly, the combination of improvement in systolic function and the reversal of remodeling are unique to $\beta$-blockade among drug treatment of heart failure. Recently, these changes have been seen with device therapy, notably bi-ventricular pacing [127]. Although inhibitors of the renin–angiotensin system (such as ACE inhibitors, angiotensin receptor blockers [ARB's] and aldosterone) can attenuate the remodeling process, they do not typically reverse it and do not typically produce improvement in intrinsic systolic function [1].

Because these changes in myocardial function and structure geometry amount to a partial reversal of the dilated cardiomyopathy phenotype, they would be expected to produce favorable effects on the natural history of heart failure, and this has been proven to be the case. This is typified in the now numerous randomized, placebo-controlled trials involving large numbers of patients showing a mortality benefit in nearly all studies of appropriate sample size (Table 5.3). Although there are quantitative differences in results among some of these trials, as discussed in detail later, all $\beta$-blockers that can be tolerated by heart failure patients in at least moderate $\beta_1$-receptor occupancy doses have demonstrated favorable effects on major heart failure clinical endpoints.

In addition, there exists a select-group of patients (approximately one-third) who do not appear to respond to chronic $\beta$-blocker therapy in terms of this reverse remodeling effect, and it appears it is

**Table 5.3** Multicenter placebo-controlled trials with beta-blocking agents in CHF.

| Trial | Year | Agent target dose (mg/day) | NYHA class | Sample size, n | Primary endpoint (PEP) | PEP Yes/No | Mortality reduction (%) |
|---|---|---|---|---|---|---|---|
| MDC [154] | 1993 | Metoprolol tartrate 100–150 | II–IV | 383 | Mortality and need for transplantation | $p = 0.058$ | — |
| CIBIS-I [160] | 1994 | Bisoprolol 5 | III–IV | 641 | Mortality | No | 20 (NS) |
| US Carvedilol Trials [62] (Mild, MOCHA, precise, severe) | 1996 | Carvedilol 50–100 | II–IV | 1094 | Mortality, exercise tolerance, quality of life, progression of disease | $\frac{3}{4}$ No Mild, Yes | 65 (not ITT) |
| MERIT-HF [59] | 1999 | Metoprolol succinate 200 | II–IV | 3991 | Mortality | Yes | 35 |
| CIBIS-II [58] | 1999 | Bisoprolol 10 | III–IV | 2446 | Mortality | Yes | 34 |
| BEST [64] | 2001 | Bucindolol 100(<75 kg) 200(>75 kg) | III–IV | 2708 | Mortality | No | 10 (NS) |
| COPERNICUS [63] | 2001 | Carvedilol 50 | "Severe" HF | 2289 | Mortality | Yes | 35 |
| SENIORS [112] | 2005 | Nebivolol 20 | I–IV | 2128 | Mortality and cardiovascular hospital | Yes | 12 (NS) |

this subgroup of patients who fail to demonstrate a mortality benefit [95]. Figure 5.2 illustrates the heterogeneity of response problem from the standpoint of carvedilol, from the Multicenter Oral Carvedilol in Heart Failure Assessment (MOCHA) trial [128]. As can be observed in Figure 5.2, at low (6.25 mg bid) and high (25 mg bid) dose respectively, 55% and 67% responded to $\beta$-blocker therapy with an improvement in LVEF of at least 5 EF units, after 6 months of treatment. However, 40% and 31% of subjects in the low and high dose arms had no improvement, and a few patients (respectively 5.3% and 2.5%) actually experienced a decline in LVEF of $\geq$5 EF units. In these latter patients it is likely that $\beta$-blocker therapy was not helpful and contributed to an adverse clinical outcome [95], and so it is important to monitor the remodeling/systolic function response to $\beta$-blockade, and to potentially not to continue treatment in patients who have evidence for a decline in LVEF after several months of therapy.

In addition to the favorable effects on myocardial function and structure, the general mechanisms through which $\beta$-blocking agents reduce mortality likely involve their established antiarrhythmic and antiischemic properties. In contrast to ACE inhibitors, $\beta$-blocking agents have consistently lowered the sudden death rate in heart failure trials [5,58,59], which suggests an antiarrhythmic contribution to mortality reduction. Because of the well-established "secondary prevention" database in ischemic heart disease, it is likely that the antiischemic properties of $\beta$-blocking agents contribute to mortality reduction in subjects with heart failure from ischemic cardiomyopathy.

## Effects of long-term treatment on myocardial gene expression

The favorable phenotypic structural changes observed in treatment with $\beta$-blocking agents are likely related to their ability to favorably alter the expression of myocardial genes that regulate contractility and pathologic hypertrophy. Several categories of contractility- and hypertropy-modifying genes are thought to be involved in producing structural and functional changes in dilated cardiomyopathy, including genes involved in myosin heavy-chain (MyHC) isoforms, calcium-handling

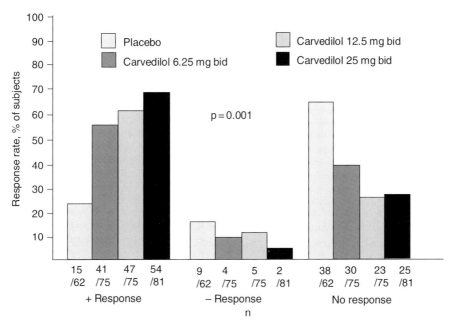

**Figure 5.2** Remodeling/systolic function responses to carvedilol in the MOCHA trial, as change in LVEF by ≥5 EF units (+Response), ≤5 EF units (−Response) and +4 to −4 EF units (No Response).

proteins, as well as other structural proteins. A pattern of abnormal myocardial gene expression in dilated cardiomyopathy has been termed the "fetal gene program" due to the profile's similarity to that seen in the fetal heart [28]. This same gene expression profile can be induced in the models of dilated cardiomyopathy produced via overexpression of the adrenergic system as previously discussed and it appears the pathologic pathway is primarily linked to $\beta_1$-receptor signaling, with the $\beta_2$- and $\alpha_1$-adrenergic pathways likely playing smaller roles.

It has been shown that patients deemed responders to treatment with $\beta$-blockers display a reversal of induction of the "fetal" gene program, with favorable changes in the expression of genes encoding sarcoplasmic-reticulum calcium ATPase, and in the $\alpha$-and $\beta$-MyHC isoforms [28]. Patients who were not phenotypic responders to $\beta$-blocker treatment failed to show these same favorable changes. This suggests that the favorable phenotypic response to $\beta$-blockers treatment is mediated through effects on myocardial gene expression, specifically on genes related to contractile proteins and calcium handling.

## Metabolic effects of $\beta$-blockade

### Cardiac metabolism

There is an emerging body of evidence that $\beta$-blockers may exert some of their beneficial effects in heart failure via beneficial modifications in cardiac metabolism. There is a substantial body of literature to show that the failing heart operates in an energy-inefficient manner and there are numerous disrupted metabolic pathways that contribute to this [129–131]. One important factor in the efficiency of cardiac metabolism is substrate utilization. Fatty acid oxidation (FAO) is less efficient, from an oxygen-utilization standpoint, than is glucose oxidation. The relative substrate utilization of the chronically failing heart remains controversial, but some evidence points to an increased relative utilization of FAO, and the chronic, catecholamine-induced elevation in free fatty acids (FFA) levels has been well-established in heart failure patients [132]. Inhibiting this catecholamine-induced increase in FFA may be beneficial. In fact, preliminary studies have shown that inhibition of FAO may be a treatment for heart failure [133–138].

## Systemic metabolism

Traditionally, chronic $\beta$-blocker use as therapy for hypertension in population-based studies has been associated with a worsening of serum glucose levels, a 22–28% increased incidence of diabetes, and worsening of glycemic control in patients with established type II diabetes mellitus (DM), all indicative of increased insulin resistance [139–144]. However, these studies used first- and second-generation $\beta$-blocking agents. Studies evaluating the third-generation compounds carvedilol and bucindolol have failed to show this same pattern. In fact, small comparative trials between carvedilol and both atenolol and metoprolol in patients with type II DM have shown that, in comparison to these second-generation compounds, carvedilol appears to provide an improvement in insulin resistance [145,146], and in COMET carvedilol exhibited evidence of a more favorable effect on insulin resistance and glucose metabolism than did metoprolol tartrate [65]. Bucindolol also exhibited evidence of increasing insulin sensitivity in BEST [86].

The effect on systemic FFA levels and the effect on insulin resistance may be interrelated, although this has yet to be shown. Taken together, though, it is clear that both of these modifications may contribute to the improved myocardial energy efficiency seen with $\beta$-blockade, and possibly to their positive effects on myocardial function [147–151]. It has been shown that at least one $\beta$-blocking agent, carvedilol, was associated with reduced myocardial FFA utilization and an associated improvement in LV systolic function in a small study of patients suffering from ischemic cardiomyopathy [148]. This lends further support to the possibility that at least one of the mechanisms by which $\beta$-blockers exert their positive influence in the improvement on myocardial function may be through altered myocardial energetics by shifting substrate utilization to a more oxygen-efficient pathway, glucose oxidation.

## Clinical outcome studies of various $\beta$-blocking agents

Table 5.3 is a summary of the placebo-controlled trials involving at least 100 patients with a minimum follow-up of 3 months. These trials have all been conducted since 1985 and with background therapy of diuretics, ACE inhibitors, and digoxin. Under pooled analysis, $\beta$-blockers appear to lower all-cause mortality in patients with widely varying degrees of heart failure and systolic function by approximately 30%. In comparison, ACE inhibitors reduce mortality by approximately 16%, aldosterone antagonists by 30% [33], and Cardiac resynchronization (CRT) device therapy in patients with infraventricular conduction devices (IVCDs) by an average of 30% [152,153]. However, the clinical trial experience with these other forms of therapy does not begin to approach the number of patients enrolled in heart failure trials, where over 15 000 patients have been randomized in placebo-controlled clinical trials where mortality effects were was reported as an endpoint (Table 5.3).

### Metoprolol

The first placebo-controlled multicenter trial with a $\beta$-blocking agent was the Metoprolol in Dilated Cardiomyopathy (MDC) trial [154], planned in 1982–3 and conducted in European and US centers between 1985 and 1991 (Table 5.3). This trial compared metoprolol tartrate to placebo in patients with symptomatic heart failure from idiopathic dilated cardiomyopathy. The primary endpoint was the combination of all-cause mortality and deterioration of the patient to the point of requiring listing for cardiac transplantation [154]. In the MDC trial, treatment with metoprolol with a twice-daily or thrice-daily dosing regimen at an average dose of 108 mg/day reduced the prevalence of the primary endpoint by 34%, which did not quite reach statistical significance ($p = 0.058$). This benefit was driven entirely by a reduction in the morbidity endpoint (reduced 90% by treatment with metoprolol) as all-cause mortality actually trended higher in the metoprolol arm [154].

This led to the larger Metoprolol CR/XL Randomized Intervention Trial in Congestive Heart Failure (MERIT-HF) trial, which began enrolling patients in early 1997, and was stopped prematurely for a 34% relative risk reduction in mortality in the metoprolol arm [59]. Unlike the MDC trial, MERIT-HF utilized the long-acting, once-daily, dosage form of metoprolol, or metoprolol succinate, and enrolled patients with both ischemic and nonischemic cardiomyopathies. The MERIT-HF trial enrolled 3991 subjects who had NYHA class II through IV heart failure, though 97% were class II and III [59]. Importantly, the average daily dose of metoprolol achieved in MERIT-HF was larger then MDC, 159 mg/day versus 108 mg/day. Mortality from both pump failure and sudden death was reduced in this trial. Additionally, the large sample size allowed for some subgroup analysis, and it appeared the mortality benefit extended across most demographic groups, including older versus younger patients, ischemic versus nonischemic etiologies, and lower versus higher ejection fractions [59]. However there was almost no mortality reduction in the female patients (23% of the total), suggesting sex may play a role in the response to $\beta$-blockade. In addition, the large ($n = 1071$, 27% of the total) subgroup enrolled in the United States failed to show any beneficial response to metoprolol CR/XL (mortality hazard ratio of 1.05, mortality plus heart failure hospitalization hazard ratio approximately 0.84, both $p = $ NS) [155].

Especially in light of the recent results of the Carvedilol or Metoprolol European Trial (COMET) trial [65], discussed later in the section on carvedilol, the differential properties of the short-acting metoprolol tartrate, formulation and the long-acting, metoprolol succinate, formulation require further discussion. The long-acting CR preparation used in MERIT-HF study produces a relatively constant blood level over 24 h [32,156]. The bioavailability of the CR preparation is approximately 70% of the short-acting, conventional formulation [156]. However, it is important to note that compared with 50 mg twice daily of the short-acting formulation, 100 mg of the CR preparation produces similar trough levels and degrees of reduction in exercise heart rate, indicating bioequivalency of the two compounds [32,156]. The MERIT-HF study protocol allowed for uptitration to a maximal dose of 200 mg/day, and, as stated above, this led to an average daily dosage of 159 mg/day, significantly greater than the 108 mg/day achieved in the MDC trial, providing indirect evidence of a lack of bioequivalency of $\beta_1$-blockade across these two trials.

Apart from the large discrepancy in dosing between the two studies to account for a difference in outcomes, there are theoretical reasons why the CR preparation may have greater tolerability than the conventional preparation in heart failure patients. The reduced fluctuation in blood levels for the CR compared with the conventional formulation provides for the potential for improved tolerability of the CR preparation in heart failure patients. In addition, the shallower slope of the CR plasma concentration curve at the end of the dosing interval would at least theoretically reduce the potential of producing a $\beta$-blocker withdrawal effect if doses are missed or dosing intervals are prolonged [32]. However, although no direct comparison of equivalency has ever been conducted, at this point, the differences observed across trials are at least suggestive that the two preparations are not equivalent. Currently, in the United States only carvedilol and metoprolol CR/XL are FDA-approved for treatment of patients with heart failure, while in Europe these agents plus bisoprolol are approved for this indication.

## Bucindolol

The third generation nonselective, sympatholytic compound bucindolol was the first $\beta$-blocking agent shown to improve LV function in a placebo-controlled trial [81]. The second multicenter trial performed with a $\beta$-blocking agent was the Bucindolol Multicenter trial [157], a phase 2 trial. The favorable results of this trial led to a phase 3 trial, the $\beta$-Blocker Evaluation of Survival Trial (BEST) [64]. The NHLBI and VA Cooperative Studies Program cosponsored BEST Trial was the first $\beta$-blocker mortality trial to be designed and to begin, and it is the "only intention to treat mortality trial" testing the effects of a $\beta$-blocker to be conducted in a predominately US population. The BEST trial included 2708 patients with advanced (NYHA class III and IV) heart failure randomized to either placebo or bucindolol (Table 5.3). The BEST Trial was stopped early on recommendation of the Data and Safety Monitoring Committee, because of positive data in the clinical subgroups (class III, European/Caucasian) that had already been reported in the MERIT-HF and CIBIS-II Trials and an increasing loss of equipoise by investigators [64,86]. The primary endpoint was all-cause mortality, which was reduced by a nonsignificant 10% ($p = 0.10$) in patients treated with bucindolol [64]. However, there were highly statistically significant reductions ($p < 0.001$) in mortality plus heart failure hospitalizations, and in heart failure hospitalizations alone [64,86], and most other secondary endpoints, such as cardiovascular mortality and mortality plus cardiac transplantation, were statistically significantly reduced by bucindolol [64]. In addition, bucindolol reduced (by 43%, $p = 0.024$) the incidence of myocardial infarction in BEST, the only $\beta$-blocker to do so in a CHF study.

This effect on mortality by bucindolol in BEST [64] was less than that observed in MERIT-HF [59], CIBS-II [58], or COPERNICUS [63]. This was initially felt to indicate either (1) that patients with more advanced heart failure may respond less favorably to $\beta$-blockade, or (2) that bucindolol is less efficacious than metoprolol, bisoprolol, or carvedilol. However, there were substantial differences between the BEST Trial population and those studied in the other three mortality trials, including more advanced heart failure in BEST compared to MERIT-HF and CIBIS-II, and a large percentage of African Americans in BEST (24%) compared to all the other trials. When the BEST Trial population was reconstituted to resemble MERIT-HF and CIBIS-II [158], the reduction in mortality and other major clinical endpoints in the "BEST Comparison Group" were quite similar to the other three trials. In addition, further review of the data and an analysis of the amount of sympatholysis observed within certain subgroups indicated that a subset of patients treated with bucindolol had an increased risk of death as the result of exaggerated sympatholytic properties of bucindolol [159], which compromised the efficacy of bucindolol. There is precedent that drugs with potent sympatholytic properties increase in mortality in heart failure [6], in complete contradistinction to the effects of $\beta$-blockers, which other than bucindolol do not exhibit lowering of norepinephrine as a pharmacologic property. More recent data from the BEST trial indicates that the adverse symaptholysis of bucindolol was confined to patients carrying an $\alpha_{2c}$-adrenergic receptor loss of function polymorphism ($\alpha_{2c}$ DEL322-325), and that the presence of a second receptor polymorphism, the high functioning 389Arg/Arg variant of the $\beta_1$-adrenergic receptor, conferred a hyper-response to bucindolol in terms of reductions in mortality (by 40%) and mortality plus heart failure hospitalization (by 39%) (Liggett SB, Bristow MR unpublished observations). As a result, bucindolol

has reentered drug development for treatment of heart failure patients with either wild type/wild type $\alpha_{2c}$ or $\beta_1$ 389Arg/Arg adrenergic receptor polymorphisms where major clinical responses are as good or superior to nongenetically targeted therapy with other agents.

**Bisoprolol**

The third multicenter trial planned and performed was the Cardiac Insufficiency Bisoprolol Study (CIBIS-1), which was a placebo-controlled trial of the effects of bisoprolol on mortality in symptomatic ischemic or nonischemic cardiomyopathy subjects treated for an average follow-up of 22.8 months [160]. This trial resulted in a nonsignificant 20% reduction in mortality, unfortunately adversely affected by a lower-than expected event rate in the placebo arm [160]. This prompted a larger follow-up trial, CIBIS-II, to address the issue of sample size and with a more conservative effect-size estimate.

The CIBIS-II trial was stopped early at 18 months because of a highly significant ($p < 0.001$), 32% relative risk reduction in all-cause mortality [58]. CIBIS-II enrolled 2647 patients with NYHA class III or IV heart failure from ischemic or nonischemic cardiomyopathies, with a median follow-up of 1.3 years. Treatment with bisoprolol also significantly reduced hospitalizations (by 20%) and cardiovascular deaths (by 29%) [58]. Besides sample size, one important difference between CIBIS-I and CIBIS-II was the average target dose of bisoprolol used: 10 mg/day in CIBIS-II [58] and 5 mg/day in CIBIS-I [160].

**Carvedilol**

The US Carvedilol Heart Failure Trials program consisted of four separate, prospective, randomized, placebo-controlled trials [62,128,161–163], which included patients with ischemic or nonischemic cardiomyopathies and NYHA class II–IV heart failure symptoms. These four trials are listed in Table 5.3. Although all-cause mortality was not an independent primary or secondary endpoint in any of the four trials, two of the trials, (the Mild Heart Failure Carvedilol Study [161] and the Severe Heart Failure Carvedilol Study [163] were stopped early by the data and safety monitoring committee due to, on grouped analysis, the presence of a highly significant ($p < 0.0001$) reduction in all-cause mortality across all four trials [62]. In addition, one of the trials, MOCHA, did produce a statistically significant reduction in mortality in favor of carvedilol [128]. Though across all four trials there were only 53 deaths in all treatment groups and the trials were not conducted according to intention-to-treat, the overall reduction in mortality was by 65%. [62]. In addition, there was a significant ($p = 0.036$) 27% relative risk reduction in cardiovascular hospitalizations. A major criticism of the trial analysis was that three of the four individual trials did not achieve statistical significance in their primary endpoints. The primary endpoint in two (MOCHA [128] and the Prospective Randomized Evaluation of Carvedilol in Symptoms and Exercise (PRECISE) [162]) of the three trials that did not achieve significance was improvement in submaximal exercise tolerance, and in the third (the Severe trial) it was quality of life [162]. The only trial that reached statistical significance in its primary endpoint was the Mild trial, which showed an improvement in the combined endpoint of total mortality, cardiovascular hospitalization, or increasing heart failure medication [161]. Nevertheless, in early 1997 the FDA used these data, in addition to phase 2 data from the Australia–New Zealand trial [164], to approve carvedilol for delaying the progression of the myocardial disease process and lowering the combined risk of morbidity and mortality [165,166].

In part, in response to the concerns above, the Carvedilol Prospective Randomized Cumulative Survival Trial (COPERNICUS) [63] was designed and conducted. This trial enrolled 2289 patients with ischemic or nonischemic cardiomyopathies, heart failure symptoms at rest or on minimal exertion, and an LVEF ≤25%. The randomization was to either carvedilol (target dose of 25 mg twice daily) or placebo [63], this time by intention-to-treat. The results showed a highly significant ($p = 0.0014$), 35% reduction in all-cause mortality, the primary endpoint [63], as well as reductions in mortality plus hospitalizations [166]. As for the MERIT-HF and CIBIS-II Trials, the majority of patients enrolled in COPERNICUS were of European descent.

The only comparative $\beta$-blocker trial to date, the Carvedilol or Metoprolol European Study (COMET) [65], has caused considerable debate regarding trial design, generalizability, and interpretation of results [32,70,71,167,168]. COMET was designed as a superiority trial to compare the efficacy of a selective $\beta_1$-blocking agent, metoprolol tartrate (IR metoprolol), to a nonselective agent with vasodilating properties, carvedilol, in the chronic treatment of heart failure. COMET enrolled 3029 subjects with ischemic or nonischemic cardiomyoapthies, NYHA class II–IV symptoms, and an LVEF ≤35% [65]. The coprimary endpoints were all-cause mortality and the composite of all-cause mortality or all-cause hospital admission. Patients were randomized to carvedilol 3.125 mg twice daily or IR metoprolol 5 mg twice daily. Each drug was to be titrated every 2 weeks to a target dose of 25 mg twice daily for carvedilol and 50 mg twice daily for IR metoprolol [65].

After a mean study duration of 58 months, all-cause mortality was 34% in the carvedilol group and 40% in the IR metoprolol group, representing a highly significant ($p = 0.0017$) relative risk reduction of 17% by treatment with carvedilol [65]. There was no statistically significant reduction in the other composite primary endpoint of all-cause mortality or all-cause hospital admission. The study investigators concluded that carvedilol extended survival compared with IR metoprolol tartrate [65]. Consistent with the study target doses for the two compounds, the mean daily dose achieved was 42 mg of carvedilol and 85 mg of IR metoprolol. Importantly, this dose of metoprolol was lower than that achieved in the MDC trial of 108 mg/day, and significantly lower than the mean daily dose achieved in MERIT-HF of 159 mg/day, a trial which utilized the long-acting preparation, metoprolol succinate [59,65,156]. These inherently difficult cross-trial comparisons aside, it is important to note in the COMET trial at 4, 8, and 16 months carvedilol treatment resulted in a statistically significantly greater reduction in resting heart rate (13.3 bpm versus 11.7 bpm reduction at 4 months) than did IR metoprolol [32,65]. This has been attributed to the lack of $\beta_1$-blocker equivalency of these two compounds at the doses prescribed and has sparked a discussion that questions the claim of superiority for carvedilol, which the investigators of COMET make as a result of this trial [32,65,70,71,167,168].

## Nebivolol

The first large, multicenter, randomized control trial of nebivolol treatment in heart failure patients was reported in early 2005 [112]. The Study of the Effects of Nevibolol Intervention on Outcomes and Rehospitalisation in Seniors with Heart Failure (SENIORS) trial [112] was designed to determine the effect of nebivolol therapy on morbidity and mortality in elderly patients (age ≤70) with heart failure, regardless of systolic function. About 2128 patients in 11 countries with NYHA class I–IV heart failure symptoms (approximately 95% with class II or III) were randomized to either nebivolol treatment or placebo and followed for a minimum of 12 months. Nebivolol treatment resulted in a 14% relative risk reduction in the primary endpoint ($p = 0.039$), which consisted of all-cause mortality and cardiovascular hospital admission [112]. Results of the primary outcome were not different when stratified between subgroups, including gender, age, ischemic etiology, or ejection fraction, though there was little power to do so. Of note, approximately one-third of patients had an ejection fraction at enrollment of at least 35% [112]. This was the first trial to specifically enroll only elderly patients and included patients with heart failure symptoms with preserved systolic function.

Nevertheless, there was a statistically significant reduction in the primary endpoint. However, there was no statistically significant effect on the secondary endpoints of total 12% reduction ($p = 0.21$) or cardiovascular ($p = 0.17$) mortality.

## Summary of clinical results with β-blockers in CHF

In summary, the collective interpretation of the placebo-controlled β-blocker data in the treatment of heart failure is that the consistently demonstrated favorable effects on ventricular function and remodeling [1,34] are translated into significant clinical benefits, with consistent findings of a reduction in morbidity and mortality across all trials as summarized in Table 5.4. In this Table 5.4, metoprolol (second generation compound) and bucindolol (third generation) appear in five of the six categories of major clinical benefit, carvedilol (third generation) and bisoprolol (second generation) in four, and nebivolol (third generation) in one. The average reduction in mortality in the trials listed Table 5.3 is by approximately 30%, with a similar degree of reduction in hospitalizations. These effects represent a significant impact in this devastating illness. The clinical benefits are evident in nearly all degrees of heart failure, with the large majority of data from patients with mild to severe heart failure and an LV ejection fraction <40%. But, as we have seen, the expansion of these data to include more and more patient subsets,

Table 5.4 Favorable major clinical effects of β-adrenergic blockade in CHF.

| Effect | Trials | β-blockers |
|---|---|---|
| Reduction in total mortality | CIBIS, MERIT-HF, COPERNICUS | metoprolol , bisoprolol, carvedilol |
| Reduction in CV mortality | CIBIS, MERIT-HF, COPERNICUS, BEST | metoprolol, bisoprolol carvedilol, bucindolol |
| Reduction in CV or CHF hospitalizations | MDC, US Carvedilol, CIBIS-II, MERIT-HF, BEST, SENIORS | metoprolol, bisoprolol, carvedilol, bucindolol, nebivolol |
| Improved CHF symptoms or QOL | MDC, CIBIS-II, MERIT-HF, US Carvedilol, COPERNICUS | metoprolol, bisoprolol, carvedilol |
| Reduced need for cardiac transplantation | MDC, MERIT-HF, BEST | metoprolol, bucindolol |
| Reduction in myocardial infarction | BEST | bucindolol |

Note: The listings under the first column are class effects due to $\beta_1$-AR blockade.
Source: Adapted from [169].

including the elderly and even to those with normal LV systolic function, is continuing. However, it is evident that more data are needed in certain demographic groups, particularly women, as well as in racial subsets.

## Controversies with the choice of $\beta$-blocking agent

As stated previously, the reduction in morbidity and mortality seen with $\beta$-blocking agents is consistent across multiple clinical trials, and thus is consistent with a class effect of blocking $\beta_1$-adrenergic receptors (Table 5.4). However, this should not lead to the gross over-generalization that all $\beta$-blockers work equally or to the same degree in the treatment of heart failure; there may be differences between the agents studied thus far that need to be investigated further. In addition to the selectivity for $\beta_1$-receptor blockade, other differences in $\beta$-blocking agents (Tables 5.1 and 5.2) used to treat heart failure are the presence or absence of sympatholysis, degree of binding, and activation or inhibition of $\beta_3$-receptors, NO generation, degree of $\alpha_1$-receptor blockade, antioxidant properties, and other effects. Some of these properties, such as sympatholysis [159], have already been shown to impact treatment effects, and almost certainly other properties will as well.

A major problem in the comparative interpretation of $\beta$-blocker trials is the potential for differences between study populations. A graphic example of this is the BEST Trial, which was conducted almost entirely in the United States in a population that was 24% black, and the COPERNICUS, MERIT-HF, and CIBIS-II Trials conducted almost entirely in European populations. As has been extensively documented, there are major differences between blacks and European Caucasians with regard to heart failure baseline characteristics and response to therapy, and when these differences and other trial-specific confounders were eliminated by normalizing the study populations, there were no differences in treatment response among the BEST, COPERNICUS, MERIT-HF, and CIBIS-II Trials [158].

Regardless of the arguments for or against comparative differences between agents of proven benefit, it is safe to say that in choosing a $\beta$-blocker for the treatment of heart failure, one should choose an agent that has been shown to be effective in reducing mortality and morbidity in a large, prospective, randomized-controlled trial. In addition, it should be emphasized that the choice of target dose should follow that used in the trials, which showed a clinical benefit. Even though there is somewhat limited data directly comparing the effects of high-dose versus low-dose $\beta$-blockade in this clinical scenario, the dose-ranging bucindolol study appeared to supply evidence that high-level $\beta$-blockade is better than low-level [157], and MOCHA appeared to show a dose-related reduction in mortality [128]. These are the most important messages when discussing $\beta$-blocker choices: to use proven agents at proven dosages. With specific regard to the relatively limited number of agents that have shown clinical outcomes benefit, the discussion of which agent is superior is far from clear and a source of on-going debate. It remains possible that different $\beta$-blocking agents have differential effects on important clinical outcomes, but further comparative trials between clinically proven agents with appropriate dose equivalency are needed. At the current time, the most important message is to use proven agents at proven target doses.

## Current guideline recommendations

A combined task force involving the ACC/AHA updated the 1995 Clinical Guidelines for the evaluation and management of Chronic Heart Failure in the Adult in 2001 [168]. This was done in collaboration with the International Society for Heart and Lung Transplantation and was endorsed by the Heart Failure Society of America. A review of their recommendations as they relate to the use of $\beta$-blocker therapy in the management of CHF is given below.

The levels of evidence on which these recommendations were based were then ranked and the discussion of this ranking has been described elsewhere [170]. We will limit our discussion to patients either with symptoms of heart failure (Stage C and D) or with documented LV systolic dysfunction (Stage B, C, or D). These statements are taken directly from the executive summary portion of the recommendations and referral to the discussion portion for details is appropriate.

*Stage B patients.* It is a class I recommendation to use $\beta$-blocker therapy in patients with a recent myocardial infarction regardless of ejection fraction (Level of Evidence: A). It is a class I recommendation to use $\beta$-blocker therapy in patients with reduced ejection fraction, whether or not they have experienced a myocardial infarction (Level of Evidence: B).

*Stage C patients.* Measures listed as class I recommendations for patients in Stage B are also appropriate for class C patients. It is a class I recommendation to use $\beta$-blocker therapy in all stable patients unless contraindicated. Patients should have no or minimal evidence of fluid retention and should not have required treatment recently with an intravenous positive inotropic agent (Level of Evidence: A). In addition, it should be noted that it is currently considered a class III recommendation to use an angiotension receptor blocker before a $\beta$-blocker in patients with heart failure who are taking an ACE inhibitor.

*Stage D patients.* There are no specific recommendations for the use of $\beta$-blocker therapy in this very sick patient population. It should be noted that it is considered a class I recommendation to refer these patients to a heart failure program with expertise in the management of refractory heart failure and consideration of cardiac transplantation in eligible patients.

## Limitations of $\beta$-blocker therapy in CHF

Despite their proven efficacy in a wide range of patients with the clinical syndrome of heart failure from primary or secondary cardiomyopathies, it is important to emphasize that $\beta$-blockers have limitations in their general application to all heart failure patients. First and foremost is that some heart failure patients have contraindications to $\beta$-blockade, such as sinus node or conduction system disease with bradycardia, advanced heart failure with hemodynamic decompensation, and to a milder degree, patients with true (as opposed to cardiac asthma) reactive airways disease. It should be pointed out, though, that most patients with

a history of COPD as well as "asthma" can be safely started on $\beta$-blockade utilizing the very low doses typically used for initiation in heart failure patients. This requires careful monitoring and should be done in a controlled setting to monitor for respiratory decompensation, and should not be attempted in patients with known adverse reactions to previous therapeutic trials of $\beta$-blocking agents. Another problem is that even in mild to moderate heart failure, initiation of therapy and uptitration of $\beta$-blockade agents can be difficult, requiring both persistence and knowledge of management maneuvers [104] that allow target doses to be achieved.

A third problem, and possibly the most important from both a health care and a scientific standpoint, is that for reasons that are not yet clear, some individuals do not respond to $\beta$-blocker therapy in terms of favorable effects on myocardial function or clinical endpoints, and as discussed earlier, these individuals may have worse outcomes than patients treated with placebo [93]. As discussed earlier for bucindolol, it is likely that pharmacogenomic targeting can improve the likelihood of favorable response to that agent, but it remains to be seen whether this is a general phenomenon that extends to other $\beta$-blockers.

Finally and most importantly, $\beta$-blockers continue to be underutilized in heart failure populations, and this inadequacy needs to be addressed and corrected. Recent data from community heart failure populations indicate a utilization rate of around 40% [171], whereas the maximum theoretical rate based on clinical trials data is more like 85%. In addition to general educational measures, the development of better tolerated $\beta$-blockers or combinations of $\beta$-blockers with other agents, or pharmacogenomic selection of individual's less likely to have difficulty with initiation of therapy and more likely to have favorable responses would presumably lead to a higher rate of utilization.

## Future directions

Some but not all of the problems mentioned earlier might be overcome by (1) the further development of heart-failure-designed "fourth-generation" $\beta$-blockers [34], (2) $\beta$-blockers combined with positive inotropic agents, or (3) the appropriate tailoring of certain therapies to given subsets of patients known or predicted to have a favorable response and avoidance in subsets known to either not respond or to respond unfavorably. This latter development is now within our grasp, using adrenergic receptor pharmacogenomic targeting.

# References

1 Eichhorn EJ, Bristow MR. Medical therapy can improve the biologic properties of the chronically failing heart: a new era in the treatment of heart failure. *Circulation* 1996;**94**:2285–2296.

2 Stephen SA. Unwanted effects of propranolol. *Am J Cardiol* 1966;**18**:463–472.

3 Epstein SE, Braunwald EB. The effect of beta adrenergic blockade on patterns of urinary sodium excretion; studies in normal subjects and in patients with heart disease. *Ann Intern Med* 1968;**65**:20–27.

4 Gaffney TE, Braunwald EB. Importance of the adrenergic nervous system in the support of circulatory function in patients with congestive heart failure. *Am J Med* 1963;**34**:320–324.

5 Bristow MR. β-adrenergic receptor blockade in chronic heart failure. *Circulation* 2000;**101**:558–569.

6 Bristow MR. Antiadrenergic therapy of chronic heart failure: surprises and new opportunities. *Circulation* 2003;**107**:1100–1102.

7 Bristow MR, Ginsburg R, Fowler M *et al.* β1- and β2-adrenergic receptor subpopulations in normal and failing human ventricular myocardium: coupling of both receptor subtypes to muscle contraction and selective β1-receptor downregulation in heart failure. *Circ Res* 1986;**59**:297–309.

8 Brodde OE, Schuler S, Kretsch R *et al.* Regional distribution of β-adrenoceptors in the human heart: coexistence of functional β1- and β2-adrenoceptors in both atria and ventricles in severe congestive cardiomyopathy. *J Cardiovasc Pharmacol* 1986;**8**:1235–1242.

9 Bristow MR. Changes in myocardial and vascular receptors in heart failure. *J Am Coll Cardiol* 1993;**22**:61A–71A.

10 Lim HW, De Windt LJ, Steinberg L *et al.* Calcineurin expression, activation, and function in cardiac pressure-overload hypertrophy. *Circulation* 2000;**101**:2431–2437.

11 Kirchhefer U, Schmitz W, Scholz H *et al.* Activity of cAMP-dependent protein kinase and Ca2+/calmodulin-dependent protein kinase in failing and nonfailing human hearts. *Cardiovasc Res* 1999;**42**:254–261.

12 Lips DJ, Bueno OF, Wilkins BJ *et al.* MEK1-ERK2 signaling pathway protects myocardium from ischemic injury in vivo. *Circulation* 2004;**109**:1938–1941.

13 Communal C, Colucci WS, Remondino A *et al.* Reciprocal modulation of mitogen-activated protein kinases and mitogen-activated protein kinase phosphatase 1 and 2 in failing human myocardium. *J Card Fail* 2002;**8**:86–92.

14 Newton GE, Packer JD. Acute effects of β1-selective and nonselective β-adrenergic receptor blockade on cardiac sympathetic activity in congestive heart failure. *Circulation* 1996;**94**:353–358.

15 Gauthier C, Tavernier G, Charpentier F, Langin D, LeMarec H. Functional β3-adrenoceptor in the human heart. *J Clin Invest* 1996;**98**:556–562.

16 Kaumann AJ, Molenaar P. Modulation of human cardiac function through 4 beta-adrenergic populations. *Naunyn Schmiedebergs Arch Pharmacol* 1997;**355**:667–681.

17 Haber HL, Christopher LS, Gimple LW *et al.* Why do patients with congestive heart failure tolerate the initiation of β-blocker therapy? *Circulation* 1993;**88**:1610–1619.

18 Swedberg K, Viquerat C, Rouleau JL *et al.* Comparison of myocardial catecholamine balance in chronic congestive heart failure and in angina pectoris without heart failure. *Am J Cardiol* 1984;**54**:783–786.

19 Hasking GJ, Esler MD, Jennings GL, Burton D, Korner PI. Norepinephrine spillover to plasma in patients with congestive heart failure: evidence of increased overall and cardiorenal sympathetic nervous activity. *Circulation* 1986;**73**:615–621.

20 Goldsmith SR, Francis GS, Cohn JN. Norepinephrine infusions in congestive heart failure. *Am J Cardiol* 1985;**56**:802–804.

21 Bristow MR, Minobe W, Rasmussen R *et al.* β-Adrenergic neuroeffector abnormalities in the failing human heart are produced by local rather than systemic mechanisms. *J Clin Invest* 1992;**89**:803–815.

22 Kaye DM, Lefkovits J, Jennings GL, Bergin P, Broughton A, Esler D. Adverse consequences of high sympathetic nervous activity in the failing human heart. *J Am Coll Cardiol* 1995;**26**:1257–1263.

23 Mann DL, Kent RL, Parsons P, Cooper G IV. Adrenergic effects on the biology of the adult mammalian cardiomyocyte. *Circulation* 1992;**85**:790–804.

24 Esposito G, Rapacciuolo A, Naga Prasad SV *et al.* Genetic alterations that inhibit in vivo pressure-overload hypertrophy prevent cardiac dysfunction despite increased wall stress. *Circulation* 2002;**105**:85–92.

25 Communal C, Singh K, Sawyer DB, Colucci WS. Opposing effects of beta(1)- and beta(2)-adrenergic receptors on cardiac myocyte apoptosis: role of a pertussis toxin-sensitive G protein. *Circulation* 1999;**100**:2210–2212.

26  Schomig A, Richardt G. Cardiac sympathetic activity in myocardial ischemia: release and effects of noradrenaline. *Basic Res Cardiol* 1990;**85**:9–30.

27  Colucci WS, Sawyer DB, Singh K, Communal C. Adrenergic overload and apoptosis in heart failure: implication for therapy. *J Card Fail* 2000;**6**:1–7.

28  Lowes BD, Gilbert EM, Abraham WT *et al.* Myocardial gene expression in dilated cardiomyopathy treated with beta-blocking agents. *N Engl J Med* 2002;**346**:1357–1365.

29  Esler M, Kaye D, Lambert G, Esler D, Jennings G. Adrenergic nervous system in heart failure. *Am J Cardiol* 1997;**80**:7L–14L.

30  Ungerer M, Bohm M, Elce JS, Erdmenn E, Lohse MJ. Altered expression of beta-adrenergic receptor kinase and beta-1-adrenergic receptors in the failing human heart. *Circulation* 1993;**87**:454–463.

31  Dorn GW. Adrenergic pathways and left ventricular remodeling. *J Card Fail* 2002;**8**:S370–S373.

32  Bristow MR, Feldman AM, Adams KF, Goldstein S. Selective Versus Nonselective $\beta$-Blockade for Heart Failure Therapy – Are There Lessons to Be Learned From the COMET Trial? *J Card Fail* 2003;**9**: 444–453.

33  Bristow MR, Port JD, Kelly R. Pharmacologic management of congestive heart failure. In: Antam EM, Colucci WS, Gotto AM Jr, *et al.*, eds. *Cardiovascular Therapeutics: A Companion to Braunwald's Heart Disease*, W.B. Saunders Co, Philadelphia, PA, 2001.

34  Bristow MR. Mechanism of action of beta-blocking agents in heart failure. *Am J Cardiol* 1997;**80**: 26L–40L.

35  Abraham WT, Lowes BD, Roden RL *et al.* Mechanism of increased cardiac adrenergic activity in heart failure: evidence for decreased cardiac neuronal norepinephrine reuptake. *Circulation* 1997;**96**:I-92.

36  Kaye DM, Lofkovits J, Cox H *et al.* Regional epinephrine kinetics in human heart failure: evidence for extra-adrenal, nonneural release. *Am J Physiol* 1995;**269**:H182–H188.

37  Engelhadt S, Hein L, Wiesmann F, Lohse MJ. Progressive hypertrophy and heart failure in $\beta$1-adrenergic receptor transgenic mice. *Proc Natl Acad Sci USA* 1999;**96**:7059–7064.

38  Bisognano JD, Weinberger HD, Bohlmeyer TJ *et al.* Myocardial-directed overexpression of the human $\beta$1-adrenergic receptor in transgenic mice. *J Mol Cell Cardiol* 2000;**32**:817–830.

39  Freeman K, Lerman I, Kranias EG *et al.* Alterations in cardiac adrenergic signaling and calcium cycling differentially affect the progression of cardiomyopathy. *J Clin Invest* 2001;**107**:967–974.

40  Liggett SB, Tepe NM, Lorenz JN *et al.* Early and delayed consequences of $\beta(2)$-adrenergic receptor overexpression in mouse hearts: critical role for expression level. *Circulation* 2000;**101**:1707–1714.

41  Lemire I, Ducharme A, Tardif JC *et al.* Cardiac-directed overexpression of wild-type $\alpha$1b-adrenergic receptor induces dilated cardiomyopathy. *Am J Physiol Heart Circ Physiol* 2001;**281**:H931–H938.

42  Milano CA, Dolber PC, Rockman HA *et al.* Myocardial expression of a constitutively active $\alpha$1b-adrenergic receptor in transgenic mice induces cardiac hypertrophy. *Proc Natl Acad Sci USA* 1994;**91**:10109–10113.

43  Mialet Perez J, Rathz DA, Petrashevskaya NN *et al.* Beta 1-adrenergic receptor polymorphisms confer differential function and predisposition to heart failure. *Nat Med* 2003;**9**:1300–1305.

44  Gonzalez-Juanatey JR, Iglesias MJ, Alcaide C, Pineiro R, Lago F. Doxazosin induces apoptosis in cardiomyocytes cultured in vitro by a mechanism that is independent of $\alpha$1-adrenergic blockade. *Circulation* 2003;**107**:127–131.

45  Singh K, Communal C, Sawyer DB, Colucci WS. Adrenergic regulation of myocardial apoptosis. *Cardiovasc Res* 2000;**45**:713–719.

46  Sabbah HN, Sharov VG, Gupta RC, Todor A, Singh V, Goldstein S. Chronic therapy with metoprolol attenuates cardiomyocyte apoptosis in dogs with heart failure. *J Am Coll Cardiol* 2000;**36**:1698–1705.

47  Ungerer M, Parruti G, Bohn M, *et al.* Expression of $\beta$-arrestins and $\beta$-adrenergic receptor kinases in the failing human heart. *Circ Res* 1994;**74**:206–213.

48  Tan LB, Benjamin IJ, Clark WA. B-adrenergic receptor desensitization may serve a cardioprotective role. *Cardiovasc Res* 1992;**26**:608–614.

49  Bristow MR. The adrenergic nervous system in heart failure. *N Engl J Med* 1984;**311**:850–851.

50  Bristow MR, Kantrowitz NE, Ginsburg R, Fowler MB. $\beta$-Adrenergic function in heart muscle disease and heart failure. *J Mol Cell Cardiol* 1985;**17**:41–52.

51  Fowler MB, Bristow MR. Rationale for beta-adrenergic blocking drugs in cardiomyopathy. *Am J Cardiol* 1985;**55**:D120–D124.

52  Dunlop D, Shanks RG. Selective blockade of adrenoceptive beta receptors in the heart. *Br J Pharmacol Chemother* 1968;**32**:201–218.

53  Bristow MR, Sherrod TR, Green RD. Analysis of beta receptor drug interactions in isolated rabbit atrium, aorta, stomach and trachea. *J Pharmacol Exp Ther* 1970;**171**:52–61.

54  Kobilka BK, Dixon RAF, Frielle T *et al.* cDNA for the human beta 2-adrenergic receptor: a protein with multiple membrane spanning domains and encoded by a gene whose chromosomal location is shared with that

of the receptor for platelet-derived growth factor. *Proc Natl Acad Sci USA* 1987;**84**:46–50.

55 Frielle T, Collins S, Danial KW, Caron MG, Lefkowitz RJ, Kobilka BK. Cloning of the cDNA for the human β1-adrenergic receptor. *Proc Natl Acad Sci USA* 1987;**84**:7920–7924.

56 Emorine LJ, Marullo S, Briend-Sutren MM *et al.* Molecular characterization of the human β3-adrenergic receptor. *Science* 1989;**245**:1118–1121.

57 Waagstein F, Hjalmarson A, Varnauskas E, Wallentin I. Effect of chronic beat-adrenergic receptor blockade in congestive cardiomyopathy. *Br Heart J* 1975;**37**:1022–1036.

58 CIBIS-II Investigators and Committees, The Cardiac Insufficiency Bisoprolol Study II (CIBIC-II): a randomized trial. *Lancet* 1999;**353**:9–13.

59 MERIT-HF Study Group. Effect of metoprolol CR/XL in chronic heart failure: Metoprolol CR/XL Randomized Intervention Trial in Congestive Heart Failure (MERIT-HF). *Lancet* 1999;**353**: 2001–20006.

60 Richards DA, Prichard BNC. Clinical pharmacology of labetalol. *Br J Clin Pharmacol* 1979;**8**:89S–93S.

61 Johnson LL, Cubbon J, Escala E *et al.* Hemodynamic effects of labetolol in patients with combined hypertension and left ventricular failure. *J Cardiovasc Pharmacol* 1988;**12**:350–356.

62 Packer M, Bristow MR, Cohn JN *et al.* The effect of carvedilol on morbidity and mortality in patients with chronic heart failure: US Carvedilol Heart Failure Study Group. *N Engl J Med* 1996;**334**: 1349–1355.

63 Packer M, Coats AJS, Fowler MB *et al.* Effect of carvedilol on survival in severe chronic heart failure. *N Engl J Med* 2001;**344**:1651–1658.

64 BEST Investigators. A trial of the beta blocker bucindolol in patients with advanced chronic heart failure. *N Engl J Med* 2001;**344**:1659–1667.

65 Poole-Wilson PA, Swedberg K, Cleland JGF *et al.* For the COMET Investigators. Comparison of carvedilol and metoprolol on clinical outcomes in patients with chronic heart failure. Results of the Carvedilol or Metoprolol European Trial. *Lancet* 2003;**362**:7–13.

66 Cockgroft JR, Chowienczyk PJ, Brett SE *et al.* Nebivolol vasodilates human forearm vasculature: evidenve for an L-arginine/NO-dependent mechanism. *J Pharmacol Exp Ther* 1995;**274**:1067–1071.

67 Bristow MR, Abraham WT, Gilbert EM, Yoshikawa T, Port JD. Relationships between carvedilol stereoisomer plasma concentrations and β-receptor occupancies in subjects in chronic heart failure in the Multicenter Oral Carvedilol Heart Failure Assessment (MOCHA) trial. *Eur Heart J* 1996;**17**:135.

68 Yoshikawa T, Port JD, Asano K *et al.* Cardiac adrenergic receptor effects of carvedilol. *Eur Heart J* 1996;**17**:B8–B16.

69 Stroe AF, Gheorghiade M. Carvedilol: beta-blockade and beyond. *Rev Cardiovasc Med* 2004;**5**:S18–S27.

70 Metra M, Dei Cas L, di Lenarda A, Poole-Wilson P. Beta-blockers in heart failure: are pharmacologic differences clinically important? *Heart Fail Rev* 2005;**9**:123–130.

71 Packer M. Do β-blockers prolong survival in heart failure only by inhibiting the β1-receptor? A perspective on the results of the COMET trial. *J Card Fail* 2003;**9**:429–443.

72 Kindermann M, Maack C, Schaller S *et al.* Carvedilol but not metoprolol reduces beta-adrenergic responsiveness after complete elimination from plasma in vivo. *Circulation* 2004;**109**:3182–3190.

73 Wolfel EE, Lowes BD, Shakar S *et al.* Lack of effect of acute withdrawal of either carvedilol or metoprolol therapy on peak and submaximal capacity in nonischemic cardiomyopathy patients with chronic heart failure. *Circulation* 1999;**100**:I-202.

74 Asano K, Zisman LS, Yoshikawa T, Bristow MR, Port DJ. Bucindolol, a nonselective $\beta_1$- and $\beta_2$-adrenergic receptor antagonist, decreases β-adrenergic receptor density in cultured embryonic chick cardiac myocyte membranes. *J Cardiovasc Pharmacol* 2001;**37**: 678–691.

75 Bristow MR, Abraham Wt, Yoshikawa T *et al.* Second and third beta blocking agents in the treatment of chronic heart failure. *Cardiovasc Drugs Ther* 1997;**11**: 291–296.

76 Hershberger RE, Wynn JR, Sundberg L, Bristow MR. Mechanism of action of bucindolol in human ventricular myocardium. *J Cardiovasc Pharmacol* 1990;**15**:959–967.

77 Deitchman D, Perhach JL, Snyder RW. β-Adrenoceptor and cardiovascular effects of MJ 13105 (bucindolol) in anesthetized dogs and rats. *Eur J Pharmacol* 1980;**61**:263–277.

78 Rimele TJ, Aarhus LL, Lorenz RR, Rooke TW, Van Houtte PM. Pharmacology of bucindolol in isolated canine vascular smooth muscle. *J Pharmacol Exp Ther* 1984;**231**:317–325.

79 Lowes BD, Chidiac P, Olsen S *et al.* Clinical relevance of inverse agonism and guanine nucleotide modulatable binding properties of β-adrenergic receptor blocking agents. *Circulation* 1994;**90**:I-543.

80 Bristow MR, Roden RL, Lowes BD, Gilbert EM, Eichhorn EJ. The role of third generation β-blocking agents in chronic heart failure. *Clin Cardiol* 1998;**21**: I3–I13.

81 Gilbert EM, Anderson JL, Deitchman D *et al*. Chronic β-blocker-vasodilator therapy improves cardiac function in idiopathic dilated cardiomyopathy: a double-blind, randomized study of bucindolol versus placebo. *Am J Med* 1990;**88**:223–229.

82 Bristow MR, Krause-Steinrauf H, Nuzzo R *et al*. Effect of Baseline or changes in adrenergic activity on clinical outcomes in the beta-blocker evaluation of survival trial (BEST). *Circulation* 2004;**110**:1437–1442.

83 Bristow MR, Larrabee P, Minobe W *et al*. Receptor pharmacology of carvedilol in the human heart. *J Cardiovasc Pharmacol* 1992;**19**:S68–S80.

84 Sederberg J, Wichman SE, Lindenfeld J *et al*. Bucindolol has no sympathomimetic activity in non-failing ventricular preparations. *J Am Coll Cardiol* 2000;**35**:1137–1147.

85 Strosberg AD. Structure and function of the beta 3-adrenergic receptor. *Annu Rev Pharmacol Toxicol* 1997;**37**:421–450.

86 Domanski M, Krause-Steinrauf H, Deedwania P *et al*. The effect of diabetes on outcome of advanced heart failure patients in the BEST Trial. *J Am Coll Cardiol* 2003;**42**:914–922.

87 Ignarro LJ. Experimental evidence of nitric oxide-dependent vasodilatory activity of nebivolol, a third generation β-blocker. *Blood Press* 2004;**13**:3–17.

88 Zanchetti A. Clinical pharmacodynamics of nebivolol. *Blood Press* 2004;**13**:18–33.

89 Kuroedov A, Cosentino F, Luscher TF. Pharmacologic mechanisms of clinically favorable properties of a selective β1-adrenoceptor antagonist, nebivolol. *Cardiovasc Drug Rev* 2004;**22**:155–168.

90 Gilbert EM, Abraham WT, Olsen S *et al*. Comparative hemodynamic, left ventricular functional, and antiadrenergic effects of chronic treatment with metoprolol versus carvedilol in the failing heart. *Circulation* 1996;**94**:2817–2825.

91 Metra M, Nodari S, Garbellini M *et al*. Comparative effects of metoprolol and carvedilol on resting and peak exercise hemodynamics and functional capacity in patients with chronic heart failure. *Circulation* 1997;**96**:I-578.

92 Wisenbaugh T, Katz I, Davis J *et al*. Long-term (3 months) effects of a new beta-blocker (nebivolol) on cardiac performance in dilated cardiomyopathy. *J Am Coll Cardiol* 1993;**21**:1094–1100.

93 Eichhorn EJ, Bedotto JB, Malloy CR *et al*. Effect of beta-adrenergic blockade on myocardial function and energetics in heart failure. *Circulation* 1990;**82**:473–483.

94 Eichhorn EJ, Heesch CM, Barnett JH *et al*. Effect of metoprolol on myocardial function and energetics in patients with nonischemic dilated cardiomyopathy. *J Am Coll Cardiol* 1994;**24**:1310–1320.

95 Lechat P, Escolano S, Golmard JL *et al*. Prognostic value of bisoprolol-induced hemodynamic effects in heart failure during the Cardiac Insufficiency Bisoprolol Study (CIBIS). *Circulation* 1997;**96**:2197–2205.

96 Hall SA, Cigarroa CG, Marcoux L, Risser RC, Grayburn PA, Eichhorn EJ. Time course of improvement in left ventricular function, mass, and geometry in patients with congestive heart failure treated with β-adrenergic blockade. *J Am Coll Cardiol* 1995;**25**:1154–1161.

97 Quaife RA, Gilbert EM, Christian PE *et al*. Effects of carvedilol on systolic and diastolic left ventricular performance in idiopathic dilated cardiomyopathy. *Am J Cardiol* 1996;**78**:779–784.

98 Doughty RN, Whalley GA, Gamble G, MacMahon S, Sharpe N, for the Australia–New Zealand Heart Failure Research Collaborative Group. Left ventricular remodeling with carvedilol in patients with congestive heart failure due ischemic heart disease. *J Am Coll Cardiol* 1997;**29**:1060–1066.

99 Lowes BD, Gill EA, Abraham WT *et al*. The effect of carvedilol on left ventricular mass, chamner geometry and mitral regurgitation in chronic heart failure. *Am J Cardiol* 1999;**83**:1201–1205.

100 Komajda M, Lutiger B, Madeira H *et al*. Tolerability of carvedilol and ACE-Inhibition in mild heart failure. Results of CARMEN (Carvedilol ACE-Inhibitor Remodelling Mild CHF EvaluatioN). *Eur J Heart Fail* 2004;**6**:467–475.

101 Gattis WA, O'Connor CM, Gallup DS *et al*. Predischarge initiation of carvedilol in patients hospitalized for decompensated heart failure: results of the Initiation Management Predischarge: Process for Assessment of Carvedilol Therapy in Heart Failure (IMPACT-HF) trial. *J Am Coll Cardiol* 2004;**43**:1534–1541.

102 Vantrimpont P, Rouleau JL, Wun CC *et al*. Additive beneficial effects of beta-blockers to angiotensin-converting enzyme inhibitors in the Survival and Ventricular Enlargement (SAVE) Study. SAVE Investigators. *J Am Coll Cardiol* 1997;**29**:229–236.

103 Dargie HJ. Effect of carvedilol on outcome after myocardial infarction in patients with left-ventricular dysfunction: the CAPRICORN randomised trial. *Lancet* 2001;**357**:1385–1390.

104 Eichhorn EJ, Bristow MR. Practical guidelines for initiation of beta-adrenergic blockade in patients with chronic heart failure. *Am J Cardiol* 1997;**79**:794–798.

105 Swedberg K, Hjalmarson A, Waagstein F *et al*. Adverse effects of beta-blockade withdrawal in patients with congestive cardiomyopathy. *Br Heart J* 1980;**44**:134–142.

106 Metra M, Nodari S, D'Aloia A *et al*. Beta-blocker therapy influences the hemodynamic response to inotropic agents in patients with heart failure: a randomized comparison of dobutamine and enoximone before and after

chronic treatment with metoprolol or carvedilol. *J Am Coll Cardiol* 2002;**40**:1248–1258.

107 Lowes BD, Tsvetkova T, Eichhorn EJ *et al.* Milrinone versus dobutamine in heart failure subjects treated chronically with carvedilol. *Int J Cardiol* 2001;**81**:141–149.

108 Talwar KK, Bhargava B, Upasani PT *et al.* Hemodynamic predictors of early intolerance and long-term effects of propranolol in dilated cardiomyopathy. *J Card Fail* 1996;**2**:273–277.

109 Armstrong PW, Chiong MA, Parker JO. Effects of propranolol on the hemodynamic, coronary sinus blood flow and myocardial metabolic response to atrial pacing. *Am J Cardiol* 1977;**40**:83–89.

110 Newton GE, Azevedo ER, Parker JD. Inotropic and sympathetic responses to the intracoronary infusion of a beta2-receptor agonist: a human in vivo study. *Circulation* 1999;**99**:2402–2407.

111 Di Lenarda A, Gilbert EM, Olsen SL, Mealey PC, Bristow MR. Acute hemodynamic effects of carvedilol versus metoprolol in idiopathic dilated cardiomyopathy. *J Am Coll Cardiol* 1991;**17**:142A.

112 Flather MD, Shibata MC, Coats AJ *et al.* Randomized trial to determine the effect of nebivolol on mortality and cardiovascular hospital admission in elderly patients with heart failure (SENIORS). *Eur Heart J* 2005;**26**:215–225.

113 Kumar A, Choudhary G, Antonio C *et al.* Carvedilol titration in patients with congestive heart failure receiving inotropic therapy. *Am Heart J* 2001;**142**:512–515.

114 Shakar SF, Abraham WT, Gilbert EM *et al.* Combined oral positive inotropic and beta-blocker therapy for treatment of refractory class IV heart failure. *J Am Coll Cardiol* 1998;**31**:1336–1340.

115 Olsen SL, Gilbert EM, Renlund DG, Taylor DO, Yanowitz FD, Bristow MR. Carvedilol improves left ventricular function and symptoms in heart failure: a double-blind randomized study. *J Am Col Cardiol* 1995;**25**:1225–1231.

116 Hryniewicz K, Androne AS, Hudaihed A, Katz SD. Comparative effects of carvedilol and metoprolol on regional vascular responses to adrenergic stimuli in normal subjects and patients with chronic heart failure. *Circulation* 2003;**108**:971–976.

117 Borchard U. Pharmacokinetics of beta-adrenoceptor blocking agents: clinical significance of hepatic and/or renal clearance. *Clin Physiol Biochem* 1990;**8**:28–34.

118 De Mey C, Brendel E, Enterling D. Carvedilol increases the systemic bioavailability of oral digoxin. *Br J Clin Pharmacol* 1990;**29**:486–490.

119 Lennard MS, Tucker GT, Woods HF. The polymorphic oxidation of beta-adrenoceptor antagonists. Clinical pharmacokinetic considerations. *Clin Pharmacokinet* 1986;**11**:1–17.

120 Neugebauer G, Akpan W, Kaufmann B *et al.* Stereoselective disposition of carvedilol in man after intravenous and oral administration of the racemic compound. *Eur J Clin Pharmacol* 1990;**38**:S108–S111.

121 Ruffolo RR, Jr., Gellai M, Hieble JP *et al.* The pharmacology of carvedilol. *Eur J Clin Pharmacol* 1990;**38**:S82–S88.

122 Basu S, Senior R, Raval U *et al.* Beneficial effects of intravenous and oral carvedilol treatment in acute myocardial infarction. A placebo-controlled, randomized trial. *Circulation* 1997;**96**:183–191.

123 Zhou HH, Wood AJ. Stereoselective disposition of carvedilol is determined by CYP2D6. *Clin Pharmacol Ther* 1995;**57**:518–524.

124 Lennard MS, Tucker GT, Silas JH *et al.* Differential stereoselective metabolism of metoprolol in extensive and poor debrisoquin metabolizers. *Clin Pharmacol Ther* 1983;**34**:732–737.

125 Silas JH, McGourty JC, Lennard MS *et al.* Polymorphic metabolism of metoprolol: clinical studies. *Eur J Clin Pharmacol* 1985;**28**:85–88.

126 Bristow MR, Gilbert EM. Improvement in cardiac myocyte function by biological effects of medical therapy: a new concept in the treatment of heart failure. *Eur Heart J* 1995;**16**:20–31.

127 St John Sutton MG, Plappert T, Abraham WT *et al.* Multicenter InSync Randomized Clinical Evaluation (MIRACLE) Study Group. Effect of cardiac resynchronization therapy on left ventricular size and function in chronic heart failure. *Circulation* 2003;**107**: 1985–1990.

128 Bristow MR, Gilbert EM, Abraham WT *et al.* For the MOCHA Investigators. Carvedilol produces dose-related improvements in left ventricular function and survival in subjects with chronic heart failure. *Circulation* 1996;**94**:2807–2816.

129 Ventura-Clapier R, Garnier A, Veksler V. Energy metabolism in heart failure. *J Physiol* 2004;**555**:1–13.

130 Taegtmeyer H. Metabolism – the lost child of cardiology. *J Am Coll Cardiol* 2000;**36**:1386–1388.

131 Dzeja PP, Pucar D, Redfield MM *et al.* Reduced activity of enzymes coupling ATP-generating with ATP-consuming processes in the failing myocardium. *Mol Cell Biochem* 1999;**201**:33–40.

132 Lommi J, Kupari M, Yki-Jarvinen H. Free fatty acid kinetics and oxidation in congestive heart failure. *Am J Cardiol* 1998;**81**:45–50.

133 Hasenfuss G, Maier LS, Hermann HP *et al.* Influence of pyruvate on contractile performance and Ca(2+) cycling in isolated failing human myocardium. *Circulation* 2002;**105**:194–199.

134 Hermann HP, Arp J, Pieske B *et al.* Improved systolic and diastolic myocardial function with intracoronary

pyruvate in patients with congestive heart failure. *Eur J Heart Fail* 2004;**6**:213–218.

135 Hermann HP, Pieske B, Schwarzmuller E *et al*. Haemodynamic effects of intracoronary pyruvate in patients with congestive heart failure: an open study. *Lancet* 1999;**353**:1321–1323.

136 Hermann HP, Zeitz O, Keweloh B *et al*. Pyruvate potentiates inotropic effects of isoproterenol and Ca(2+) in rabbit cardiac muscle preparations. *Am J Physiol Heart Circ Physiol* 2000;**279**:H702-H708.

137 Hermann HP, Zeitz O, Lehnart SE *et al*. Potentiation of beta-adrenergic inotropic response by pyruvate in failing human myocardium. *Cardiovasc Res* 2002;**53**:116–123.

138 Di Napoli P, Taccardi AA, Barsotti A. Long term cardioprotective action of trimetazidine and potential effect on the inflammatory process in patients with ischaemic dilated cardiomyopathy. *Heart* 2005;**91**: 161–165.

139 Lithell HO. Effect of antihypertensive drugs on insulin, glucose, and lipid metabolism. *Diabetes Care* 1991;**14**:203–209.

140 Dornhorst A, Powell SH, Pensky J. Aggravation by propranolol of hyperglycaemic effect of hydrochlorothiazide in type II diabetics without alteration of insulin secretion. *Lancet* 1985;**1**:123–126.

141 Holzgreve H, Nakov R, Beck K *et al*. Antihypertensive therapy with verapamil SR plus trandolapril versus atenolol plus chlorthalidone on glycemic control. *Am J Hypertens* 2003;**16**:381–386.

142 Lind L, Pollare T, Berne C *et al*. Long-term metabolic effects of antihypertensive drugs. *Am Heart J* 1994;**128**:1177–1183.

143 Pollare T, Lithell H, Selinus I *et al*. Sensitivity to insulin during treatment with atenolol and metoprolol: a randomised, double blind study of effects on carbohydrate and lipoprotein metabolism in hypertensive patients. *Br Med J* 1989;**298**:1152–1157.

144 Dahlof B, Devereux RB, Kjeldsen SE *et al*. Cardiovascular morbidity and mortality in the Losartan Intervention For Endpoint reduction in hypertension study (LIFE): a randomised trial against atenolol. *Lancet* 2002;**359**:995–1003.

145 Giugliano D, Acampora R, Marfella R *et al*. Metabolic and cardiovascular effects of carvedilol and atenolol in non-insulin-dependent diabetes mellitus and hypertension. A randomized, controlled trial. *Ann Intern Med* 1997;**126**:955–959.

146 Bakris GL, Fonseca V, Katholi RE *et al*. Metabolic effects of carvedilol vs metoprolol in patients with type 2 diabetes mellitus and hypertension: a randomized controlled trial. *J Am Med Assoc* 2004;**292**: 2227–2236.

147 Beanlands RS, Nahmias C, Gordon E *et al*. The effects of beta(1)-blockade on oxidative metabolism and the metabolic cost of ventricular work in patients with left ventricular dysfunction: a double-blind, placebo-controlled, positron-emission tomography study. *Circulation* 2000;**102**:2070–2075.

148 Wallhaus TR, Taylor M, DeGrado TR *et al*. Myocardial free fatty acid and glucose use after carvedilol treatment in patients with congestive heart failure. *Circulation* 2001;**103**:2441–2446.

149 Hara Y, Hamada M, Shigematsu Y *et al*. Effect of beta-blockers on insulin resistance in patients with dilated cardiomyopathy. *Circ J* 2003;**67**:701–704.

150 Heesch CM, Marcoux L, Hatfield B *et al*. Hemodynamic and energetic comparison of bucindolol and metoprolol for the treatment of congestive heart failure. *Am J Cardiol* 1995;**75**:360–364.

151 Eichhorn EJ, Heesch CM, Risser RC *et al*. Predictors of systolic and diastolic improvement in patients with dilated cardiomyopathy treated with metoprolol. *J Am Coll Cardiol* 1995;**25**:154–162.

152 Bristow MR, Saxon LA, Boehmer J *et al*. Cardiac-resynchronization therapy with or without an implantable defibrillator in advanced chronic heart failure. *N Engl J Med* 2004;**350**:2140–2150.

153 Cleland JG, Daubert JC, Erdmann E *et al*. Cardiac Resynchronization-Heart Failure (CARE-HF) Study Investigators. *N Engl J Med* 2005;**352**:1539–1549.

154 Waagstein F, Bristow MR, Swedberg K *et al*. Beneficial effects of metoprolol in idiopathic dilated cardiomyopathy. Metoprolol in Dilated Cardiomyopathy (MDC) Trial Study Group. *Lancet* 1993;**342**:1441–1446.

155 Wedel H, DeMets D, Deedwania P *et al*. Challenges of subgroup analyses in multinational clinical trials: Experiences from the MERIT-HF trial. *Am Heart J* 2001;**142**:502–511.

156 Sandberg A, Blomqvist I, Jonsson UE *et al*. Pharmacokinetic and pharmacodynamic properties of a new controlled-release formulation of metoprolol: a comparison with conventional tablets. *Eur J Clin Pharmacol* 1988;**33**:S9–S14.

157 Bristow MR, O'Connell JB, Gilbert EM *et al*. Dose–response of chronic beta-blocker treatment in heart failure from either idiopathic dilated or ischemic cardiomyopathy. Bucindolol Investigators. *Circulation* 1994;**89**:1632–1642.

158 Domanski MJ, Krause-Steinrauf H, Massie BM *et al*. BEST Investigators. A comparative analysis of the results from 4 trials of beta-blocker therapy for heart failure: BEST, CIBIS-II, MERIT-HF, and COPERNICUS. *J Card Fail* 2003;**9**:354–363.

159 Bristow MR, Krause-Steinrauf H, Nuzzo R *et al*. Effect of baseline or changes in adrenergic activity on clinical

outcomes in the beta-blocker evaluation of survival trial. *Circulation* 2004;**110**:1437–1442.

160 CIBIS Investigators and Committees. A randomized trial of beta-blockade in heart failure. The Cardiac Insufficiency Bisoprolol Study (CIBIS). *Circulation* 1994;**90**:1765–1773.

161 Colucci WS, Packer M, Bristow MR *et al*. Carvedilol inhibits clinical progression in patients with mild symptoms of heart failure. US Carvedilol Heart Failure Study Group. *Circulation* 1996;**94**:2800–2806.

162 Packer M, Colucci WS, Sackner-Bernstein JD *et al*. Double-blind, placebo-controlled study of the effects of carvedilol in patients with moderate to severe heart failure. The PRECISE Trial. Prospective Randomized Evaluation of Carvedilol on Symptoms and Exercise. *Circulation* 1996;**94**:2793–2799.

163 Cohn J, Fowler MB, Bristow MR *et al*. For the Carvedilol Heart Failure Study Group. Effect of carvedilol in severe chronic heart failure. *J Am Coll Cardiol* 1996;**27**:169A.

164 Australia/New Zealand Heart Failure Research Collaborative Group. Randomised, placebo-controlled trial of carvedilol in patients with congestive heart failure due to ischaemic heart disease. *Lancet* 1997;**349**:375–380.

165 Coreg finally approved in the US. *SCRIP World Pharmaceutical News* 1997;**2238**:17.

166 Packer M, Fowler MB, Roecker *et al*. Effect of carvedilol on the morbidity of patients with severe chronic heart failure: results of the carvedilol prospective randomized cumulative survival (COPERNICUS) study. *Circulation* 2002;**106**:2194–2199.

167 Massie BM. A comment on COMET: how to interpret a positive trial? *J Card Fail* 2003;**9**:425–428.

168 Shepherd AM. A clinical pharmacologist's response to Dr Milton Packer's perspective on the results of the COMET trial. *J Card Fail* 2003;**9**:454–457.

169 Mann DL, Bristow MR. Mechanisms and models in heart failure: the biochemical model and beyond. *Circulation* 2005;**111**:2837–2849.

170 Hunt SA, Baker DW, Chin MH *et al*. ACC/AHA guidelines for the evaluation and management of chronic heart failure in the adult: executive summary. A report of the American College of Cardiology/American Heart Association Task Force on Practice Guidelines (Committee to revise the 1995 Guidelines for the Evaluation and Management of Heart Failure). *J Am Coll Cardiol* 2001;**38**: 2101–2113.

171 Stafford RS, Radley DC. The underutilization of cardiac medications of proven benefit, 1990 to 2002. *J Am Coll Cardiol* 2003;**41**:56–61.

**CHAPTER 6**

# Aldosterone antagonism in the pharmacological management of chronic heart failure

*Biykem Bozkurt,* MD

## Introduction

Almost half a century ago, the urinary extracts from patients with chronic heart failure were found to contain aldosterone, a substance with sodium retaining activity [1]. In the years that followed it's recognition in heart failure in 1954 [1], aldosterone was considered a target for therapy in heart failure because of its role in sodium retention [2]. In the last two decades, with the growing emphasis on angiotensin-converting enzyme (ACE) inhibitors and their presumptive elimination of angiotensin II, the focus had shifted away from aldosterone. However, recent evidence has revived interest in aldosterone and its role in congestive heart failure [2–6].

## Aldosterone production and mechanisms of action

Aldosterone is predominantly produced by the adrenal glands, but recent evidence suggests that to a small degree it can also be produced by endothelial and vascular smooth muscle cells in the heart and the blood vessels [7–9] implying a potential autocrine and paracrine action in addition to its endocrine action [2]. The two primary regulators of aldosterone secretion are potassium [10] and the renin–angiotensin system. Angiotensinogen, the precursor of all angiotensin peptides, is synthesized by the liver. It is cleaved by renin, which is secreted into the lumen of renal afferent arterioles by juxtaglomerular cells, forming angiotensin I.

Angiotensin II, formed from angiotensin I by ACE, is the principal stimulator of aldosterone in the zona glomerulosa of the adrenal cortex [2,10] (Figure 6.1). Additional simulators of aldosterone production include corticotropin, catecholamines (e.g. norepinephrine), and endothelins [2]. High salt intake suppresses the renin–angiotensin system and aldosterone levels, and the low salt intake has the opposite effect [11]. If the production of aldosterone is inappropriate for the level of sodium intake, hyperaldosteronism emerges to be detrimental resulting in excessive renal sodium retention, potassium wasting, hypertension, and cardiovascular damage [11]. In addition to salt and water retention, the deleterious effects of raised aldosterone include arteriolar vasoconstriction, upregulation of inflammatory mediators, platelet aggregation, and stimulation of fibroblasts and development of fibrosis [2]. These effects are summarized in Table 6.1.

Aldosterone acts through mineralocorticoid receptors that are ligand-dependent transcription factors. The mineralocorticoid receptor was cloned and sequenced in 1987 [12], enabling detailed study of regulatory DNA sequences, hormone response elements, and the ability to influence transcription/translation of inducible protein elements. Corticosterone and aldosterone bind equally well to the mineralocorticoid receptor. Thus, the selectivity of this receptor for mineralocorticoids does not occur at the receptor level but is conferred by the presence of the 11β-hydroxysteroid dehydrogenase enzyme [13]. In those tissues possessing this enzyme in close proximity to the

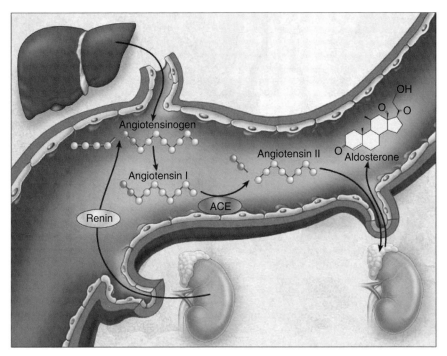

**Figure 6.1** The renin–angiotensin–aldosterone system. Angiotensinogen, the precursor of all angiotensin peptides, is synthesized by the liver. In the circulation it is cleaved by renin, which is secreted into the lumen of renal afferent arterioles by juxtaglomerular cells. Renin cleaves four amino acids from angiotensinogen, thereby forming angiotensin I. In turn, angiotensin I is cleaved by ACE, an enzyme bound to the membrane of endothelial cells, to form angiotensin II. In the zona glomerulosa of the adrenal cortex, angiotensin II stimulates the production of aldosterone. Aldosterone production is also stimulated by potassium, corticotropin, catecholamines (e.g. norepinephrine), and endothelins. (Reproduced with permission from [2].)

receptor (e.g. epithelial cells in kidney, bladder, gastrointestinal tract, sweat and saliva glands, smooth muscle, and vascular endothelium) only mineralocorticoids can activate the receptor. In other tissues (e.g. brain and myocytes) that do not possess this enzyme, glucocorticoids, because of their higher concentration, likely are the principle activators of the mineralocorticoid receptor [13].

Like the other steroid hormones, aldosterone has a dual mechanism of action. It affects the transcriptional modulation of target genes via intracellular receptors, but also elicits rapid effects on second messenger signaling cascades similar to those initiated by peptide hormones or catecholamines. Aldosterone membrane steroid binding sites have been identified, but none of the postulated membrane steroid receptors has yet been purified to homogeneity and cloned [14]. Nongenomic actions of aldosterone have been described in a number of cell culture and *in vivo* systems. In contrast to

the classical genomic effects on gene transcription, which occur at a very slow rate, the nongenomic actions of aldosterone occur rapidly – within minutes of aldosterone administration [14]. The primary effector is still unknown. Whether it is a so far unidentified membrane-bound aldosterone receptor or the classical mineralocorticoid receptor or both is under debate.

The human mineralocorticoid receptor, a ligand-dependent transcription factor (NR3C2) that belongs to the nuclear receptor superfamily, mediates most of the known effects of aldosterone. After aldosterone is bound to its high-affinity corticoid receptor component of the receptor protein complex, the activated receptor moves from the cytosol into the nucleus via exposure of its DNA-binding domain or zinc fingers and positions itself for binding in major grooves of DNA. DNA binding changes the transcriptional rate of specific genes, such as type I or III collagen genes [3]. Subsequently

**Table 6.1** Effects of raised levels of plasma aldosterone.

*Salt and water retention*
  Sodium retention [2]
  Potassium depletion or prevention of hyperkalemia [2]

*Circulatory Vasoconstriction and Upregulation of Norepinephrine*
  Arteriolar vasoconstriction [2]
  Catecholamine potentiation by prevention of norepineprine uptake [17]
  Stimulation of overexpression of cardiac angiotensin-1 receptors [20]

*Modulation of Parasympathetic tone*
  Blunting of baroreflex response [21]

*Upregulation of Inflammatory Mediators*
  Stimulation of cytokine and chemokine production [2,85]
  Activation of macrophages [2]
  Fibrinoid necrosis [19]
  Myocyte necrosis and microscopic scarring [19]

*Development of Fibrosis*
  Stimulation of growth of fibroblasts and synthesis of collagen [3,24,28,86;87]

*Hypercoagulability*
  Increased production of plasminogen activator inhibitor-1 [23]
  Aggregation and activation of platelets [23]

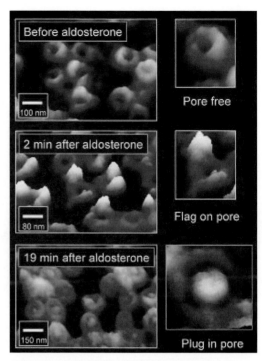

**Figure 6.2** Atomic force microscopic images of nuclear envelope cytoplasmic surfaces before and after aldosterone injection depicting the signaling pathway of aldosterone across the nuclear envelope [15]. Top panel: Before aldosterone injection, nuclear pore complexes are clearly visible. Middle panel: 2 min after aldosterone, most nuclear pore complexes are flagged. After aldosterone is bound to its the receptor protein complex, the activated receptor will move from the cytosol into the nucleus via exposure of its DNA binding domain or zinc fingers and will position itself for binding in major grooves of DNA. The flags represent aldosterone receptors on their way into the cell nucleus. Lower panel: 19 min after aldosterone, most nuclear pore complexes are plugged. Plugs represent ribonucleoproteins carrying aldosterone-induced mRNA from the nucleoplasm into the cytoplasm. (Reproduced with permission from [15].)

messenger RNA will be expressed leading to enhanced protein synthesis. The signaling pathway of aldosterone across the nuclear envelope has recently been described by a novel technology called the atomic force microscopy. Schafer and colleagues [15] described that cells microinjected with aldosterone demonstrated an immediate early change in the nucleus (Figure 6.2). Within 2 min of the injection, they described the appearance of small molecules (called flags) attached to the nuclear pore surface (Figure 6.2). Investigators identified these flags as aldosterone receptors on their way into the cell nucleus. Large molecules were detected inside the nuclear pore central channels, 20 min after injection, which obliterated the nuclear pore complex channel and hence were termed 'plugs' (Figure 6.2). These plugs represent ribonucleoproteins carrying aldosterone-induced mRNA from the nucleoplasm into the cytoplasm [15]. Coinjection of aldosterone with its competitive inhibitor spironolactone eliminated the flag and plug

formation at the cellular level. The investigators envision that since these plugs can be mechanically harvested with the atomic force microscopy stylus, these cells could serve as a bioassay system for identifying aldosterone-induced early genes [15].

## Aldosterone in heart failure

The activity of the renin–angiotensin–aldosterone system is increased in most patients with heart

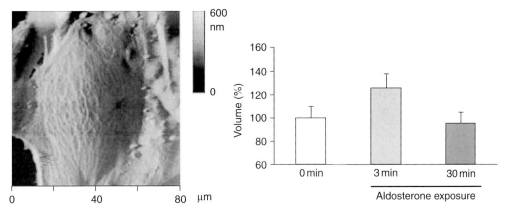

**Figure 6.3** Acute, nongenomic direct effects of aldosterone on endothelial cells. Left panel: three-dimensional image of living endothelial cell exposed to aldosterone, imaged in buffered solution by atomic force microscopy. Cytoskeletal and plasma membrane attached elements can be visualized without damaging the cell. Shown on the left panel are the measurements of individual endothelial cell dimension along two planes ($x$ and $y$ plane). The height of the cell is coded shown by a tint bar in nanometer range. Volume measurements are computed after measurement of the height ($z$ plane). Right panel: graph demonstrating % volume increase of endothelial cells induced by aldosterone. A 28% increase of cell volume was observed 5 min after aldosterone addition. Cell volume returned to normal 25 min later (mean and SEM, $n = 7$). (Reproduced with permission from [22].)

failure and plasma levels of aldosterone may increase to 20 times the normal in these patients [2,16]. This increase is mainly due to the increased synthesis of aldosterone in response to increased levels of angiotensin II and partially to the decreased hepatic clearance by the liver in heart failure [2].

Aldosterone was originally thought to be important in the progression of heart failure because of its role in sodium and water retention. However, recent research has suggested that elevated levels of aldosterone can contribute directly to the pathophysiology of heart failure. Aldosterone levels inversely relate to the compliance of the large arteries and to left ventricular function [9]. In experimental models, aldosterone has been shown to result in direct vascular damage [17], arteriolar vasoconstriction [18], myocyte necrosis, and microscopic scarring [19]. It potentiates the effects of norepinephrine by inhibition of reuptake of norepinephrine by the myocardium [2,17], it stimulates the overexpression of cardiac angiotensin-1 receptors [20], modulates parasympathetic tone, and results in baroreceptor dysfunction [21]. Aldosterone is also known to have acute, nongenomic direct effects on intracellular pH, intracellular electrolytes, and

inositol-1,4,5-triphosphate production. As seen in Figure 6.3, aldosterone results in acute swelling of endothelial cells and individual endothelial cell volume increases by 28% within 5 min after aldosterone exposure. After 25 min, cell volume returns back to normal despite the continuous presence of aldosterone in the medium [22]. Additionally, aldosterone has been demonstrated to promote aggregation and activation of platelets and regulate expression of plasminogen activator inhibitor, thus along with angiotensin II provides a potential link between the renin–angiotensin system and thrombosis [23]. (Table 6.1)

In the early 1990s, Weber and colleagues [3,24,25] documented that chronic aldosterone excess in the presence of salt loading caused cardiac fibrosis in experimental animals (Figure 6.4). Interestingly, the same type of change was not seen on low salt diet. Additional animal studies demonstrated that uni-nephrectomized rats fed a high salt diet and aldosterone were protected from development of cardiac fibrosis with the administration of spironolactone [26]. Subsequently, these findings were further supported by the observation that patients with primary hyperaldosteronism had significantly higher severity of left ventricular hypertrophy as compared to those

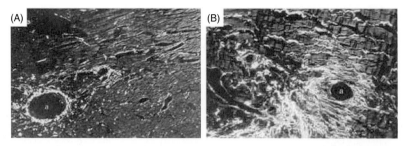

**Figure 6.4** Coronary vascular remodeling in hyperaldosteronism in rats. Panel A shows a section from a normal heart with a normal intramural coronary artery (a) surrounded by yellow-stained fibrillar collagen. A small amount of collagen is also present between the muscle fibers. In panel B, a section from the heart of a rat given aldosterone (plus salt) shows marked perivascular fibrosis of coronary vessels (a) and the contiguous interstitial space between muscle fibers. (Sirius red staining and polarized light, ×40.) (Reproduced with permission from [2].)

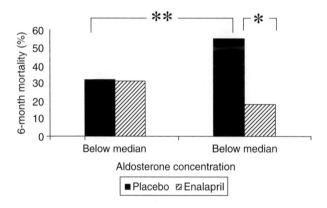

**Figure 6.5** Six-month mortality rates for patients enrolled in the CONSENSUS trial, by median (1395 pmol/L) aldosterone concentration at baseline, **$p < 0.001$, *$p < 0.01$. (Reproduced with permission from [30].)

with essential hypertension despite controlling for age, duration of hypertension, gender, and severity of hypertension [27].

Aldosterone-induced fibrosis has been implicated in the development of remodeling of the atria, ventricles and great vessels [28], increase in left ventricular and vascular stiffness, development of systolic and diastolic dysfunction [29], and increase in risk for arrhythmia. In addition to myocardial fibrosis causing heterogeneous intra cardiac conduction defects, the arrhythmogenic properties of aldosterone have also been attributed to potassium and magnesium depletion, augmentation of sympathetic activity by inhibition of cardiac norepinephrine uptake [18].

## Prognostic role of aldosterone levels in patients with heart failure

Raised aldosterone levels along with other neurohormones indicate worse prognosis and worse survival in patients with heart failure [30]. The prognostic role of serum aldosterone levels have been examined in several clinical studies. The first of these was a study of 23 patients with varying degrees of heart failure [21]. The serum aldosterone levels were highest among the patients with acute and recent onset heart failure compared with chronic heart failure patients [21]. Subsequently, in 119 patients enrolled in First Cooperative North Scandinavian Enalapril Survival Study (CONSENSUS) [30], serum aldosterone levels were significantly higher among patients who died at 6 months compared to survivors (Figure 6.5). Similarly, in 4300 patients enrolled in the Valsartan Heart Failure Trial (Val-HeFT), baseline aldosterone levels above the median significantly related to mortality [Simple-regression-hazard ratio 2.56, 95% confidence interval (CI) 2.28–2.89] [19]. However, when the hazard ratios were adjusted for the other three neurohormones including brain natriuretic peptide, norepinephrine, and plasma

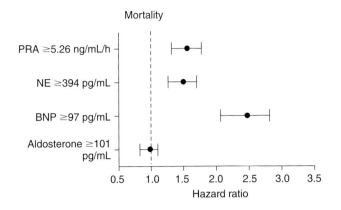

Figure 6.6 Hazard ratios and 95% CI for all-cause mortality according to baseline neurohormones in the Valsartan Heart Failure Trial (Val-HeFT), *high* (≥median) versus *low* (<median), using Cox simple-regression-analysis. Results for each of the four neurohormones analyzed include adjustments for each of the other three neurohormones. (Reproduced with permission from [19].)

renin activity or for demographic, clinical, and echocardiographic data, aldosterone was no longer predictive of mortality, whereas the other three neurohormones remained significantly associated with increased mortality [19] (Figure 6.6).

Thus, there is evidence that plasma aldosterone levels are an indicator of a worse prognosis in heart failure but the association does not appear to be as strong as for some of the other neurohormones in patients with mild to moderate heart failure [19]. However, it should be kept in mind that the patients enrolled in the CONSENSUS trial had severe heart failure [New York Heart Association (NYHA) class IV not treated with ACE-inhibitors or β-blockers] whereas the patients enrolled in the Val-HeFT trial had mild to moderate heart failure (most NYHA class II–IV on ACE-inhibitors and ß-blockers). Therefore, the median aldosterone levels in the CONSENSUS trial were much higher (1305 pmol/L ≈ 471 ng/mL) [30] than the levels in the Val-HeFT trial (101 pg/mL) [19] This may explain why the aldosterone levels did not appear to be a significant risk for mortality in patients with mild to moderate heart failure in the Val-HeFT trial [19].

Another observation from the Val-HeFT trial is the discordance between total mortality and the aldosterone levels in a subgroup of patients receiving ACE-inhibitors and β-blockers. In 1226 patients receiving background therapy with ACE-inhibitor and β-blockers, valsartan increased mortality, resulted in a trend for worse mortality or morbidity [31], and did not confer any benefit in left ventricular remodeling [32] but produced sustained reductions in plasma aldosterone levels when compared to placebo [33]. The discordance between the clinical outcomes or the changes in left ventricular remodeling and the plasma aldosterone levels in the Val-HeFT trial challenged the formerly accepted hypotheses which proposed elevated aldosterone levels predicted worse prognosis in heart failure and that aldosterone antagonism reduced mortality via a favorable effect on left ventricular structure [33]. This is further supported by the finding that, despite significantly elevated aldosterone levels, aldosterone-induced injury was not observed in animals with low salt intake [26]. Thus, we can conclude that the level of aldosterone alone may not be useful in determining its potential causative role in heart failure [11].

There is also evidence that local or 'extra-adrenal' production of aldosterone may contribute to the systemic levels of aldosterone in heart failure. Aldosterone can be produced and extracted by the failing human heart. In fact, local production of aldosterone in heart failure may lead to myocardial aldosterone levels that are several times higher than in the periphery [9,20]. Cardiac production of aldosterone can be induced by angiotensin II or dietary sodium/potassium manipulations [34]. Quantitatively, the transcardiac gradient in aldosterone levels correlate with rise in left ventricular filling pressures and with decline in left ventricular ejection fraction [9]. These suggest a potential autocrine and paracrine action for aldosterone in the failing heart.

## Aldosterone 'escape'

In chronic heart failure, treatment with ACE inhibitors result in an acute reduction in

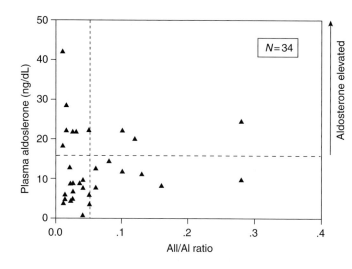

**Figure 6.7** Degree of ACE inhibition and plasma aldosterone levels. An angiotensin II/angiotensin I (AII/AI) ratio >0.05 indicates incomplete inhibition of the vascular converting enzyme. Triangles indicate study subjects, dashed horizontal line indicates upper normal value for aldosterone (15 ng/dL), and vertical dashed line an AII/AI ratio of 0.05. (Reproduced with permission from [38].)

aldosterone levels. Long-term ACE inhibition, however, is associated with aldosterone suppression that is weak, variable, and unsustained. This phenomenon is identified as aldosterone 'escape.'

A reduction in plasma aldosterone levels during ACE inhibitor therapy is associated with a favorable impact on survival [30] (Figure 6.5). Although ACE inhibitors might be expected to reduce aldosterone levels by reducing the stimulating effect of angiotensin II (AII) on aldosterone production, there is increasing evidence that standard doses of ACE inhibitors only transiently suppress the production of aldosterone [35–38]. In a study of 24 patients with heart failure, 11 subjects had elevated plasma aldosterone levels, that is, >15.0 ng/dL [38]. Four of these 11 subjects (36%) had an angiotensin II/angiotensin I (AII /AI) ratio >0.05, which indicated incomplete inhibition of the vascular converting enzyme (Figure 6.7). Other studies have reported that up to 40% of patients on ACE inhibitors have persistently elevated concentrations of serum aldosterone via breakthrough generation of angiotensin II.

Several mechanisms have been proposed to explain this escape phenomenon, which include angiotensin II production through ACE-independent mechanisms, ACE production that is not inhibited by ACE inhibitors due to different ACE-inhibitor genotypes [33], and angiotensin II independent production of aldosterone through the actions of atrial natriuretic factor, endothelin, corticotropin, or serum potassium concentrations

[4,38]. Changes in serum potassium concentrations by 0.1 mmol/L have been shown to change aldosterone secretion. This mechanism comes to play in patients with diuretic-induced kaliuresis treated with oral potassium supplementation. Similarly ACE inhibitors may cause hyperkalemia and thus decrease aldosterone secretion by suppressing angiotensin II. Furthermore, local production of aldosterone in the heart that is not totally regulated by AT-II [9,39] may also have a role in progression of heart failure. Nevertheless, the exact mechanisms underlying incomplete aldosterone suppression with ACE inhibitors have not been adequately investigated.

Compared to ACE inhibitors, the effects of angiotensin receptor blocker treatment on aldosterone are even less clear. In the Randomized Evaluation of Strategies for Left Ventricular Dysfunction (RESOLVD) pilot study [40], high dose of the candesartan or a combination of candesartan and enalapril suppressed plasma aldosterone levels at 17 weeks but the levels of aldosterone returned to pretreatment values at 43 weeks [33]. In Val-HeFT, valsartan added to background therapy for heart failure produced sustained reduction in plasma aldosterone when compared to placebo [33].

Subsequently, to counteract the harmful effects of the residual aldosterone in the circulation, and potentially of the local aldosterone, aldosterone antagonism combined with ACE inhibition was studied in heart failure. These studies will be reviewed in the next section.

## Aldosterone antagonists

Amphenone was the first investigational agent identified to blunt mineralocorticoid action by inhibiting aldosterone biosynthesis [13,41]. The ability of amphenone to alter urinary sodium excretion enabled description of secondary hyperaldosteronism in congestive heart failure and cirrhosis. Subsequently, 17-spirolactone steroids or spirolactones were developed to antagonize aldosterone and the activity of other sodium-retaining hormones at the renal distal tubule [13]. In the late 1950s, this led to the development of spironolactone the first clinically approved aldosterone receptor antagonist for use as a potassium-sparing diuretic in the treatment of volume overloaded states and primary hyperaldosteronism [13].

Spironolactone has been in clinical use for hypertensive conditions for more than 20 years. It acts as a competitive receptor antagonist to aldosterone. At high concentrations, it can also inhibit the biosynthesis of aldosterone. However, spironolactone is not very selective for the mineralocorticoid receptor over other steroid receptors. Its affinity for progesterone and androgen receptors is reflected by side effects such as menstrual irregularity in women and gynecomastia in men. These side effects limited its widespread use and have encouraged the development of more selective mineralocorticoid receptor antagonists, such as eplerenone [42].

Eplerenone is the first *selective* aldosterone receptor antagonist. It is a derivative of spironolactone that is more selective for the aldosterone receptor [43,44]. The presence of the 9,11-epoxy group reduces the progestagenic and antiandrogenic action of eplerenone, but maintains the aldosterone-blocking properties. Compared with spironolactone, eplerenone is 1000-fold less binding to the androgen receptor and 100-fold less binding to the progesterone receptor, while having only a 20-fold reduction in binding to the mineralocorticoid-receptor that blocks the effects of aldosterone [42,43]. This results in effective aldosterone blockade without the attendant side effects often seen with the chronic administration of spironolactone.

The pharmacokinetic parameters of eplerenone were determined in humans who received a single dose of 100 mg of eplerenone [45].

Its bioavailability is greater than that of spironolactone, probably because of its lower protein binding capacity [46]. Unlike spironolactone, eplerenone does not appear to have an active metabolite and its half-life is 3.5–5 h [45]. The drug is a substrate of the CYP3A4 isoenzyme but its effect on the cytochrome P-450 is not clinically relevant. It is excreted in urine (66%) and in feces (32%) [46,47].

## Preclinical studies with aldosterone antagonists

In animal models, the use of spironolactone or eplerenone results in prevention or attenuation of development of myocardial, interstitial, or vascular fibrosis [48,49], and neointimal proliferation [50]. These changes are accompanied by an improvement in arterial stiffness [51], reduction in arterial wall stress [51], improvement in left ventricular systolic and diastolic function, reduction in left ventricular mass as well as reduction in plasma levels of markers for myocardial fibrosis [52,53]. Furthermore, spironolactone has been shown to prevent the elevation of ventricular angiotensin II and AT1 receptor density induced by aldosterone [54], suppress vascular AT-II conversion, increase nitric oxide bioactivity, attenuate platelet aggregation, and attenuate and improve endothelial dysfunction induced by aldosterone [55].

## Early clinical studies with aldosterone antagonists

Until the 1990s, aldosterone antagonists were not used or studied widely in patients with heart failure. This was due to the fact that ACE inhibitors were believed to suppress the formation of aldosterone, that aldosterone antagonists had relatively weak diuretic effects, and that an aldosterone receptor blocker in conjunction with an ACE inhibitor would cause serious hyperkalemia [5]. However, some clinicians had recognized earlier that aldosterone antagonists appeared to benefit patients with hepatic congestion and ascites secondary to right heart failure and advocated the use of spironolactone in such patients.

In the early heart failure clinical trials with ACE inhibitors, use of aldosterone antagonists was not controlled by trial design but a significant number of patients in these trials were on potassium-sparing diuretics including spironolactone. Approximately half of the patients in the CONSENSUS trial were on background therapy with spironolactone [30]. In the Studies of Left Ventricular Dysfunction (SOLVD), reduction in mortality was more pronounced in patients receiving a potassium-sparing diuretics than in those receiving a non-potassium sparing diuretic [56].

The first small-scale study of the randomized addition of spironolactone (50 to 100 mg/day, titrated to blood pressure and plasma potassium) or placebo to ACE inhibitors, in 42 patients with NYHA II to III congestive heart failure [57] demonstrated a significant increase in the cardiac norepinephrine uptake with spironolactone. Also, 4 of 28 patients developed significant hyperkalemia and elevation of plasma creatinine and two of them needed discontinuation of the drug [57].

In other small clinical studies of patients with heart failure, the addition of aldosterone receptor blockers to ACE inhibitors, resulted in reduction in left ventricular volumes and left ventricular mass [58,59], improvement in left ventricular ejection fraction [58–61], improvement in NYHA functional class [60,61], reduction in serum brain-natriuretic peptide [59,61], improvement in exercise capacity and peak oxygen consumption [58], increase in cardiac norepinephrine uptake [57], reduction in ventricular arrhythmias [57], improvement in heart rate variability, improvement in baroreceptor dysfunction [62,63], and reduction in circulating levels of markers of vascular collagen turnover [62].

In a pilot dose escalation study of 214 patients with NYHA class II–IV heart failure, the RALES investigators [64], studied the efficacy and safety of four doses of spironolactone at 12.5, 25, 50, or 75 mg/day versus placebo added to background standard therapy with an ACE inhibitor and a loop diuretic over 12 weeks. The incidence of hyperkalemia (serum potassium $\leq$5.5 mmol/L) was 5% for the placebo group, whereas it was 5%, 13%, 20%, and 24% for the 12.5-, 25-, 50- and 75-mg spironolactone treatment groups, respectively. Thus, the investigators concluded that daily doses of 12.5 to 25 mg of spironolactone coadministered with conventional therapy of ACE inhibitors

were relatively safe, provided that serum potassium levels were closely monitored. There was no change in body weight, sodium retention score, or urinary sodium. It was also noted that the 25-mg dose had no apparent diuretic effect. These studies culminated in two multicenter, large-scale, randomized, placebo-controlled trials that will be reviewed in the next section.

## The randomized aldactone evaluation study

The RALES was a study of 1663 patients with severe heart failure and left ventricular ejection fraction less than 35% who were randomized to 25 mg spironolactone versus placebo, in a double-blind fashion [5]. Patients were eligible if they had had NYHA class IV heart failure symptoms within the 6 months before enrollment and were in NYHA class III or IV at the time of enrollment. All patients were already being treated with ACE inhibitors and loop diuretics. Treatment with Digitalis and vasodilators was allowed, but potassium-sparing diuretics were not permitted. Oral potassium supplements were not recommended unless hypokalemia (defined as a serum potassium concentration of less than 3.5 mmol/L) developed. Patients with serum creatinine concentration of more than 2.5 mg/dL or a serum potassium concentration of more than 5.0 mEq/L were excluded. Serum potassium was closely monitored after initiation of the drug and at follow-up. The mean dose of spironolactone used in the trial was 26 mg/day [5].

After a mean follow-up of 24 months, there was a 30% reduction in the primary endpoint of all-cause mortality (relative risk 0.70, 95% CI, 0.60–0.82, $p < 0.001$). In addition, (Figure 6.8) there was a 30% reduction in the frequency of hospitalizations for cardiac causes and a 35% reduction in hospitalizations for heart failure in the spironolactone group compared to placebo. The reductions in risk of death and hospitalization were observed after 2 to 3 months of treatment and persisted throughout the study. The reduction in the risk of death among patients in the spironolactone group was similar in analyses of all six prespecified subgroups of sex, NYHA class, baseline serum potassium concentration, use of potassium supplements, and use of $\beta$-blockers. A significant improvement in

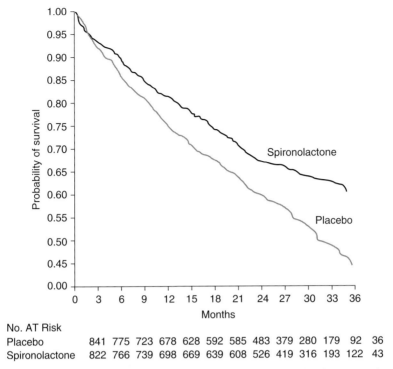

**Figure 6.8** Kaplan–Meier analysis of the probability of survival among patients in the placebo group and patients in the spironolactone group. Randomized Aldactone Evaluation Study (RALES). (Reproduced with permission from [5].)

symptoms as assessed by functional class was also observed. Based on this study, low dose spironolactone (25 mg/day) was recommended for patients with recent or current symptoms of heart failure at rest despite the use of ACE inhibitors, diuretics, digoxin and a β-blocker assuming close follow-up of renal function and serum potassium [65].

In the RALES trial, gynecomastia or breast pain was reported in 10% of the men. Discontinuation of study drug due to side effects occurred in 2% of patients in the spironolactone group compared with 0.2% in the placebo arm ($p = 0.006$). The incidence of serious hyperkalemia, defined as serum potassium >6.0 mEq/L, was 2% and 1% respectively ($p = 0.42$). During the study period, the median creatinine concentration increased more in the spironolactone group (approximately 0.05 to 0.10 mg/dL) than the placebo group ($P < 0.001$).

The reduction in risk of death with spironolactone treatment was attributed to significant reductions in the risk of both death from progressive heart failure and sudden death from cardiac causes. It did not appear to be related to the effect of spironolactone on sodium retention or potassium loss. This is supported by the fact that 25 mg spironolactone daily had no apparent diuretic effect [64]. and spironolactone did not have a clinically significant hemodynamic effect. Subsequently, in a substudy of RALES of 261 patients [52], the baseline serum values of markers of collagen synthesis correlated with disease severity and mortality. In the spironolactone-treated subjects, survival benefit correlated with reduced collagen synthesis markers at 6 months. The investigators indicated that down-regulation of the excessive extracellular matrix turnover could be one of the various extra-renal mechanisms to explain the beneficial effects of spironolactone in the RALES trial [52]. Other mechanisms such as regression of hypertrophy, improvement of endothelial function, reduced arterial stiffness, enhanced renal sodium excretion, and antiarrhythmic actions may also have played a role, but currently there are no other substudies to elucidate the potential beneficial role of these mechanisms in the RALES trial.

It should be noted that only approximately 10% of the patients in the RALES trial were receiving a β-blocker and the reduction in risk of death did not differ in this subgroup. Furthermore, the patients studied in the RALES trial were at higher risk than those studied in the β-blocker heart failure trials. Thus, it is not clear whether spironolactone would have conferred similar benefit if the majority of the patients had been on β-blocker therapy. Another criticism for the RALES trial was that the doses of ACE inhibitors were not maximized to the target doses. The mean dose of ACE inhibitors in the RALES trial was approximately 40–80% of the target dose. Therefore, further studies are needed to examine the tolerability and effectiveness of the concomitant use of β-blockers, ACE inhibitors, and spironolactone in such high-risk populations at target doses. Similarly, additional clinical trials will be necessary to assess the effect of spironolactone on morbidity and mortality in patients with lesser degrees of heart failure and also in asymptomatic patients with left ventricular dysfunction.

## Clinical experience in the aftermath of RALES trial

After the report of the RALES trial, it was noted that spironolactone was being used widely in heart failure without consideration of the NYHA class and ejection fraction, without optimization of background treatment with ACE inhibitors and β-blockers, and without close monitoring of serum potassium levels [66,67]. Many patients who received new prescriptions for spironolactone after the publication of RALES did not have severe heart failure, had renal insufficiency, and simultaneously received prescriptions for potassium supplements [66].

In a cohort of 110 patients with heart failure studied after the RALES trial publication, the mean daily dose of spironolactone administered to heart failure patients was 41 mg, much higher than the dose used in the RALES trial (26 mg) [66]. Only a quarter of the patients were documented to have NYHA class III to IV heart failure and approximately half of the patients had documented

left ventricular ejection fraction (LVEF) of >35% before beginning spironolactone. Of these patients 35% were on β-blockers and 40% of the patients were continued on potassium supplements despite absence of hypokalemia. At baseline, one-third of the patients had renal insufficiency and 46% had diabetes mellitus. Approximately two-thirds of the patients did not have appropriate laboratory and clinical follow-up [66]. The development of adverse events in this cohort was much higher than in the RALES trial. The incidences of hyperkalemia (levels ≥5.2 mEq/L) and serious hyperkalemia (levels ≥6 mEq/L) were 24% and 12% respectively. One-fourth of the patients developed renal insufficiency and 3% of the patients required temporary pacemaker insertion for hemodynamically unstable bradyarrhythmia related to serious hyperkalemia. Twenty-one percent of these patients were subsequently discontinued from spironolactone, whereas this number was 8% in the RALES trial [66].

A larger population-based time-series analysis, linking prescription-claims data and hospital-admission records for more than 1.3 million adults in Canada [67], demonstrated that among patients treated with ACE inhibitors who had recently been hospitalized for heart failure, the spironolactone-prescription rate increased immediately after the publication of RALES, from 34 to 149 per 1000 patients ($P < 0.001$). The rate of hospitalization for hyperkalemia rose from 2.4 in 1994 to 11.0 per 1000 patients in 2001 ($P < 0.001$), and the associated mortality rose from 0.3 per 1000 to 2.0 per 1000 patients ($P < 0.001$). (Figure 6.9) The investigators concluded that the publication of RALES was not associated with significant decreases in the rates of readmission for heart failure or death from all causes in their population [67]. The investigators attributed the increased risk of hyperkalemia to the reasons that were identified in the earlier cohort study [66], that physicians may not monitor potassium levels closely in patients receiving spironolactone, may neglect baseline attributes that predispose patients to hyperkalemia such as diabetes mellitus, may overlook conditions that develop during therapy such as renal dysfunction, may prescribe inappropriately high doses of spironolactone or other medications that contribute to hyperkalemia, and may extend the RALES findings

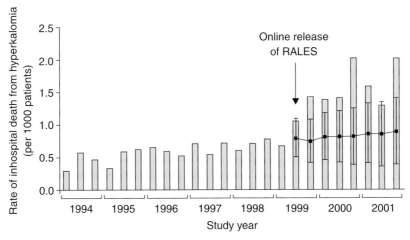

**Figure 6.9** Rate of inhospital death associated with hyperkalemia among patients recently hospitalized for heart failure who were receiving ACE inhibitors. Each bar shows the rate of inhospital death associated with hyperkalemia per 1000 patients during one 4-month interval. The line beginning in the second interval of 1999 shows projected death rates derived from interventional ARIMA models, with 'I' bars representing the 95% CI. (Reproduced with permission from [67].)

to patients who, unlike the patients in that study, do not have left ventricular systolic dysfunction or severe heart failure [66].

## Hyperkalemia with aldosterone receptor blockade

Hyperkalemia is an uncommon complication of therapy with ACE inhibitors, aldosterone antagonists, or angiotensin-receptor blockers in patients *without* comorbities of diabetes or renal insufficiency. The low incidence of hyperkalemia in the controlled trials involving these drugs, such as RALES, can be attributed to the enrollment of patients at low risk, frequent follow-up, and intensive monitoring [68]. The mean serum creatinine concentration in major trials involving patients with congestive heart failure range from 1.2–1.4 mg/dL [69]. Since one-third to one-half of patients with congestive heart failure have renal insufficiency, in actual practice a large proportion of patients being treated with these drugs are at increased risk for hyperkalemia [69]. The development of hyperkalemia as a result of decreased aldosterone concentrations is usually seen when aldosterone concentrations have already decreased before the administration of the drugs. Decreased aldosterone concentrations

can result from disturbances that originate at any point in the renin–angiotensin–aldosterone system, from a disease state, or from the effects of other drugs such as the normal aging process, adrenal disease, diabetic nephropathy, type IV renal tubular acidosis, nonsteroidal anti-inflammatory drugs, β-adrenergic blocking agents, heparin, and ketoconazole [68].

## Clinical experience with eplerenone prior to the EPHESUS trial

Prior to its evaluation in post-myocardial patients, eplerenone had been evaluated in numerous hypertension trials involving more than 3000 patients, including subgroups of patients with low plasma renin activity, diabetes, left ventricular hypertrophy, uncontrolled blood pressure while receiving monotherapy with ACE inhibitors, angiotensin-receptor blockers, calcium channel blockers, or β-blockers [44,70–72], and had been approved for the treatment of systemic hypertension. Results of these trials indicated that eplerenone lowered blood pressure and reduced end-organ damage in hypertensive patients with doses ranging from 50–200 mg/day [44,70,71]. The most effective dose of eplerenone for hypertension was 100 mg once daily [71,73]. Of note, eplerenone performed better than losartan in African American patients and lowered blood pressure regardless of initial plasma renin activity [74].

The risk of hyperkalemia in these hypertension trials was relatively low, similar to that of enalapril, or placebo, and approximately 1% of patients had to be withdrawn from studies because of elevated serum potassium levels. In fact, the incidence of all adverse events in the entire eplerenone hypertension clinical trial database was not significantly different from the incidence of adverse events reported on placebo. In an overview of all patients studied in the hypertension clinical trials eplerenone was associated with hyperkalemia ($\geq$5.5 mmol/L) in 0.7% of patients, an incidence that was not significantly greater than the 0.3% reported in placebo patients (44,70,71). Increases in serum aldosterone levels were related to dose but not to reductions in 24-h blood pressure.

Even though the safety profile of eplerenone is acceptable in patients with hypertension (with normal kidney function), the risk of hyperkalemia appears to be higher in patients with concomitant diabetes and/or heart failure. In the one trial involving diabetic hypertensive patients with proteinuria [75], the incidence of elevated plasma potassium (>5.5 mmol/L) was 8% on eplerenone monotherapy compared to 4% on enalapril monotherapy. The incidence of hyperkalemia on the combination of these two agents was 14% [75]. In a dose ranging study, eplerenone in patients with congestive heart failure [76], hyperkalemia (potassium level $\geq$6 mEq/L) was seen in 12% of patients receiving eplerenone 100 mg/day and in 8.7% of patients receiving spironolactone 25 mg/day.

## Eplerenone post–acute myocardial infarction heart failure efficacy and survival study

The experimental and clinical data demonstrating attenuation of left ventricular remodeling [77], reduction in cardiac fibrosis [49], and prevention of left ventricular dysfunction [49] after myocardial infarction with aldosterone blockers when added to ACE inhibitors, led to the design of the Eplerenone Post-Acute Myocardial Infarction Survival and Efficacy study (EPHESUS) trial. In the earlier studies, left ventricular end-diastolic pressure and wall stress were both reduced significantly with doses of spironolactone or eplerenone that did *not* affect blood pressure or heart rate indicating a therapeutic effect of these agents independent of the antihypertensive effect. This, and the safety concern of increased hyperkalemia risk with higher doses, culminated in selection of a lower dose of eplerenone (25 mg/day) in the EPHESUS trial [6].

In the EPHESUS trial, a total of 6632 patients were randomized to placebo or eplerenone following an acute myocardial infarction with signs and symptoms of heart failure and left ventricular systolic dysfunction (LVEF <40%) [6]. Nearly three-quarters of the study population were male and the mean LVEF was 33%. Study drug was initiated at 25 mg and then increased to 50 mg daily if tolerated, average dose received in the active group was 43 mg eplerenone per day. The primary endpoint was all-cause mortality and death from cardiovascular causes or hospitalization for a cardiovascular event, which included heart failure, recurrent myocardial infarction, stroke, or ventricular arrhythmia. All-cause mortality was reduced by 15% ($p = 0.008$). Cardiovascular death or hospitalization for cardiovascular events was reduced by 13% ($p = 0.002$) [6] (Table 6.2). Importantly, there was again a significant reduction in the rate of sudden death from cardiac causes (21% reduction, $p = 0.03$).

Serious hyperkalemia was increased in the eplerenone group, but the incidence of gynecomastia was not higher in the eplerenone group. (Table 6.2) The beneficial effects of eplerenone were consistent across patient subgroups. In the subgroup of patients already receiving ACE inhibitors and $\beta$-blockers, the addition of eplerenone further reduced mortality by 27% [6]. Serious hyperkalemia occurred in 5.5% of patients in the eplerenone group, compared with 3.9% of patients in the placebo group (Table 6.2). There was a greater increase in the serum creatinine concentration in the eplerenone group (0.06 mg/dL) than in the placebo (0.02 mg/dL) group ($p < 0.001$). No significant increase in gynecomastia was seen. Based on this trial, the US Food and Drug Administration approved the use of eplerenone

**Table 6.2** Comparison of patient demographics, concurrent medications, and side effects in the RALES and EPHESUS trials.

|  | RALES [5]<br>Spironolactone | EPHESUS [6]<br>Eplerenone |
|---|---|---|
| **Baseline Characteristics** | | |
| Symptoms | Chronic | Acute, post-MI |
| NYHA Class | III (79%), IV (21%) | N/A |
| Ischemic | 55% | 100% |
| Female | 27% | 29% |
| LVEF (mean) | 25% | 33% |
| Study drug dose (mean) | 26 mg | 43 mg |
| **Concurrent medications** | | |
| Loop diuretics | 100% | 60 % |
| ACE inhibitors or ARB | 95 % | 87% |
| Digitalis | 75 % | 60% |
| β-blockers | 10% | 75% |
| **Outcomes** | Relative risk (95% CI) | |
| Death from any cause | 0.70 (0.60–0.82)*¥ | 0.85 (0.75–0.96)** |
| Death from cardiac cause or cardiovascular<br>  hospitalization | 0.68 (0.59–0.78)* | 0.87 (0.79–0.95)** |
| Death from any cause or any hospitalization | 0.77 (0.68–0.86)* | 0.92 (0.86–0.98)* |
| Sudden cardiac death | 0.71 (0.59–0.82)* | 0.79 (0.64–0.97)* |
| HF hospitalization | 0.65 (0.54–0.77)* | 0.85 (0.74–0.99)* |
| **Adverse Reactions** | | |
| Serious hyperkalemia | 2% | 5.5%* |
| Gynecomastia | 10%* | 0.5% |
| Median serum creatinine increase (mg/dL) | 0.05–0.10* | 0.06* |
| Discontinuation of study drug | 2%* | unknown |

N/A = not applicable; NYHA class = New York Heart Association Class; HF = Heart failure; MI = Myocardial infarction; LV = Left ventricular ejection fraction; ACE = Angiotensin-converting enzyme; ARB = Angiotensin receptor blocker; Serious hyperkalemia = serum potassium >6.0 mEq/L.
* $p < 0.05$ when compared to placebo
¥ Primary endpoint
** Coprimary endpoint

to improve survival of stable patients with left ventricular systolic function and clinical evidence of heart failure following an acute myocardial infarction [78].

The package insert for eplerenone (Inspra®) points out that hyperkalemia can occur in 2.6% of patients with normal renal function and in more than 10% in patients with mild renal dysfunction [79]. As with spironolactone, hyperkalemia occurs more frequently in persons with diabetes particularly when eplerenone is given with ACE inhibitors, 38% receiving this combination had hyperkalemia [79]. Eplerenone is

category B in pregnancy. It is contraindicated in patients with hyperkalemia (serum potassium more than 5.5 mEq/L), type 2 diabetes with microalbuminuria, or moderate renal dysfunction, (creatinine clearance <50 mL/min, serum creatinine >2.0 mg/dL in men or >1.8 mg/dL in women, and in those taking potassium supplements or with other potassium-sparing diuretics (amiloride, triamterene, or spironolactone) [79]. Eplerenone serum levels are increased when taken with detoconazole, erythromycin, saquinavir, verapamil, fluconazole, and grapefruit juice [79].

## Which patients should be treated with an aldosterone blocker?

As reviewed earlier, two large-scale, randomized clinical trials suggest that aldosterone blockade is effective in patients with severe heart failure caused by systolic left ventricular dysfunction (RALES) [5], or in patients with clinical evidence of heart failure and left ventricular systolic function following an acute myocardial infarction (EPHESUS) [6], provided that patients have normal baseline renal function and normal potassium. There is no prospective evidence from randomized studies on the effect of aldosterone blockade on mortality and morbidity in mild to moderate chronic heart failure (NYHA class II–III), in patients with asymptomatic left ventricular systolic dysfunction, or in patients with preserved left ventricular function. Although small-scale studies suggest that surrogate markers such as ventricular remodeling, endothelial function, heart rate variability, baroreceptor function, and myocardial collagen formation improve with aldosterone antagonism [80] in patients with mild to moderate heart failure, without prospective randomized trials powered to evaluate clinical events, these results cannot be safely extrapolated to definitive clinical benefit in patients with mild to moderate heart failure (NYHA class II–III). Further definitive randomized clinical studies are also needed to study the effect of aldosterone antagonism in patients with asymptomatic left ventricular systolic dysfunction or in patients with preserved left ventricular function.

### Which aldosterone receptor blocker?

Although it may be logical to assume that the beneficial effects of aldosterone blockade may be a class effect, spironolactone and eplerenone differ in pharmacokinetics, bioavailability, metabolism, potency of mineralocorticoid receptor blockade, and effects on androgen and protestogen receptors [43,46,47,80]. Thus, evidence-based approach would require spironolactone to be considered in patients with severe chronic heart failure caused by systolic dysfunction, according to the dosing regimen recommended in the RALES [5]. Currently low-dose spironolactone is recommended for patients with recent or current symptoms of heart failure at rest despite the use of

ACE inhibitors, diuretics, digoxin, and a β-blocker [65]. Though not reflected in the ACC/AHA heart failure guidelines, which predates the publication of the EPHESUS trial, it would be reasonable to add eplerenone to background therapy in patients with clinical evidence of heart failure and left ventricular systolic function following an acute myocardial infarction according to the dosing regimen suggested in EPHESUS [6]. However, there is equipoise in the cardiology community as to which agent is appropriate for specific patient populations. For example, the 2005 Guideline Update from the ACC/AHA notes that the 'addition of an aldosterone antagonist is reasonable in selected patients with mild to moderate symptoms of heart failure and reduced left ventricular ejection fraction who can be carefully monitored for preserved renal function and normal potassium concentration' with a class IIA recommendation; therefore, leaving the choice of the agent to the practicing clinician [81]. However, information other than simply efficacy (i.e. cost) should be part of the decision-making process for any clinician. For example, a 1-month supply of eplerenone will cost patients $113. This price is significantly higher than the cost of spironolactone, which is approximately $30/month [82]. When cost is a major factor and relatively short-term use of aldosterone blockade is anticipated, one might consider administering spironolactone according to the dosing regimen in RALES. Since there are insufficient data at this time to be confident about relative effectiveness and risk/benefit ratio of these two agents routine interchangeable use cannot be justified [80]. In the interim, it would be prudent to use the drug regimen and indications proven by the pivotal prospective randomized studies [80].

## Aldosterone antagonism or angiotensin receptor blockade as an add-on therapy?

In the last decade, several studies have shown that angiotensin receptor blockers (ARBs), when added to background therapy with ACE inhibitors, can result in improvement in combined morbidity and mortality in patients with chronic heart failure [31,83], similar to the benefit shown with spironolactone [5]. The role of angiotensin

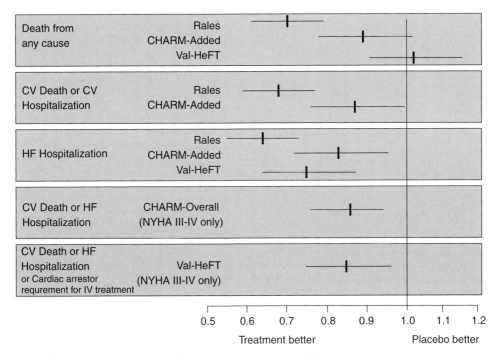

**Figure 6.10** Effect of aldosterone receptor blocker (spironolactone in RALES trial) or angiotensin receptor blocker (valsartan in Val-HeFT trial or candesartan in CHARM trial) treatment compared with placebo on different outcomes. Point estimates of hazard ratios given with 95% CI. CV = Cardiovascular; HF = Heart Failure; IV = Intravenous treatment (for heart failure without admission or cardiac arrest with resuscitation); NYHA = New York Heart Association; RALES = Randomized Aldactone Evaluation Study [5]; CHARM-added = Candesartan in Heart failure: Assessment of Reduction in Mortality and morbidity (CHARM)-added trial [83]; VAL-HeFT = Valsartan Heart Failure Trial [31]; CHARM-Overall = The Candesartan in Heart failure Assessment of Reduction in Mortality and morbidity (CHARM) programme [88]. (Adapted with permission from Pitt B *et al*. [5]; Cohn JN *et al*.[31]; Pfeffer MA *et al* the CHARM-Overall programme [88]; McMurray JJ *et al*. the CHARM-added trial [83].)

receptor blockade in the treatment of heart failure is reviewed in detail in other chapters. In this section, we will review the question whether ARBs versus aldosterone receptor antagonists, or both, should be added to background therapy with ACE inhibitors and β-blockers. A summary of aldosterone antagonists and ARB clinical trials are found in Figure 6.10 [5,31,83–88].

It is important to recognize that in chronic heart failure, the ARB [31,82,83] were conducted predominantly in patients with mild to moderate heart failure (NYHA class II–III), whereas the RALES trial [5], (the only aldosterone receptor antagonist trial in chronic heart failure), was conducted in patients with severe heart failure (NYHA class III–IV) (Table 6.3). At present time, there are no large-scale, prospective, randomized clinical trials with aldosterone receptor blockers in *mild to*

*moderate* chronic heart failure patients and there are no head-to-head trials comparing ARBs and aldosterone receptor blockers in the treatment of heart failure. Thus, it is not feasible to compare the efficacy or safety of these two treatment strategies in mild to moderate heart failure at present time.

One might question then whether a comparison between these two groups of agents can be performed for the treatment of *severe* heart failure from the existing data. The representation of NYHA class III/IV heart failure patients in the ARB trials is of substantial size, allowing subgroup analysis for prespecified endpoints for these subgroups in these trials [31,82]. As seen in Figure 6.10, in NYHA class III/IV heart failure patients, there is significant risk reduction (approximately 14–16%) in the combined endpoints of cardiovascular death or heart failure hospitalization with candesartan [83]

**Table 6.3** Comparison of baseline characteristics in the RALES, CHARM-added, and Val-HeFT trials.

|  | RALES | | CHARM Add-on | | VAL-HeFT | |
|---|---|---|---|---|---|---|
|  | Spironolactone | Placebo | Candesartan | Placebo | Valsartan | Placebo |
| NYHA III (%) | 72* | 69* | 73 | 73 | 36.1 | 36.2 |
| NYHA IV (%) | 27 | 31 | 2.6 | 3.5 | 1.7 | 2.2 |
| LVEF (%±SD) | 25.6 ± 6.7 | 25.2 ± 6.8 | 28 ± 7.5 | 28 ± 7.5 | 26.6 ± 7.3 | 26.9 ± 7.0 |
| ACE inhibitors (%) | 95 | 94 | 100 | 99.8 | 92.6 | 92.8 |
| β-blockers (%) | 11 | 10 | 55 | 55.9 | 34.5 | 35.3 |
| Spironolactone (%) | N/A | N/A | 17.4 | 16.9 | 5 | unknown |

*Patients had to have history of NYHA class IV heart failure within 6 months of enrollment

N/A = Not applicable; SD = standard deviation;

RALES = Randomized Aldactone Evaluation Study (RALES) [5];

CHARM Add-on = Candesartan in Heart failure: Assessment of Reduction in Mortality and morbidity (CHARM)-added trial [83];

VAL-HeFT = Valsartan Heart Failure Trial [31].

and mortality and morbidity (defined as hospitalization for heart failure, requirement for intravenous treatment with inotropes or vasodilator, or cardiac arrest requiring resuscitation) with valsartan [31]. The risk reduction in the combined endpoint of cardiovascular death or hospitalization for cardiovascular causes is 32% with spironolactone (relative risk 0.68, CI, 0.59–0.78, $p < 0.001$) [5] (Figure 6.10).

Since the subgroup analyses were not reported for other endpoints in the ARB trials, a comparison for all-cause mortality cannot be provided. Though there appears to be a difference in the magnitude of risk reduction in combined endpoints between the two treatment strategies, such an extrapolation would not be advisable because of the major differences in the background therapy, patient population, and trial design between these studies. First of all, the background therapy with ACE inhibitors and β-blockers is quite different in these trials. As can be seen in Table 6.3, only 10% of the patients in the RALES trial were on β-blockers, whereas approximately 35% of the patients in the Val-HeFT and 55% of the patients in the CHARM-added trial were on β-blockers. Second, the primary endpoints for these trials were different, making comparison of different endpoints unreliable. Third, the RALES [5] and CHARM-added [83] trials were designed to examine the effect of addition of these agents to ACE inhibitors. Thus, patients had to be on background therapy with ACE inhibitors by trial design. In the Val-HeFT trial [31], the background

therapy was left to the discretion of the primary care provider. Thus the trials differ significantly not allowing a direct comparison.

The safety profile of the aldosterone antagonists or ARBs seems to be comparable in patients with heart failure. Of interest is that the incidence of serious hyperkalemia is around 2–3% with either aldosterone or ARBs when added to ACE inhibitors in these trials. However, in population-based cohorts this number is reported to be as high as 12% for reasons explained in the earlier sections [66,67]. Similarly, the rise in creatinine is comparable between the ARB and RALES trials [31,83] but again this risk appears to be much higher when used in the general population not limited to trial inclusion or exclusion criteria [66]. Hypotension, though mild, is reported to be a significant adverse effect for candesartan in CHARM-added trial [83] and a trend for adverse event for valsartan in the VAL-HeFT trial [31]. Again, even though blood pressure changes were not significant between the spironolactone and placebo groups in the RALES trial, there have been reports of hypotension with spironolactone when added to ACE inhibitors in heart failure patients [66].

At present time, there are no large-scale, prospective trials directly comparing these two treatment strategies for the same target patient population. Both strategies have been shown to be beneficial in different severity of heart failure patients and the data do not support superiority of one treatment modality over the other as an 'add-on' therapy for the same target population. Current 'ACC/AHA Guidelines for the Evaluation and Management of Chronic Heart Failure in the Adult' recommends initiation of low-dose spironolactone for patients with recent or current symptoms of heart failure at rest despite the use of ACE inhibitors, diuretics, digoxin and a β-blocker [65]. The guidelines have not changed substantially since the publication of the CHARM trial as the addition of an aldosterone antagonist is considered as reasonable in selected patients who are still symptomatic despite optimal pharmacologic therapy with a β-blocker and ACE inhibitor (or ARB) – class IIa.

The efficacy and more importantly *safety* of combined treatment with ACE inhibitors, ß-blockers, aldosterone, *and* angiotensin receptor antagonists remain to be examined. Five percent of the patients in Val-HeFT and 17 % of the patients in CHARM-added trial were also on spironolactone. Due to small numbers, the safety and efficacy of valsartan when given in combination with ACE inhibitors and spironolactone could not be evaluated [31]. In the CHARM-added trial, the risk of serious hyperkalemia (4% versus 1% in placebo) and the risk of development of renal insufficiency (serum creatinine at least doubled from baseline in 11% in the candesartan group versus 4% in the placebo, $p = 0.21$) appeared to be higher in the candesartan group compared to placebo, when candesartan was given in combination with ACE inhibitors and spironolactone. Therefore, until further safety and efficacy data are available the combined use of 'all' of these agents are not recommended in treatment of heart failure.

## Conclusion

Over the last 20 years, aldosterone antagonism has emerged as an important modality in treatment of heart failure and left ventricular dysfunction. Experimental data suggest aldosterone plays a significant role in left ventricular remodeling, vascular stiffness, endothelial function, heart rate variability, baroreceptor function, myocardial collagen formation, potentiation of myocardial catecholamine expression, and upregulation of inflammatory mediators (Table 6.1). Increased aldosterone levels are associated with poor prognosis and increased mortality in patients with

heart failure [30]. ACE inhibitor therapy is not adequate to completely and chronically suppress production of aldosterone, resulting in aldosterone 'escape' [4]. This has led to the studies with combination of aldosterone antagonists with ACE inhibitors in patients with heart failure [64]. Two large-scale, randomized clinical trials demonstrated that aldosterone blockade is effective in patients with severe heart failure caused by systolic left ventricular dysfunction (RALES) [5], or in patients with clinical evidence of heart failure and left ventricular systolic function following an acute myocardial infarction (EPHESUS) [6], provided that patients have normal baseline renal function and normal potassium, and are followed very closely. Currently low-dose spironolactone (25 mg/day) is recommended for patients with recent or current symptoms of heart failure at rest despite the use of ACE inhibitors, diuretics, digoxin, and a β-blocker [65], and eplerenone has been approved for patients with left ventricular systolic function and clinical evidence of heart failure following an acute myocardial infarction [78]. After the report of the RALES trial [5], several population-based cohort studies reported that there was broad use of spironolactone in patients with heart failure without consideration of the severity of heart failure or left ventricular dysfunction, without optimization of background treatment with ACE inhibitors and/or β-blockers, and without close monitoring of serum potassium levels [66,67]. Indiscriminate use of spironolactone has been implicated in hyperkalemia-associated morbidity and mortality in heart failure patients [67]. Appropriate selection of patients similar to trial populations, closer laboratory monitoring, and adherence to the trial guidelines may allow more judicious use of these agents and prevent such complications [66,67].

Although small-scale studies suggest that aldosterone antagonism may be beneficial in patients with *mild to moderate chronic* heart failure [80], without prospective, large-scale, randomized trials powered to evaluate clinical events these results cannot be safely extrapolated for use in these populations. The efficacy and safety of aldosterone antagonism in patients with mild to moderate heart failure, asymptomatic left ventricular systolic dysfunction, or patients with preserved left ventricular function remain to be evaluated.

Furthermore, aldosterone receptor blockers will need to be compared against the ARBs for the benefit or the risk conferred when added to background therapy with ACE inhibitors, β-blockers, or even device therapy in management of heart failure. In the interim, it would be prudent to use these agents according to the regimen proven to be beneficial by the pivotal prospective randomized studies.

# References

1 Luetscher JA, Jr., Johnson BB. Observations on the sodium-retaining corticoid (aldosterone) in the urine of children and adults in relation to sodium balance and edema. *J Clin Invest* 1954;**33**:1441–1446.

2 Weber KT. Aldosterone in congestive heart failure. *N Engl J Med* 2001;**345**:1689–1697.

3 Weber KT, Brilla CG. Pathological hypertrophy and cardiac interstitium. Fibrosis and renin–angiotensin–aldosterone system. *Circulation* 1991;**83**:1849–1865.

4 Struthers AD. Aldosterone escape during angiotensin-converting enzyme inhibitor therapy in chronic heart failure. *J Card Fail* 1996;**2**:47–54.

5 Pitt B, Zannad F, Remme WJ et al. The effect of spironolactone on morbidity and mortality in patients with severe heart failure. Randomized Aldactone Evaluation Study Investigators. *N Engl J Med* 1999;**341**:709–717.

6 Pitt B, Remme W, Zannad F. Eplerenone, a selective aldosterone blocker, in patients with left ventricular dysfunction after myocardial infarction. *N Engl J Med* 2003;**348**:1309–1321.

7 Takeda Y, Miyamori I, Yoneda T et al. Production of aldosterone in isolated rat blood vessels. *Hypertension* 1995;**25**:170–173.

8 Silvestre JS, Robert V, Heymes C et al. Myocardial production of aldosterone and corticosterone in the rat. Physiological regulation. *J Biol Chem* 1998;**273**:4883–4891.

9 Mizuno Y, Yoshimura M, Yasue H et al. Aldosterone production is activated in failing ventricle in humans. *Circulation* 2001;**103**:72–77.

10 Giroud CJ, Stachenko J, Venning EH. Secretion of aldosterone by the zona glomerulosa of rat adrenal glands incubated in vitro. *Proc Soc Exp Biol Med* 1956;**92**:154–158.

11 Dluhy RG, Williams GH. Aldosterone – villain or bystander? *N Engl J Med* 2004;**351**:8–10.

12 Arriza JL, Weinberger C, Cerelli G et al. Cloning of human mineralocorticoid receptor complementary DNA: structural and functional kinship with the glucocorticoid receptor. *Science* 1987;**237**:268–275.

13 Williams JS, Williams GH. 50th anniversary of aldosterone. *J Clin Endocrinol Metab* 2003;**88**:2364–2372.

14 Boldyreff B, Wehling M. Rapid aldosterone actions: from the membrane to signaling cascades to gene transcription and physiological effects. *J Steroid Biochem Mol Biol* 2003;**85**:375–381.

15 Schafer C, Shahin V, Albermann L et al. Aldosterone signaling pathway across the nuclear envelope. *Proc Natl Acad Sci USA* 2002;**99**:7154–7159.

16 Francis GS, Benedict C, Johnstone DE et al. Comparison of neuroendocrine activation in patients with left ventricular dysfunction with and without congestive heart failure. A substudy of the Studies of Left Ventricular Dysfunction (SOLVD). *Circulation* 1990;**82**:1724–1729.

17 Weber MA, Purdy RE, Drayer JI. Interactions of mineralocorticoids and pressor agents in vascular smooth muscle. *Hypertension* 1983;**5**:I41–I46.

18 Weber MA, Purdy RE. Catecholamine-mediated constrictor effects of aldosterone on vascular smooth muscle. *Life Sci* 1982;**30**:2009–2017.

19 Latini R, Masson S, Anand I et al. The comparative prognostic value of plasma neurohormones at baseline in patients with heart failure enrolled in Val-HeFT. *Eur Heart J* 2004;**25**:292–299.

20 Hayashi M, Tsutamoto T, Wada A et al. Relationship between transcardiac extraction of aldosterone and left ventricular remodeling in patients with first acute myocardial infarction: extracting aldosterone through the heart promotes ventricular remodeling after acute myocardial infarction. *J Am Coll Cardiol* 2001;**38**:1375–1382.

21 Dzau VJ, Colucci WS, Hollenberg NK, Williams GH. Relation of the renin–angiotensin–aldosterone system to clinical state in congestive heart failure. *Circulation* 1981;**63**:645–651.

22 Schneider SW, Yano Y, Sumpio BE et al. Rapid aldosterone-induced cell volume increase of endothelial cells measured by the atomic force microscope. *Cell Biol Int* 1997;**21**:759–768.

23 Vaughan DE, Lazos SA, Tong K. Angiotensin II regulates the expression of plasminogen activator inhibitor-1 in cultured endothelial cells. A potential link between the renin-angiotensin system and thrombosis. *J Clin Invest* 1995;**95**:995–1001.

24 Brilla CG, Weber KT. Reactive and reparative myocardial fibrosis in arterial hypertension in the rat. *Cardiovasc Res* 1992;**26**:671–677.

25 Brilla CG, Pick R, Tan LB, Janicki JS, Weber KT. Remodeling of the rat right and left ventricles in experimental hypertension. *Circ Res* 1990;**67**:1355–1364.

26 Rocha R, Chander PN, Khanna K, Zuckerman A, Stier CT, Jr. Mineralocorticoid blockade reduces vascular

injury in stroke-prone hypertensive rats. *Hypertension* 1998;**31**:451–458.

27 Napoli C, Di Gregorio F, Leccese M *et al.* Evidence of exercise-induced myocardial ischemia in patients with primary aldosteronism: the Cross-sectional Primary Aldosteronism and Heart Italian Multicenter Study. *J Investig Med* 1999;**47**:212–221.

28 Sun Y, Ramires FJ, Weber KT. Fibrosis of atria and great vessels in response to angiotensin II or aldosterone infusion. *Cardiovasc Res* 1997;**35**:138–147.

29 Young M, Fullerton M, Dilley R, Funder J. Mineralocorticoids, hypertension, and cardiac fibrosis. *J Clin Invest* 1994;**93**:2578–2583.

30 Swedberg K, Eneroth P, Kjekshus J, Wilhelmsen L. Hormones regulating cardiovascular function in patients with severe congestive heart failure and their relation to mortality. CONSENSUS Trial Study Group. *Circulation* 1990;**82**:1730–1736.

31 Cohn JN, Tognoni G. A randomized trial of the angiotensin-receptor blocker valsartan in chronic heart failure. *N Engl J Med* 2001;**345**:1667–1675.

32 Wong M, Staszewsky L, Latini R *et al.* Valsartan benefits left ventricular structure and function in heart failure: Val-HeFT echocardiographic study. *J Am Coll Cardiol* 2002;**40**:970–975.

33 Cohn JN, Anand IS, Latini R, Masson S, Chiang YT, Glazer R. Sustained reduction of aldosterone in response to the angiotensin receptor blocker valsartan in patients with chronic heart failure: results from the Valsartan Heart Failure Trial. *Circulation* 2003;**108**:1306–1309.

34 Silvestre JS, Heymes C, Oubenaissa A *et al.* Activation of cardiac aldosterone production in rat myocardial infarction: effect of angiotensin II receptor blockade and role in cardiac fibrosis. *Circulation* 1999;**99**:2694–2701.

35 Duprez DA, De Buyzere ML, Rietzschel ER *et al.* Inverse relationship between aldosterone and large artery compliance in chronically treated heart failure patients. *Eur Heart J* 1998;**19**:1371–1376.

36 Borghi C, Boschi S, Ambrosioni E, Melandri G, Branzi A, Magnani B. Evidence of a partial escape of renin-angiotensin-aldosterone blockade in patients with acute myocardial infarction treated with ACE inhibitors. *J Clin Pharmacol* 1993;**33**:40–45.

37 Staessen J, Lijnen P, Fagard R, Verschueren LJ, Amery A. Rise of plasma aldosterone during long-term captopril treatment. *N Engl J Med* 1981;**304**:1110.

38 Jorde UP, Vittorio T, Katz SD, Colombo PC, Latif F, Le Jemtel TH. Elevated plasma aldosterone levels despite complete inhibition of the vascular angiotensin-converting enzyme in chronic heart failure. *Circulation* 2002;**106**:1055–1057.

39 Aldigier JC, Huang H, Dalmay F *et al.* Angiotensin-converting enzyme inhibition does not suppress plasma angiotensin II increase during exercise in humans. *J Cardiovasc Pharmacol* 1993;**21**:289–295.

40 McKelvie RS, Yusuf S, Pericak D *et al.* Comparison of candesartan, enalapril, and their combination in congestive heart failure: randomized evaluation of strategies for left ventricular dysfunction (RESOLVD) pilot study. The RESOLVD Pilot Study Investigators. *Circulation* 1999;**100**:1056–1064.

41 Tullner WW, Graff MM, Hertz R. Amphenone inhibition of adrenal corticosteroid output in the hypophysectomized dog. *Endocrinology* 1956;**58**:802–807.

42 de Gasparo M, Joss U, Ramjoue HP *et al.* Three new epoxy-spirolactone derivatives: characterization in vivo and in vitro. *J Pharmacol Exp Ther* 1987;**240**: 650–656.

43 Zillich AJ, Carter BL. Eplerenone – a novel selective aldosterone blocker. *Ann Pharmacother* 2002;**36**:1567–1576.

44 Stier CT, Jr. Eplerenone: a selective aldosterone blocker. *Cardiovasc Drug Rev* 2003;**21**:169–184.

45 Delyani JA. Mineralocorticoid receptor antagonists: the evolution of utility and pharmacology. *Kidney Int* 2000;**57**:1408–1411.

46 Delyani JA, Rocha R, Cook CS *et al.* Eplerenone: a selective aldosterone receptor antagonist (SARA). *Cardiovasc Drug Rev* 2001;**19**:185–200.

47 Tolbert D, Karim A, Cook C. SC-66110 (Eplerenone): a selective antialdosterone antagonist. Disposition kinetics in man and identification of its major CYP450 isoenzyme in its biotransformation. *AAPS PharmSci* 1998;Abstract 1155.

48 Brilla CG, Matsubara LS, Weber KT. Antifibrotic effects of spironolactone in preventing myocardial fibrosis in systemic arterial hypertension. *Am J Cardiol* 1993;**71**: 12A–16A.

49 Suzuki G, Morita H, Mishima T *et al.* Effects of long-term monotherapy with eplerenone, a novel aldosterone blocker, on progression of left ventricular dysfunction and remodeling in dogs with heart failure. *Circulation* 2002;**106**:2967–2972.

50 Van Belle E, Bauters C, Wernert N *et al.* Neointimal thickening after balloon denudation is enhanced by aldosterone and inhibited by spironolactone, and aldosterone antagonist. *Cardiovasc Res* 1995;**29**:27–32.

51 Lacolley P, Labat C, Pujol A, Delcayre C, Benetos A, Safar M. Increased carotid wall elastic modulus and fibronectin in aldosterone-salt-treated rats: effects of eplerenone. *Circulation* 2002;**106**:2848–2853.

52 Zannad F, Alla F, Dousset B, Perez A, Pitt B. Limitation of excessive extracellular matrix turnover may contribute to survival benefit of spironolactone therapy in patients with congestive heart failure: insights from the randomized aldactone evaluation study (RALES). Rales Investigators. *Circulation* 2000;**102**:2700–2706.

53 Querejeta R, Varo N, Lopez B *et al.* Serum carboxy-terminal propeptide of procollagen type I is a marker of myocardial fibrosis in hypertensive heart disease. *Circulation* 2000;**101**:1729–1735.

54 Robert V, Heymes C, Silvestre JS, Sabri A, Swynghedauw B, Delcayre C. Angiotensin AT1 receptor subtype as a cardiac target of aldosterone: role in aldosterone-salt-induced fibrosis. *Hypertension* 1999;**33**:981–986.

55 Bauersachs J, Heck M, Fraccarollo D *et al.* Addition of spironolactone to angiotensin-converting enzyme inhibition in heart failure improves endothelial vasomotor dysfunction: role of vascular superoxide anion formation and endothelial nitric oxide synthase expression. *J Am Coll Cardiol* 2002;**39**:351–358.

56 Domanski M, Norman J, Pitt B, Haigney M, Hanlon S, Peyster E. Diuretic use, progressive heart failure, and death in patients in the Studies Of Left Ventricular Dysfunction (SOLVD). *J Am Coll Cardiol* 2003;**42**: 705–708.

57 Barr CS, Lang CC, Hanson J, Arnott M, Kennedy N, Struthers AD. Effects of adding spironolactone to an angiotensin-converting enzyme inhibitor in chronic congestive heart failure secondary to coronary artery disease. *Am J Cardiol* 1995;**76**:1259–1265.

58 Cicoira M, Zanolla L, Rossi A *et al.* Long-term, dose-dependent effects of spironolactone on left ventricular function and exercise tolerance in patients with chronic heart failure. *J Am Coll Cardiol* 2002;**40**:304–310.

59 Tsutamoto T, Wada A, Maeda K *et al.* Effect of spironolactone on plasma brain natriuretic peptide and left ventricular remodeling in patients with congestive heart failure. *J Am Coll Cardiol* 2001;**37**:1228–1233.

60 Korkmaz ME, Muderrisoglu H, Ulucam M, Ozin B. Effects of spironolactone on heart rate variability and left ventricular systolic function in severe ischemic heart failure. *Am J Cardiol* 2000;**86**:649–653.

61 Feola M, Menardi E, Ribichini F *et al.* Effects of the addition of a low dose of spironolactone on brain natriuretic peptide plasma level and cardiopulmonary function in patients with moderate congestive heart failure. *Med Sci Monit* 2003;**9**:CR341–CR345.

62 MacFadyen RJ, Barr CS, Struthers AD. Aldosterone blockade reduces vascular collagen turnover, improves heart rate variability and reduces early morning rise in heart rate in heart failure patients. *Cardiovasc Res* 1997;**35**:30–34.

63 Yee KM, Pringle SD, Struthers AD. Circadian variation in the effects of aldosterone blockade on heart rate variability and QT dispersion in congestive heart failure. *J Am Coll Cardiol* 2001;**37**:1800–1807.

64 The Randomized Aldactone Evaluation Study (RALES). Effectiveness of spironolactone added to an angiotensin-converting enzyme inhibitor and a loop diuretic for severe chronic congestive heart failure. *Am J Cardiol* 1996;**78**:902–907.

65 Hunt SA, Baker DW, Chin MH *et al.* ACC/AHA Guidelines for the Evaluation and Management of Chronic Heart Failure in the Adult: Executive Summary A Report of the American College of Cardiology/American Heart Association Task Force on Practice Guidelines (Committee to Revise the 1995 Guidelines for the Evaluation and Management of Heart Failure): Developed in Collaboration With the International Society for Heart and Lung Transplantation; Endorsed by the Heart Failure Society of America. *Circulation* 2001;**104**: 2996–3007.

66 Bozkurt B, Agoston I, Knowlton AA. Complications of inappropriate use of spironolactone in heart failure: when an old medicine spirals out of new guidelines. *J Am Coll Cardiol* 2003;**41**:211–214.

67 Juurlink DN, Mamdani MM, Lee DS *et al.* Rates of hyperkalemia after publication of the Randomized Aldactone Evaluation Study. *N Engl J Med* 2004;**351**: 543–551.

68 Palmer BF. Managing hyperkalemia caused by inhibitors of the renin–angiotensin–aldosterone system. *N Engl J Med* 2004;**351**:585–592.

69 Shlipak MG. Pharmacotherapy for heart failure in patients with renal insufficiency. *Ann Intern Med* 2003;**138**:917–924.

70 Burgess E. Eplerenone in hypertension. *Expert Opin Pharmacother* 2004;**5**:2573–2581.

71 White WB, Carr AA, Krause S, Jordan R, Roniker B, Oigman W. Assessment of the novel selective aldosterone blocker eplerenone using ambulatory and clinical blood pressure in patients with systemic hypertension. *Am J Cardiol* 2003;**92**:38–42.

72 Weinberger MH. Eplerenone: a new selective aldosterone receptor antagonist. *Drugs Today (Barc)* 2004;**40**: 481–485.

73 Burgess ED, Lacourciere Y, Ruilope-Urioste LM *et al.* Long-term safety and efficacy of the selective aldosterone blocker eplerenone in patients with essential hypertension. *Clin Ther* 2003;**25**:2388–2404.

74 Flack JM, Oparil S, Pratt JH *et al.* Efficacy and tolerability of eplerenone and losartan in hypertensive black and white patients. *J Am Coll Cardiol* 2003;**41**: 1148–1155.

75 Epstein M, Buckalew V, Martinez F. Antiproteinuric efficacy of eplerenone, enalapril, and eplerenone/enalapril combination therapy in diabetic hypertensives with microalbuminuria. *Am J Hypertens* 2002;**15**:A24.

76 Pitt B, Roniker B. Eplerenone a novel selective aldosterone receptor antagonist (SARA): dose finding study in patients with heart failure. *J Am Coll Cardiol* 1999;**33**:188A–189A.

77 Hayashi M, Tsutamoto T, Wada A et al. Immediate administration of mineralocorticoid receptor antagonist spironolactone prevents post-infarct left ventricular remodeling associated with suppression of a marker of myocardial collagen synthesis in patients with first anterior acute myocardial infarction. Circulation 2003;107:2559–2565.

78 FDA Talk Paper. FDA Approves Inspra for Improving Survival of Congestive Heart Failure Patients After a Heart Attack. FDA Talk Paper. 8 October 2003. Ref Type: Electronic Citation.

79 Inspra [package insert]. http://www.inspra.com/inspra.pdf. [III]. 2003. Pharmacia.Ref Type: Electronic Citation. (Accessed 11 July 2005).

80 Pitt B. Aldosterone blockade in patients with systolic left ventricular dysfunction. Circulation 2003;108:1790–1794.

81 Hunt SA, Abraham WT, Chin MH et al. Acc/AHA 2005 Guideline update for the diagnosis and management of chronic heart failure in the adult: a report of The American College of Cardiology/American Heart Association task force on Practice guidelines (Writing Committee to update the 2001 guidelines for the evaluation and management of heart failure): developed in collaboration with the American College of Chest physicians and the International society for heart and lung transplantation: endorsed by the heart rhythm society. Circulation 2005;112:154–235.

82 Taylor CT. Eplerenone (Inspra) for hypertension. Am Fam Physician 2004;69:915–916.

83 McMurray JJ, Ostergren J, Swedberg K et al. Effects of candesartan in patients with chronic heart failure and reduced left-ventricular systolic function taking angiotensin-converting-enzyme inhibitors: the CHARM-Added trial. Lancet 2003;362:767–771.

84 Pitt B, Poole-Wilson PA, Segal R et al. Effect of losartan compared with captopril on mortality in patients with symptomatic heart failure: randomised trial–the Losartan Heart Failure Survival Study ELITE II. Lancet 2000;355:1582–1587.

85 Sun Y, Zhang J, Lu L, Chen SS, Quinn MT, Weber KT. Aldosterone-induced inflammation in the rat heart: role of oxidative stress. Am J Pathol 2002;161:1773–1781.

86 Weber KT. Extracellular matrix remodeling in heart failure: a role for de novo angiotensin II generation. Circulation 1997;96:4065–4082.

87 Syed AA, Redfern CP, Weaver JU. Aldosterone revisited. N Engl J Med 2004;351:2131–2133.

88 Pfeffer MA, Swedberg K, Granger CB et al. Effects of candesartan on mortality and morbidity in patients with chronic heart failure: the CHARM-Overall programme. Lancet 2003;362:759–766.

**CHAPTER 7**

# Inotropic therapy in clinical practice

*Sharon Rubin,* MD *& Theresa Pondok,* MD

## Introduction

For decades, inotropic therapy has been part of the pharmacologic armamentarium utilized by clinicians in the management of patients with dilated cardiomyopathy and systolic dysfunction. This approach was based on the traditional concept that heart failure was predominantly a hemodynamic problem and that impaired contractility was the underlying abnormality. Therapies directed toward improving pump function, such as inotropic agents, therefore appeared to be warranted, and these agents were evaluated in a large number of clinical trials beginning in the early 1980s. More recently, however it has been recognized that neurohormones play a pivotal role in the pathophysiology of heart failure and that blockage of neurohormonal pathways – and in particular adrenergic signaling – can improve both cardiac morphology and function [1–4].

As our understanding of the pathophysiology of heart failure has evolved, and the results of clinical trials evaluating both oral and intravenous inotropic therapy are unveiled, the role of inotropic agents in the management of the heart failure patient continues to be reevaluated. This chapter reviews both early and emerging data, evaluating the role of nonglycosidic inotropic agents in the clinical management of the heart failure patient.

## Classification of inotropes

An inotrope is defined as an agent that increases myocardial contractility resulting in a greater rate and force of contraction. The various inotropic agents under investigation or in clinical use act at key points in the complex biochemical pathways affecting the myocardial contractile state. The common mediator, which accounts for the enhancement in contractility, is an increase in the concentration or availability of calcium to the contractile proteins of the myofibril. A proposed classification scheme that categorizes inotropic therapy according to their mechanism of action on the excitation contraction pathway is given in Table 7.1. This system recognizes that an agent may possess more than one mechanism to account for their inotropic effect [5]:

| | |
|---|---|
| Class I inotropes | Increase intracellular cyclic adenosine monophosphate (cAMP) |
| Class II inotropes | Affect sarcolemmal ion, pumps, and channels |
| Class III inotropes | Increase the release or sensitization of contractile proteins to calcium. |
| Class IV inotropes | Exert multiple mechanisms of action |

## Mechanism of action and hemodynamic effects

An understanding of the mechanisms of action and hemodynamic effects of the various inotropics agents is necessary in order to apply inotropic therapy to clinical practice. Importantly, the pharmacological action of most inotropic agents also involves the peripheral vasculature, which contributes significantly to the overall hemodynamic effect produced. Intuitively, an assessment of the effects

**Table 7.1** Inotrope classification.

| Mechanism of action | Class I<br><br><br>Agents that increase cAMP | Class II<br>Agents that inhibit Na+/K+ ATPase pump | Class III<br><br>Agents that modulate intracellular calcium | Class IV<br><br>Multiple mechanisms of action |
| --- | --- | --- | --- | --- |
| Inotropic agents | Increased production of cAMP (BAR agonists)<br>Epinephrine*<br>Norepinephrine*<br>Dobutamine*<br>Dopamine*<br>Dopexamine<br>Ibopamine<br>Decreased degradation of cAMP (PDE III inhibitors)<br>amrinone<br>milrinone*<br>enoximone** | Digoxin* | Increased intracellular calcium release<br>Flosequinan<br><br>Increased calcium sensitization<br>Levosimendan** | PDE III inhibitor/Ca++ sensitizer<br>Pimobendan<br><br>PDE III inhibitor/modified rectifying K+ currents<br>Vesnarinone |

*Agents that are currently clinically used
**Agents that are currently undergoing clinical trails

of inotropic agents on cardiac hemodynamics is clinically relevant because the symptoms of heart failure are in part a reflection of altered hemodynamics and a patient's hemodynamic state is relevant to the clinical outcome, especially in hospitalized patients [6,7]. The importance of the heart failure patient's hemodynamic state is supported by data showing that an improvement in a patient's hemodynamic profile with 'tailored' medical therapy including vasodilators and diuretics is associated with improved symptoms and survival [8,9]. However, the favorable acute and chronic improvement in cardiac hemodynamics associated with the use of inotropic agents have not translated into favorable effects on morbidity or mortality [10–12]. Consequently, while an improvement in cardiac hemodynamics is important in the management of a patient with an acute exacerbation of heart failure, improved hemodynamics are not a reliable surrogate marker for long-term survival [13].

The most commonly used inotropic therapies in the heart failure patients are the class I agents, the beta-adrenergic receptor (β-AR) agonists and the phosphodiestrase (PDE) inhibitors. These agents share the common mechanism of increasing intracellular myocardial cyclic adenosine monophosphate (cAMP) levels, a second messenger in the adrenergic signaling pathway that effects both an improvement in cardiac contractility (inotropic state) and relaxation (lusitropic state). Cyclic AMP effects an increase in cardiac contractility though activation of a group of intracellular proteins including protein kinase A (PKA) and the subsequent phosphorylation of key regulatory proteins that regulate both the uptake and utilization of calcium (Figure 7.1). These proteins include the myofibril contractile protein troponin I, sarcoplasmic reticulum membrane protein phospholamban, and sarcolemmal calcium channels [14]. Phosphorylation mediated processes result in both a rise in intracellular calcium, which promotes actin and myocyte cross bridging, and the reaccummulation of calcium by the sarcoplasmic reticulum leading to an increase in the rate of myocardial relaxation [15,16].

The β-AR agonists and PDE inhibitors share a common effect on intracellular cAMP, but differ in the mechanism by which they increase levels of intracellular cAMP. The beta-adrenergic receptor pathway is initiated through agonist binding to

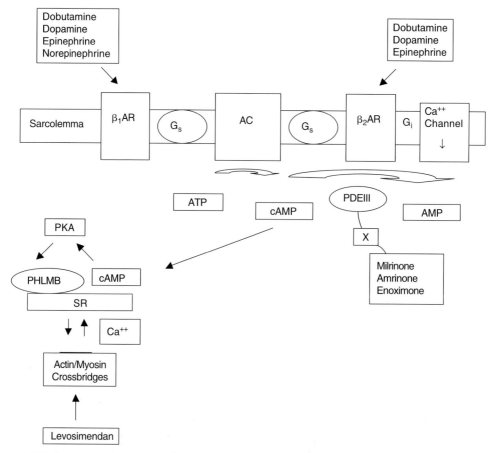

**Figure 7.1** Mechanism of action. PDE III = Phosphodiesterase III; AC = Adenylyl cyclase; cAMP = cyclic AMP; $G_s$ = G stimulatory protein; $G_i$ = G inhibitory protein; PKA = Protein kinase A; PHLMB = phosphlamban; SR = Sarcoplasmic reticulum. *Adapted from [88].

beta-receptor subtypes located on the surface of the myocyte sarcolemma (Figure 7.1). Agonist binding, mediated through guanine nucleotide-binding regulatory proteins is coupled to adenyl cyclase, the enzyme that converts ATP to cAMP resulting in increased cAMP production. In contrast, the PDE inhibitors augment intracellular cAMP by blocking cAMP degradation. PDE III inhibitors mediate this effect through inhibition of PDE III, the isoenzyme which hydrolyzes cAMP.

The overall pharmacological and hemodynamic effects of the class I inotropic agents are regulated at both the level of the heart in terms of influencing myocardial contraction as well as at the peripheral vasculature. The different β-AR agonists vary not only in their α- and β-receptor selectivity, but also in terms of their dose-dependent pharmacological responses. Importantly, in the failing heart, the pharmacological response to β-adrenergic agonists and PDE inhibitors are attenuated as compared to normals. This is a consequence of chronic adrenergic stimulation, which leads to alterations in β-receptor density, β-adrenergic responsiveness, and signal transduction [17–19].

## β-adrenergic receptor agonists

Dobutamine is one of the most commonly used inotropic agents in the treatment of patients with clinical heart failure. Dobutamine binds α- and β-receptors in the heart and peripheral vasculature; however, its predominant receptor activity is stimulation of myocardial B1 receptors. The inotropic effect of dobutamine is proportionately greater than its chronotropic effect, reflecting the stereoisomeric mixture of synthetic dobutamine and its differential binding to myocardial α- and β-receptors. Myocardial α-receptor stimulation primarily mediates an inotropic response, which in addition to the combined inotropic and chronotropic effect of β-stimulation, result in a greater increase in contractility relative to heart rate [20,21]. In the peripheral vasculature, dobutamine stimulates both α-1 and β-2 receptors, which essentially counter balance each other, resulting in minimal direct effect on systemic vascular resistance.

Hemodynamically, dobutamine effects a dose-dependent augmentation of stroke volume and cardiac index with a progressive decrease in left ventricular end-diastolic pressure and pulmonary capillary wedge pressure. Mean arterial blood pressure is usually unchanged or may slightly decrease [22–25]. This decrease in systemic vascular resistance likely reflects the withdrawal of sympathetic tone as a result of improved stroke volume [26–28]. At lower doses, dobutamine has minimal effects on heart rate; however, increases in heart rate are often seen at higher doses of dobutamine (>10 μg/kg/min) [23,28]. Although dobutamine increases coronary blood flow, in the setting of tachycardia, myocardial oxygen demand will increase and may precipitate the development of myocardial ischemia. Dobutamine increases conduction through the atrioventricular node; therefore, heart rate may increase appreciably in patients in atrial fibrillation [29]. The onset of action of dobutamine occurs within several minutes with a peak effect within 10–20 min [30]. Hemodynamic tolerance has been shown to develop with continuous dobutamine infusion after approximately 72 h [31]. In patients with chronic heart failure, the inotropic response to dobutamine may be diminished as a function of the down regulation and desensitization of myocardial β-1 adrenergic receptors as a result of prolonged receptor activation; however, improvement in cardiac function may actually decrease adrenergic drive [32,33].

Dopamine is distinct from dobutamine due to its action on dopaminergic receptors located in the renal, mesenteric, and coronary vasculature [34]. In the myocardium, dopamine stimulates both β-1 and β-2 receptors, and in the periphery dopamine acts on peripheral α-receptors.

The pharmacological effects of dopamine are highly dose dependent. At low doses (<3 μg/kg/min), dopamine primarily stimulates dopaminergic (D1) receptors found predominantly in the kidney and the splanchnic beds, thereby promoting vasodilatation and increased perfusion to vascular beds. The effect of low-dose dopamine on renal function is debatable. In the heart failure patient treated with low-dose dopamine, the improvement of renal blood flow is generally in proportion to increases in cardiac output [35–37]. At intermediate doses (2–5 μg/kg/min), dopamine stimulates β-1 receptors in the myocardium causing an increase in heart rate and contractility, which translates hemodynamically to an increase in stroke volume and cardiac output. In the periphery, higher doses of dopamine (5–15 μg/kg/min) stimulate α-receptors resulting in arterial and venous constriction. Thus, in the patient with systolic dysfunction, high concentrations of dopamine may effectively decrease stroke volume because of a marked increase in myocardial afterload [38,39].

The hemodynamic actions of dopamine and dobutamine have been compared in heart failure, and both agents have been shown to increase cardiac index. Dopamine, unlike dobutamine, produces an incremental rise in pulmonary capillary wedge pressure as the dose is increased. In addition, dopamine causes a greater increase in heart rate and systemic blood pressure as compared to dobutamine thereby increasing myocardial oxygen consumption more than dobutamine [24,28]. However, it must be noted that these studies utilized higher doses of dopamine than one might consider in practice.

Epinephrine and norepinephrine, though potent β-AR agonists, are rarely used in the management of patients with worsening heart failure. Epinephrine is a nonselective β- and α-agonist with dose-dependent receptor selectivity [14]. At low doses (0.01 to 0.05 μg/kg/min), epinephrine primarily activates β-receptors causing an increase in heart rate and contractility as well as peripheral vasodilation. Mean blood pressure is generally unchanged due to the counterbalance of the inotropic and chronotropic effects with the decrease in systemic vascular resistance. At higher doses, epinephrine stimulates peripheral α-1 receptors, which in conjunction with its agonist action on myocardial β-1 receptors will result in an increase in blood pressure. Norepinephrine, similar to epinephrine, increases heart rate and contractility via myocardial β-1 receptor activity. In the periphery, norepinephrine stimulates α-receptors, yet unlike epinephrine, lacks clinically significant peripheral β-receptor activation. Thus, the overall hemodynamic effect of norepinephrine is to increase blood pressure. In the patient with preexisting left ventricular dysfunction, the increase in afterload due to vasoconstriction is associated with a decrease in cardiac output. In patients with heart failure, the use of norepinephrine as well as epinephrine is further limited by the propensity of both agents to cause tachyarrhythmias.

## PDE inhibitors

In addition to the β-adrenergic receptor agonists, the PDE inhibitors are class I agents that are commonly used in the management of the patient with an acute exacerbation of heart failure symptoms. In cardiac myocytes and smooth muscle cells, PDE III is the isoenzyme that specifically hydrolyzes cAMP. The PDE III inhibitors block the degradation of cAMP, resulting in an increase in cAMP, a subsequent rise in intracellular calcium, and therefore an enhanced inotropic state. In vascular smooth muscle cells, the increase in cAMP results in relaxation of venous and arterial smooth muscle, which accounts for the potent vasodilatory action of PDE III inhibitors. Due to their combined inotropic and vasodilator action, the PDE III inhibitors are best characterized as inodilators. Amrinone was one of the first PDE III inhibitors evaluated in heart failure, but due to its adverse side effect profile including thrombocytopenia, gastrointestinal symptoms, and fever it has been replaced with the chemically related milrinone [40]. Enoximone, another well studied PDE III inhibitor is available in intravenous form in Europe.

The hemodynamic effects of milrinone, representative of the PDE III inhibitors, are increases in cardiac output as well as decreases in pulmonary capillary wedge pressure and pulmonary and arterial vascular resistance. Cardiac output is increased due to its direct inotropic effects as well as secondary to the decrease in afterload [41,42]. Mean blood pressure and heart rate tend to be unchanged but at higher doses (0.5 mg/kg), hypotension and tachycardia may develop [43]. Milrinone can be administered as a loading dose followed by a continuous infusion [42]. There is a dose response relationship for loading dose increments of 37.5–50 μg/kg. At higher bolus doses (50–75 μg/kg), there is less of an incremental increase in cardiac index and hypotension is more likely to occur. For this reason, milrinone is usually administered without a loading dose to avoid hypotension. Favorable hemodynamics are produced with continuous infusions of doses between 0.375 and 0.75 μg/kg/min [43]. The onset of action of milrinone is rapid: hemodynamic indices change within minutes of infusion of a bolus and the half-life is approximately 1.5–2 h [44]. Hemodynamic tolerance does not appear to occur with milrinone administered as a continuous infusion or as chronic oral therapy [45].

The hemodynamic effects of PDE III inhibitors have been compared to dobutamine. Like dobutamine, milrinone increases cardiac output and decreases pulmonary capillary wedge pressure [42]. Milrinone, as compared to dobutamine, is a more potent vasodilator and has a greater effect on lowering systemic vascular resistance, mean pulmonary artery pressure, and pulmonary capillary wedge pressure [46]. Milrinone exerts its hemodynamic effects with less effect on heart rate and myocardial oxygen demand as compared to dobutamine [45]. Dobutamine is characterized as a more powerful inotropic agent as compared to milrinone causing a greater effect on contractility as measured by changes in left ventricular pressure over time ($dP/dt$). Both agents are arrhythmogenic, similarly precipitating ventricular tachycardia [46].

The combination of dobutamine and a PDE inhibitor produce augmented hemodynamic responses – a useful effect in patients with severely compromised left ventricular function who are being bridged to either an assist device or to cardiac surgery. The addition of amrinone to dobutamine produced a higher cardiac index, and a decrease in systemic vascular resistance and left ventricular end-diastolic pressure than either agent alone [47]. Similar hemodynamic responses were seen with milrinone and enoximone in combination with dobutamine. An additional benefit of this combined therapy is a more significant decrease in pulmonary artery resistance [48,49].

## Calcium sensitizers

The class III inotropes enhance contractility through their effect on intracellular calcium homeostasis. The calcium sensitizer, levosimendan is currently approved for use in several European countries for short-term treatment of acutely decompensated heart failure. Levosimendan mediates its inotropic effect by binding and stabilizing calcium-induced conformational changes of troponin C which facilitates myofilament cross bridging and increases contractility. The advantage of this mechanism of action is that contractility is improved without the arrhythmogenic and cardiotoxic effects or increases in intracellular cAMP and calcium concentration [50,51]. Several recent reports suggest that levosimendan increases contractility without increasing myocardial oxygen demand or impairing diastolic function [51–53]. However, a well-controlled trial in a large animal model demonstrated that levosimendan effected a marked increase in oxygen consumption when compared with norepinephrine [54]. Levosimendan also functions as a vasodilator via activation of potassium dependent ATP channels and at high doses inhibits myocardial and smooth muscle PDE III [55–57]. The vasodilating property of levosimendan influence both coronary conductance and resistance arteries, and despite a decrease in coronary perfusion pressure coronary blood flow is increased. Indeed, the association of improved left ventricular systolic function and decreased myocardial oxygen extraction with levosimendan suggests improved myocardial efficiency [58].

The acute hemodynamic effects of levosimendan are a dose-dependent increase in stroke volume and cardiac index as well as decreases in pulmonary capillary wedge pressure, mean pulmonary artery pressure, and systemic vascular resistance. Increases in heart rate and decreases in mean arterial pressure may occur at higher doses ($>0.4 \, \mu g/kg/min$) [59,60]. As compared to dobutamine, levosimendan decreases pulmonary capillary wedge pressure and increases cardiac index more significantly, and is less likely to produce consequential tachycardias or hypotension [61].

Levosimendan is administered as a loading dose, followed by a continuous infusion [51]. Although the half-life of levosimendan is relatively short, the hemodynamic effects of levosimendan may be prolonged due to the presence of active metabolites [62]. In the recent SURVIVE study the drug did not improve survival at 180 days. In the REVIVE II trial, clinical signs and symptoms improved at 5 days with levosimendan; however, the number of adverse events including deaths was higher (AHA presentation). Thus, the role of levosimendan will await full publication of this data.

## Application of inotropic therapy to the heart failure patient

The spectrum of clinical manifestations of heart failure may range from shock with end-organ hypoperfusion to acute decompensated heart failure and advanced chronic refractory heart failure. Management of the heart failure patient will depend on the patient's clinical presentation and the goals of therapy. Clinical assessment of the heart failure patient is often challenged by the limited findings on physical examination [63]. The role of inotropic therapy may be viewed differently depending upon whether the goal of therapy is bridging to another therapeutic option (i.e. surgical revascularization, ventricular assist device, heart transplantation), improvement in quality of life, reduction in hospitalizations, or improving survival. Therapeutic endpoints need to be individualized and based upon the patient's personal wishes blended with medically realistic goals.

### Acute decompensated heart failure

Although inotropes have been shown to exert favorable hemodynamic effects, the role of inotropic therapy in the overall management of the patient with acute decompensated heart failure is poorly defined. Historically, inotropes have been utilized in the patient with 'acutely decompensated heart failure' with little evidence-based guidance. Whereas guidelines for the management of chronic heart failure have been established, strategies for the management of patients with acutely decompensated heart failure have not been formally agreed upon [64]. The therapeutic approach to the patient with acutely decompensated heart failure is challenged by the lack of a clear definition of this syndrome and/or an agreed upon classification system [65]. Acutely decompensated heart failure represents a heterogeneous clinical spectrum with patients presenting with a wide range of symptoms reflective of varying abnormalities of volume status and peripheral perfusion. Therefore, designing clinical trials to evaluate appropriate therapeutic options including inotropic therapy in the patient with acutely decompensated heart failure is complex. Clinical trials randomizing patients with acute decompensation to noninotropic therapy is further complicated by the potential reluctance of physicians to withhold inotropic therapy.

In clinical practice, the term 'acute decompensation' is commonly applied to the patient who presents with newly diagnosed heart failure or an acute exacerbation of chronic heart failure. The role for inotropic therapy in the patient with acute decompensation is dependent on the etiology of the decompensation and the clinical manifestations of the patient's volume status and peripheral perfusion. Characterizing the patient's presentation into a hemodynamic profile based on a clinical assessment of the patient's volume status and cardiac output provides one strategy to guide therapeutic options [66].

The decision to initiate inotropic support as well as the choice of therapy will be dependent on the presence and magnitude of end organ hypoperfusion.

In the patient who presents with acute decompensation and a maintained blood pressure, inotropic therapy is not necessarily required to preserve adequate cardiac output. Intravenous vasodilator therapy alone may improve cardiac output with a lower likelihood of precipitating arrhythmias [67–69].

In the patient with evidence of end organ hypoperfusion despite other therapeutic interventions, inotropic support will be needed. The impact of short-term inotropic therapy on long-term outcome in this clinical scenario though is unclear. Given that inotropic therapy has not been proven to have a beneficial effect on mortality, and data suggests that long-term inotropic support impacts negatively on survival, inotropic therapy in the

patient with acute decompensated heart failure is utilized as a bridge to alternative medical or surgical therapeutic measures [11].

Due to their favorable hemodynamic effects, dobutamine and milrinone are the most commonly used therapies in the patient with low cardiac output heart failure. There are no large prospective randomized trials comparing the use of dobutamine and milrinone on clinical outcomes in these patients. Both dobutamine and milrinone when used as short-term inotropic support have been shown to successfully facilitate the initiation and titration of oral vasodilator therapy [70–72]. Based on retrospective data, there are no significant differences between milrinone and dobutamine in terms of clinical outcomes such as incidence of arrhythmia, renal failure, heart transplant listing, or inhospital mortality rate [46]. Observational data suggests that milrinone may be advantageous over dobutamine in the hemodynamic support of patients waiting for heart transplantation based upon the lower likelihood of milrinone supported patients requiring mechanical support to bridge successfully to heart transplantation [73]. One small randomized prospective study, however, comparing milrinone to dobutamine in patients awaiting heart transplantation found no difference in the need for mechanical support between the two agents [74]. The combination of a PDE inhibitor and dobutamine should be considered if the hemodynamic response of either agent alone is suboptimal. This combination of inotropes results in a more significant increase in cardiac index and decrease in systemic vascular resistance [47,48].

An important point with clinical relevance is the differing duration of action between dobutamine and milrinone. The short duration of action and half-life of dobutamine is unchanged in patients with low output heart failure. Therefore, in the event of significant side effects, the adverse effects of dobutamine will dissipate quickly with discontinuation [30]. Milrinone, in contrast, has a longer duration of action than dobutamine and its effects will not be as readily reversed. Importantly, the half-life of milrinone is increased in patients with renal insufficiency and dose reductions are needed to avoid significant adverse effects such as hypotension or tachyarrhythmias. In patients with significant renal impairment (creatinine clearance <30 mL/min), milrinone infusions of <0.50 µg/min/kg are recommended [75].

The calcium sensitizer levosimendan may be an alternative to dobutamine in the treatment of patients with low output heart failure. The hemodynamic effects of levosimendan appear to be favorable compared to dobutamine. Patients with low output heart failure treated with levosimendan were shown to have a decrease in mortality at 6 months as compared to treatment with dobutamine or placebo [61,76]. However, the long half-life of levosimendan and the increased cost that will incur with a new agent may be important points to consider in choosing an inotropic agent. Furthermore, well-controlled and adequately sized clinical trials will be required to better assess its efficacy and utility in the heart failure patients. The REVIVE (Randomized Multicenter Evaluation of Intravenous Levosimendan Efficacy Versus Placebo in the Short-term Treatment of Decompensated Heart Failure) trial is currently underway in the United States to evaluate the mortality benefit of levosimendan in patients with left ventricular dysfunction and acute decompensated heart failure.

The patient with acute decompensated heart failure who is hypotensive may require alternative inotropic agents for blood pressure support. In the heart failure patient with shock, the management of inotropic therapy will be best determined by the patient's cardiac output in relation to the patient's systemic vascular resistance and filling pressures. Therefore, right heart catheterization is often necessary to optimize therapy. Although data suggest that the use of a pulmonary artery catheter in critically ill patients may increase morbidity and mortality, this may not broadly apply to the hypotensive heart failure patient [77]. Right heart catheterization is not useful for the management of patients with mild to moderate exacerbations of heart failure and should not be used routinely; however, the distinction between cardiogenic and noncardiogenic causes of hypotension as well as guidance of pharmacologic therapy are considered appropriate indications [78,79]. In the hypotensive heart failure patient, dopamine initiated at moderate doses (5 µg/kg/min) is an appropriate inotropic agent. The addition of dobutamine may need to be considered to offset the rise in left ventricular

filling pressure associated with increasing doses of dopamine [80]. Dopamine will act to support blood pressure with dobutamine minimizing the elevation in filling pressures potentially caused by dopamine alone [81]. If the patient remains hypotensive despite increasing doses of dopamine or in combination with dobutamine, a more potent vasoconstricting agent such as norepinephrine may be needed in order to support blood pressure. The consequence of the beneficial effect of norepinephrine on blood pressure is excessive vasoconstriction, which may negate the effect of enhanced contractility. Additionally, renal perfusion is often worsened by the vasoconstrictive actions of norepinephrine, which limit its use in the heart failure patient.

A large subset of patients with left ventricular dysfunction will present with acute decompensated heart failure without overt signs of end organ hypoperfusion. In clinical practice, inotropic therapy has been historically utilized without evidence-based guidance. The OPTIME-CHF (Outcomes of a Prospective Trial of Intravenous Milrinone for Exacerbations of Chronic Heart Failure) trial is the only large randomized trial published to evaluate the outcome of patients with acute decompensated heart failure treated with short-term intravenous inotropes [82]. In this trial, the use of milrinone compared to placebo had no significant effect on number of days hospitalized, mortality either in hospital or at 60 days, or the need for hospital readmission. Hypotension and atrial arrhythmias were more common in the milrinone treated patients. Based on this study, the routine use of empiric inotropic therapy in the patient with acute decompensated heart failure offered no significant benefit with the potential cost of increased morbidity. It is important to recognize that in this trial, patients were excluded if inotropic therapy was required based on the treating physician's opinion. Therefore, although OPTIME-CHF was a well-designed trial, an inherent patient selection bias existed. Interestingly, in the OPTIME-CHF trial the etiology of the patient's heart failure may have played a role in the response to milrinone. Patients with ischemic heart failure appeared to have a deleterious response to milrinone, whereas the patients with nonischemic etiology may have had a beneficial response to milrinone [83]. This study underscores both the challenge and need for well-designed clinical trials to evaluate the appropriate role of inotropic therapy in patients with acute decompensated heart failure.

An important factor that will influence the choice of inotropic therapy is the patient's background medical therapy at the time of their clinical decompensation. Based on clinical trials, which have shown a mortality benefit, β-blockers are standard of care therapy in patients with left ventricular dysfunction [3,84,85]. Given the widespread use of β-blockers, there is an increased likelihood that a patient who presents in acute decompensated heart failure will be receiving concomitant therapy with a β-blocker.

The hemodynamic response to different inotropic therapies will be altered in patients on chronic β-blocker therapy depending on the specificity of the β-blocker in use. Heart failure patients pretreated with the nonselective β-blocker carvedilol will require higher doses of dobutamine (15–20 μg/kg/min) to achieve an increase in cardiac index as compared to patients not treated with carvedilol. The high doses of dobutamine required to overcome the β-blockade results in an increase in mean arterial blood pressure and increases in systemic and pulmonary vascular resistance, which may be explained by the persistent blockade of the vascular BAR but not the α-1 adrenergic receptors by carvedilol [84]. This is related to the decrease in α-1 antagonist activity of carvedilol over time, as well the binding affinity of carvedilol to the α-receptor is less than that of the β-1 receptor [85].

The hemodynamic response to dobutamine is less affected in patients taking the β-1 selective agent metoprolol as background therapy. Dobutamine administered to these patients will cause the expected increase in the cardiac index seen in patients not receiving metoprolol. The decline in mean pulmonary artery and pulmonary capillary wedge pressures, however, will be less pronounced [86–88]. In contrast, the hemodynamic effects of the PDE inhibitor, enoximone, have been shown to be unaffected and may be enhanced in patients on concurrent β-blockers regardless of the selectivity of the β-blocker [86–88]. A PDE inhibitor, therefore, should be considered the inotropic agent of choice in the patient who presents with low output heart failure in the setting of background β-blocker therapy. The beneficial hemodynamic effects of levosimendan also appear to be unaffected by β-blocker therapy [61].

## Inotropic therapy in chronic heart failure

### Oral inotropic therapy

In patients with chronic heart failure, the ideal goal of therapy is to prolong survival. Large randomized prospective placebo-controlled trials have evaluated the survival benefit of oral nonglycosidic inotropic therapy in patients with chronic symptomatic heart failure (Table 7.2). These trials included different classes of inotropic agents and have

**Table 7.2** Oral inotropic therapy trials.

| Drug | Study | Number of patients | Mechanism | Mortality |
|------|-------|--------------------|-----------|-----------|
| Digoxin | (DIG) | 6800 | Na/K ATPase inhibitor | Neutral |
| Vesnarinone | (VEST) | 3833 | PDE inhibitor | Increased |
| Ibopamine | (PRIME II) | 1906 | Potassium channel adrenergic receptor agonist | Increased |
| Milrinone | (PROMISE) | 1088 | PDE inhibitor | Increased |
| Xamoterol | | 516 | Partial adrenergic agonist | Increased |
| Pimobendan | (PICO) | 317 | PDE inhibitor Calcium sensitizer | Increased |
| Enoximone | | 102(32) | PDE inhibitor | Increased |

demonstrated an increase in mortality attributed to proarrhythmic or potentially cardiotoxic effects [10–12,89,90]. Digoxin is the only oral inotrope that has been shown to have a neutral effect on survival in a large randomized placebo-controlled trial [91].

One issue raised from the earlier oral inotropic trials is the relationship between the dose of the inotrope studied and mortality [11,90,91]. The PDE inhibitor, enoximone was shown to increase mortality in patients treated with high doses, whereas lower doses of enoximone (25–50 mg three times a day) in previous studies appeared to be well tolerated without an adverse effect on survival [10,92,93]. This prompted a reevaluation of the role of the oral inotropic therapy enoximone in patients with severe symptomatic heart failure. The ESSENTIAL (The Studies of Oral Enoximone Therapy in Advanced Heart Failure) trials, two clinical trials, differing only in geographic location were recently completed. Preliminary data suggests that in the overall study population, enoximone neither improved nor worsened the risk of a patient either dying or being hospitalized during the course of the trial. Surprisingly, enoximone also had no effect on quality of life or symptomatology. As a result, the sponsor has discontinued its development in the United States (Bristow MR, personal communication).

## Chronic intravenous inotropic therapy

As compared to the clinical trials assessing the efficacy of oral inotropic therapy, there are no large prospective randomized placebo-controlled mortality trials evaluating the effect of intravenous inotropic therapies administered intermittently or continuously in patients with chronic heart failure. Early studies utilized intermittent dobutamine therapy based on the rationale that although dobutamine has a short half-life, the hemodynamic effects may persist up to 30 min after an infusion is discontinued and clinical improvement in terms of functional status may be sustained for at least 1 week after discontinuation [92]. Most of the published data are predominantly open-labeled observational studies utilizing intravenous dobutamine and milrinone [95–97,108,110]. Trial comparisons are difficult due to variations in the dose of

inotrope administered, duration of infusion, time interval between infusions, and patient laboratory monitoring. The largest placebo-controlled trial evaluating intermittent dobutamine included 60 patients and an increase in mortality was seen in the dobutamine treated patients [98]. Subsequent placebo-controlled trials included smaller number of patients and significant effects on mortality were not clearly evident [99–102]. Regardless of the results of these trials, the FDA recently recommended that intermittent intravenous inotropic therapy not be used in the therapy of patients with chronic heart failure and recent consensus guidelines have supported this admonition.

The effect of a chronic continuous inotropic therapy on mortality also has not been well studied in a large prospective placebo-controlled trial. A retrospective analysis of patients enrolled in the FIRST (Flolan International Randomized Survival Trial) trial who were on continuous dobutamine had an increased mortality compared to the patients who were not treated with dobutamine raising concern of the increased risk associated with chronic inotropic infusion [103]. Therefore, if an improvement in survival is the goal of treatment in patients with chronic heart failure, there is no available data to support the use of intermittent or continuous intravenous inotropic therapy as definitive therapy.

Although it has been well-established from clinical trials that β-blocker therapy prolongs survival in patients with left ventricular dysfunction, β-blockers are not always tolerated in patients with chronic heart failure. An important potential role of inotropic therapy is to stabilize patients with chronic heart failure to allow for the initiation of β-blocker therapy. This strategy offers the advantage of an inotrope to provide hemodynamic stabilization combined with the long term biologic benefits of β-blockade. Phosphodiesterase inhibitors are a rational choice of inotropic agent because they maintain their beneficial hemodynamic effect in heart failure patients treated with β-blockers [86–88]. The addition of metoprolol was shown to be well-tolerated in a group of patients with refractory severe heart failure treated with enoximone and allowed for the discontinuation of inotropic therapy in almost half of the patients [104]. The EMPOWER (Enoximone Plus Extended-Release

Metoprolol Succinate in Subjects with Advanced Chronic Heart Failure) study was a clinical trial to evaluate the potential of enoximone to increase the tolerability of continuous release metoprolol in patients previously intolerant to β-blocker therapy. Unfortunately, this trial was also stopped in response to the recent results from the ESSENTIAL trial.

Patients with severe refractory heart failure symptoms may not view survival as their primary objective, and an improvement in their quality of life may be of greater importance and worth trading for length of life [105]. The oral inotropic trials have shown inconsistent results in regard to quality of life parameters. Small, yet significant increases in exercise time was observed in patients treated with pimobendan without an improvement in overall symptoms [106]. An improvement in symptoms was seen in patients treated with xamoterol, a β blocking drug with intrinsic sympathomimetic activity, yet there was no change in exercise time [107]. Short-lived improvements in quality of life scores were observed in patients treated with vesnarinone, yet no symptom improvement was demonstrated in patients treated with oral milrinone [11,90]. Therefore, the effects of oral inotropic therapy on quality of life parameters are variable.

The impact of intermittent inotropic therapy on quality of life parameters is challenged by the lack of large-scaled prospective placebo-controlled trials. Published case studies and small placebo-controlled trials have suggested favorable results in terms of improvements in exercise tolerance and decreases in the frequency of hospitalizations [98,102,108,109]. However, as noted above, intermittent inotropic therapy is not viewed as an acceptable therapeutic intervention in patients with heart failure.

In clinical practice, continuous inotropic infusions are often utilized in patients with severe heart failure symptoms refractory to other therapies. These patients may be labeled as 'inotrope dependent' although this term is not universally defined. Many patients initially deemed inotrope dependent can be successfully transitioned to oral vasodilator therapy under careful hemodynamic guidance [110]. A potential alternative for these patients is the use of a low dose oral inotropic agent to wean a patient from intravenous therapy. Low dose enoximone therapy (EMOTE trial) improved the success of weaning patients from intravenous inotropic therapy with no significant increase in mortality and offers the advantage of eliminating catheter related morbidity [111]. Interestingly, in the EMOTE trial, nearly 50% of patients were able to be successfully weaned from continuous intravenous inotropic support in the group randomized to placebo, suggesting that physicians may overestimate the 'inotrope-dependency' of their patients.

Despite aggressive medical optimization with oral medications, a subset of patients deteriorate when inotropes are withdrawn. The patient who experiences an improvement in their quality of life with continuous inotropic therapy in the hospital therapy may wish to continue inotropic support at home. The role of inotropic therapy in this clinical scenario must be individualized and based on the patient's understanding that their perceived improvement in quality of life may be in exchange for length of life. In individual patients, when one compares the interval of time before the initiation of inotropic therapy to the period during which inotropes are administered, reductions in hospital admissions, length of stay, and cost of care as well as an improvement in functional class may be seen [108,112]. Continuous inotropic infusion in this clinical scenario is considered an accepted form of palliative care [64].

## Conclusion

The role of inotropic therapy in patients with systolic dysfunction continues to evolve as our understanding of the pathophysiology of the heart failure syndrome progresses. In the patient with severe heart failure, inotropic support may be necessary for hemodynamic stabilization. There is limited data to guide the use of inotropic therapy in the patient with acutely decompensated heart failure and chronic inotropic therapy has been associated with an increase in mortality. Novel inotropic agents are under investigation that may provide the benefit of hemodynamic improvement without adverse effects. Additionally, efforts continue at developing the 'perfect inotrope', that is, one that improves cardiac function and decreases morbidity without adversely influencing mortality. Future clinical trials may further clarify the appropriate application of inotropic therapy in the management of the heart failure patient.

## References

1 Packer, M. The Neurohormonal Hypothesis: A theory to explain the mechanism of disease progression in heart failure. *J Am Coll Cardiol* 1992;**20**:248–254.

2 The SOLVD Investigators. Effect of enalapril on survival in patients with reduced left ventricular ejection fractions and congestive heart failure. *N Engl J Med* 1991;**325**:293–302.

3 MERIT-HF Study Group. Effect of metoprolol CR/XL in chronic heart failure: Metoprolol CR/XL Randomized Intervention Trial in Congestive Heart Failure. (MERIT-HF) *Lancet* 1999;**353**:2001–2007.

4 Pitt B, Zannad F, Remme WJ *et al.* The effect of spironolactone on morbidity and mortality in patients with severe heart failure. *N Engl J Med* 1999;**341**:709–717.

5 Feldman AM. Classification of positive inotropic agents. *J Am Coll Cardiol* 1993;**22**:1223–1227.

6 Campana C, Gavazzi A, Berzuini C *et al.* Predictors of prognosis in patients awaiting heart transplantation. *J Heart Lung Transplant* 1993;**12**:756–765.

7 Unverferth DV, Magorien RD, Moeschberger ML *et al.* Factors influencing the one-year mortality of dilated cardiomyopathy. *Am J Cardiol* 1984;**54**:147–152.

8 Steimle AE, Stevenson LW, Chelimsky-Fallick C *et al.* Sustained hemodynamic efficacy of therapy tailored to reduce filling pressures in survivors with advanced heart failure. *Circulation* 1997;**96**:1165–1172.

9 Stevenson LW, Tillisch JH, Hamilton M *et al.* Importance of hemodynamic response to therapy in predicting survival with ejection fraction less than or equal to 20% secondary to ischemic or nonischemic dilated cardiomyopathy. *Am J Cardiol* 1990;**66**:1348–1354.

10 Uretsky, BF, Jessup M, Konstam MA *et al.* Multicenter trial of oral enoximone in patients with moderate to moderately severe congestive heart failure: Lack of benefit compared to placebo. *Circulation* 1990;**82**:774–780.

11 Packer M, Carver JR, Rodeheffer RJ *et al.* Effect of oral milrinone on mortality in severe chronic heart failure. *N Engl J Med* 1991;**325**:1468–1475.

12 Hampton JR, van Veldhuisen DJ, Kleber FX *et al.* Randomized study of effect of ibopamine on survival in patients with advanced severe heart failure. *Lancet* 1997;**349**:971–977.

13 Anand IS, Florea VG, Fisher L. Surrogate end points in heart failure. *J Am Coll Cardiol* 2002;**39**:1414–1421.

14 Myers CW and Rocco TP. Pharmacology of cardiac contractility. In: Golan DE, Tashjian AH, Armstrong EJ *et al.* eds. *Principals of Pharmacology.* Lippincott William & Wilkins, Philadelphia, 2005; 285–297.

15 Carroll JD, Lang RM, Neumann AL *et al.* The differential effects of positive inotropic and vasodilator therapy on diastolic properties in patients with congestive cardiomyopathy. *Circulation* 1986;**74**:815–825.

16 Monrad ES, McKay RG, Baim DS *et al.* Improvement in indexes of diastolic performance in patients with congestive heart failure treated with milrinone. *Circulation* 1984;**70**:1030–1037.

17 Feldman AM, Copelas L, Gwathmey JK *et al.* Deficient production of cyclic AMP: Pharmacologic evidence of an important cause of contractile dysfunction in patients with end-stage heart failure. *Circulation* 1987;**75**:331–339.

18 Fowler MB, Laser JA, Hopkins GL *et al.* Assessment of the beta adrenergic pathway in the intact failing heart: Progressive receptor down-regulation and sub-sensitivity to agonist response. *Circulation* 1986;**74**:1290–1302.

19 Bristow MR, Ginsburg R, Minobe W *et al.* Decreased catecholamine sensitivity and beta adrenergic receptor density in failing human hearts. *N Engl J Med* 1982;**307**:205–211.

20 Ruffolo RR, Spradlin TA, Pollack GD *et al.* Alpha and beta adrenergic effects of the stereoisomers of dobutamine. *J Pharmacol Exp Ther* 1982;**219**:447–452.

21 Lawless CE, Loeb HS. Pharmacokinetics and pharmacodynamics of dobutamine. In: Chatterjee K, ed. *Dobutamine: A Ten-Year Review.* NCM Publishers, New York, 1989:33–47.

22 Leier CV. Acute inotropic support. In: Leier CV, ed. *Cardiotonic Drugs.* Marcel Dekker, New York, 1991:63–105.

23 Biddle TL, Benotti JR, Creager MA *et al.* Comparison of Intravenous Milrinone and Dobutamine for Congestive Heart Failure Secondary to Either Ischemic or Dilated Cardiomyopathy *Am J Cardiol* 1987;**59**:1345–1350.

24 Stoner JD, Bolen JL, Harrison DC. Comparison of dobutamine and dopamine in treatment of severe heart failure. *Br Heart J* 1977;**39**:536–539.

25 Colucci WC, Wright RF, Jaski BE. Milrinone and dobutamine in severe heart failure: differing hemodynamic effects and individual patient responsiveness. *Circulation* 1986;**73**:175–183.

26 Liang CS, Hood WB Jr: Dobutamine infusion in conscious dogs with and without autonomic nervous system inhibition: Effects of systemic hemodynamics, regional blood flows and cardiac metabolism. *J Pharmacol Exp Ther* 1979;**211**:698–705.

27 Al-Hesayen A, Azeved ER, Newton GE *et al.* The effects of dobutamine n cardiac sympathetic activity in

patients with congestive heart failure. *J Am Coll Cardiol* 2002;**39**:1269–1274.

28  Leier CV, Heban PT, Huss P *et al.* Comparative systemic and regional hemodyamic effects of dopamine and dobutamine in patients with cardiomyopathic heart failure. *Circulation* 1978; 58: 466-475.

29  Bianchi C, Diaz T, Gonzales C, and Beregovich J. Effects of dobutamine on atria-ventricular conduction. *Am Heart J* 1975;**90**:474–478.

30  Kates RE, Leier CV. Dobutamine pharmacokinetics in severe heart failure. *Clin Pharmacol Ther* 1978;**24**:537–541.

31  Unverferth DV, Blanford M, Kates RE, Leier CV. Tolerance to dobutamine after 72 hour continuous infusion. *Am J Med* 1980;**69**:262–266.

32  Fowler MB, Laser JA, Hopkins GL *et al.* Assessment of the Beta adrenergic receptor pathway in the intact failing human heart: Progressive receptor down-regulation and sub-sensitivity to agonist response. *Circulation* 1986;**74**:1290–1302.

33  Bristow MR, Ginsburg R, Minobe W *et al.* Decreased catecholamine sensitivity and b-adrenergic receptor density in failing human hearts. *N Engl J Med* 1982;**307**:205–211.

34  Goldberg LI. Cardiovascular and renal applications of dopamine: Potential clinical applications. *Pharmacol Rev* 1972;**24**:1–29.

35  Leier CV, Heban PT, Huss P *et al.* Comparative systemic and regional hemodynamic effects of dopamine and dobutamine in patients with cardiomyopathic heart failure. *Circulation* 1978;**58**:466–475.

36  Beregovich J, Bianchi C, Rubler S *et al.* Dose-related hemodynamic and renal effects of dopamine in congestive heart failure. *Am Heart J* 1974;**87**:550–557

37  Stevenson LW. Clinical use of inotropic therapy for heart failure: Looking backward or forward? Part I: Intropic infusions during hospitalization. *Circulation* 2003;**108**:367–380.

38  Goldberg LI. Dopamine: clinical uses of an endogenous catecholamine. *N Engl J Med* 1974;**291**:707–710.

39  Goldberg LI, Hsieh Y, Resnekov L. Newer catecholamines for treatment of heart failure and shock: an update on dopamine and a first look at dobutamine. *Prog Cardiovasc Dis* 1977;**19**:327.

40  Wilsmhurst PT, Webb-Peploe MM. Side effects of amrinone therapy. *Br Heart J* 1983;**49**:447–451.

41  Simonton CA, Chatterjee K, Cody RJ *et al.* Milrinone in congestive heart failure: acute and chronic hemodynamic and clinical evaluation. *J Am Coll Cardiol* 1985;**6**:453–459.

42  Shipley JB, Tolman D, Hastillo A, Hess ML. Review: milrinone: basic and clinical pharmacology and acute and chronic management. *Am J Med Sci* 1996;**311**:286–291.

43  Anderson JL for the United States Milrinone Multicenter Investigators. Hemodynamic and clinical benefits with intravenous milrinone in severe chronic heart failure: Results of a Multicenter study in the United States. *Am Heart J* 1991;**121**:1956–1964.

44  Benotto JR, Lesko LJ, McCue JE *et al.* Pharmacokinetics and pharmacodynamics of milrinone in chronic congestive heart failure. *Am J Cardiol* 1985;**56**:685–689.

45  Monrad ES, Baim DS, Smith HS *et al.* Milrinone, dobutamine and nitroprusside: comparative effects on hemodynamics and myocardial energetics in patients with severe congestive heart failure. *Circulation* 1986;**74**:168–174.

46  Yomani MH, Haji SA, Starling FC *et al.* Comparison of dobutamine-based and milrinone- based therapy for advanced decompensated congestive heart failure: Hemodynamic efficacy, clinical outcome, and economic impact. *Am Heart J* 2001;**142**:998–1002.

47  Gage J, Rutman H, Lucid D, LeJemtel TH, Additive effects of dobutamine and amrinone on myocardial contractility and ventricular performance in patients with severe heart failure. *Circulation* 1986;**74**:367–373.

48  Thuillez C, Richard C, Teboul JL *et al.* Arterial hemodynamics and cardiac effects of enoximone, dobutamine and their combination in severe heart failure. *Am Heart J* 1993;**125**:799–808.

49  Meissner A, Herrman G, Gerdesmeyer L, Simon R. Additive effects of milrinone and dobutamine in severe heart failure. *Z Kardiol* 1992;**81**:266–271.

50  Haikala H , Kaivola J, Nissinen E *et al.* Cardiac troponin C as a target protein for a novel calcium sensitizing drug levosimendan. *J Mol Cell Cardiol* 1995;**27**:1859–1866.

51  Figgitt DP, Gillies PS, Goa KL. Levosimendan *Drugs* 2001;**61**:613–617.

52  Cleland JG, McGowan J. Levosimendan: a new era for inodilator therapy for heart failure? *Curr Opin Cardiol* 2002;**17**:257–265.

53  Janssen PM, Datz N, Zeitz, Hasenfuss. Levosimendan improves diastolic and systolic function in failing human myocardium. *Eur J Pharmacol* 2000;**404**:191–199.

54  Todaka K, Wang J, Yi GH *et al.* Effects of levosimendan on myocardial contractility and oxygen consumption. *J Pharmacol Exp Ther* 1996;**279**:120–127.

55  Michaels AD, McKeown B, Kostal M *et al.* Effects of intravenous levosimendan on human coronary vasomotor regulation, left ventricular wall stress, and myocardial oxygen uptake. *Circulation* 2005;**111**:1504–1509.

56  Yokoshiki H, Katsube Y, Sunagawa M *et al.* The novel calcium sensitizer levosimendan activates the ATP-sensitive $K^+$ Channels in rat ventricular cells. *J Pharmacol Exp Ther* 1997;**283**:375–383.

57 Sato S. Talukder MA, Sugawara H *et al.* Effects of levosimendan on myocardial contractility and $Ca^{2+}$ transients in aequorin-loaded right ventricular papillary muscles and indo-1-loaded single ventricular cardiomyocytes of the rabbit. *J Mol Cell Cardiol* 1998;**30**:1115–1128.

58 Gruhn N, Nielson-Kudsk JE, Theilgaard S *et al.* Coronary vasorelaxant effect of levosimendan, a new inodilator with calcium-sensitizing properties. *J Cardiovasc Pharmacol* 1998;**31**:741–749.

59 Slawsky MT, Colucci WS, Gottlieb SS *et al.* Acute hemodynamic and clinical effects of levosimendan in patients with severe heart failure. *Circulation* 2000;**102**: 2222–2227.

60 Nieminen MS, Akkila J, Hasenfuss G *et al.* Hemodynamic and neurohumeral effects of continuous infusion of levosimendan in patients with congestive heart failure. *J Am Coll Cardiol* 2000;**36**:1903–1912.

61 Follath F, Cleland JGF, Just H *et al.* Efficacy and safety of intravenous levosimendan compared with dobutamine in severe low-output heart failure (the LIDO study): a randomized double-blind trial. *Lancet* 2002;**360**: 196–202.

62 Kivikko M, Lechtonen L, Colucci WS. Sustained hemodynamic effects of levosimendan. *Circulation* 2003;**107**:81–86.

63 Stevenson, LW, Perloff JK. *JAMA* 1989;**261**:884–888.

64 Hunt SA, Baker WD, Chin MH *et al.* ACC-AHA guidelines for the evaluation and management of chronic heart failure in the adult: executive summary. *J Am Coll Cardiol* 2001;**38**:2101–2113.

65 Felker GM, Adams KF, Konstam MA. The problem of decompensated heart failure: Nomenclature, classification, and risk stratification. *Am Heart J* 2003, **145**:S18–25.

66 Stevenson LW. Tailored therapy to hemodynamic goal for advanced heart failure. *Eur Heart J* 1999, **1**: 251–257.

67 Colucci WS, Elkayam U, Horton DP *et al.* Intravenous nesiritide, a natriuretic petide, in the treatment of decompensated congestive heart failure. *NEJM* 2000;**343**:246–253.

68 Capomolla S, Pozzoli M, Opasich C *et al.* Dobutamine and nitroprusside infusion in patients with severe congestive heart failure: Hemodynamic improvement by discordant effects on mitral regurgitation, left atrial function and ventricular function. *Am Heart J* 1997;**134**:1089–1098.

69 Burger AJ, Elkayam U, Neibaur MT *et al.* Comparison of the occurrence of ventricular arrhythmias in patients with acutely decompensated congestive heart failure receiving dobutamine versus nesiritide therapy. *Am J Cardiol* 2001;**88**:35–39.

70 Levine TB, Levine AB, Elliott WG *et al.* Dobutamine as bridge to angiotensin- converting enzymes inhibitor-nitrate therapy in endstage heart heart failure. *Clin Cardiol* 2001, **24**:231–236.

71 Cusick DA, Pfeifer PB and Quigg RJ. Effects of intravenous milrinone followed by titration of high-dose oral vasodilator therapy on cinical outcome and rehospitalization rates in patients with severe heart failure. *Am J Cardiol* 1998;**82**:1060–1065.

72 Quigg, RJ. Rationale for the short-term use of intravenous milrinone under hemodynamic guidance in patients with severe systolic heart failure. *Congest Heart Fail* 2000;**6**:202–214.

73 Mehra MR, Ventura HO, Kapoor C *et al.* Safety and clinical utility of long term intravenous milrinone in advanced heart failure *Am J Cardiol* 1997;**80**:61–64.

74 Aranda JM, Schofield RS, Pauly DF *et al.* Comparison of dobutamine versus milrinone therapy in hospitalized patients awaiting cardiac transplantation: a prospective, randomized trial. *Am Heart J* 2003;**145**:324–329.

75 Woolfrey SG, Hegbrant J, Thysell H *et al.* Dose regimen adjustment for milrinone in congestive heart faillure patients with moderate and severe renal failure. *J Pharm Pharmacol* 1995; Aug;**47**:651–655.

76 Zaires MN, Apostolatos C, Anastasiadis P *et al.* The effect of a calcium sensitizer or an inotrope or none in chronic low output decompensated heart failure: results from the Calcium Sensitizer or Inotrope or None in Low Output Heart Failure Study (CASINO) Abstract 835–836. *J Am Coll Cardiol* 2004;**43**:206A.

77 Connors AF, Jr, Spleroff T, Dawson NV *et al.* The effectiveness of right heart catheterization in the initial care of critically ill patients. SUPPORT Investigators. *JAMA* 1996, **276**:889–897.

78 Mueller HS, Chatterjee K, Davis K *et al.* Present use of bedside right heart catheterization in patients with cardiac disease. *J Am Coll Cardiol* 1998;**32**: 840–864.

79 Shah, MR and Stevenson LW. Escape: Evaluation Study of Congestive Heart Failure and Pulmonary Artery Catheterization Effectiveness. Presented at American Heart Association 2004 Annual Scientific Sessions.

80 Francis GS, Sharma B and Hodges M. Comparative hemodynamic effects of dopamine and dobutamine in patients with acute cardiogenic circulatory collapse. *Am Heart J* 1982;**103**:995–1000.

81 Richard C, Ricome JL, Rimailho A *et al.* Combined hemodynamic effects of dopamine and dobutamine in cardiogenic shock. *Circulation* 1983;**67**:620–626.

82 Cuffe, MS, Califf RM, Adams KF *et al.* Short-term intravenous milrinone for the acute exacerbation of chronic heart failure: a randomized controlled trial. *JAMA* 2002;**287**:1541–1547.

83 Felker GM, Benza RL, Chandler AB *et al.* Heart failure etiology and response to milrinone in decompensated heart failure: results from the OPTIME-CHF study. *J Am Coll Cardiol* 2003;**41**:997–1003.

84 Packer M, Bristow MR, Cohn JN *et al.* The effect of carvedilol on morbidity and mortality in patients with chronic heart failure. *N Engl J Med* 1996;**334**: 1349–1355.

85 CIBIS-II Investigators and Committees: The Cardiac Insufficiency Bisoprolol Study II (CIBIS-II): A randomized trial. *Lancet* 1999;**353**:9–13.

86 Metra M, Nodari S, D 'Aloia A *et al.* Beta-blocker therapy influences the hemodynamic response to inotropic agents in patients with heart failure. *J Am Coll Cardiol* 2002;**40**:1248–1258.

87 Bristow MR. Beta-adrenergic receptor blockade in chronic heart failure. *Circulation* 2000;**101**:558–569.

88 Lowes BD, Smon MA ,Tsvetkova TO *et al.* Inotropes in the beta-blocker era. *Clin Cardiol* 2000;**23**:11–16.

89 Xamoterol in Severe Heart Failure Study Group. Xamoterol in severe heart failure. *Lancet* 1990;**336**: 1–6.

90 Feldman AM, Bristow MR, Parmley WW *et al.* Effects of vesnarinone on morbidity and mortality in patients with heart failure. *N Engl J Med* 1993;**329**: 149–155.

91 Digitalis Investigation Group. The effect of digoxin on mortality and morbidity in patients with heart failure. *N Engl J Med* 1997;**336**:525–533.

92 Lowes, BD, Higginbotham M, Petrovich L *et al.* Low dose enoximone improves exercise capacity in chronic heart failure. *J Am Coll Cardiol* 2000;**36**:501–508.

93 Naranhara KA, Western Enoximone Study Group. Oral enoximone therapy in chronic heart failure: a placebo-controlled randomized trial. *Am Heart J* 1991;**21**: 1471–1479.

94 Leier CV, Webel J and Bush CA. The cardiovascular effects of the continuous infusion of dobutamine in patients with severe cardiac failure. *Circulation* 1977;**56**:468–472.

95 Young JB and Moen EK; Outpatient parenteral inotropic therapy for advanced heart failure. *J Heart Lung Transpl* 2000;**19**:S49–S57.

96 Applefeld MM, Newman KA, Sutton FJ *et al.* Outpatient dobutamine and dopamine infusions in the management of chronic heart failure: clinical experience in 21 patients. *Am Heart J* 1987;**114**:589–595.

97 Miller LW. Outpatient dobutamine for refractory congestive heart failure: advantages, techniques and results *J Heart Lung Transpl* 1991;**10**:482–487.

98 Dies F, Krell MJ, Whitlow P *et al.* Intermittent dobutamine in ambulatory outpatients with chronic cardiac failure. *Circulation* 1986;**74**:II–38.

99 Leier CV, Webel J and Bush CA. The Cardiovascular effects of the continuous infusion of dobutamine in patients with severe cardiac failure. *Circulation* 1977;**56**:468–472.

100 Erlemeier HH, Kupper W, Bleifeld W. Intermittent infusion of dobutamine in the therapy of severe congestive heart failure-long term effects and lack of tolerance. *Cardiovasc Drugs Ther* 1992;**6**:391–398.

101 Elis A, Bental T, Kimchi O *et al.* Intermittent dobutamine treatment in patients with chronic refractory congestive heart failure: a randomized, double blind, placebo-controlled study. *Clin Pharmacol Ther* 1998;**63**: 682–685.

102 Olivia F, Latini R, Politi A *et al.* Intermittent 6-month low dose dobutamine infusion in severe heart failure: DICE Multicenter Trial. *Am Heart J* 1999;**138**: 247–253.

103 O'Connor CM, Gattis WA, Uretsky BF *et al.* Continuous intravenous dobutamine is associated with an increased risk of death in patients with advanced heart failure: Insights from the Flolan International randomized Survival Trial (FIRST). *Am Heart J* 1999;**138**: 78–86.

104 Shakar SF, Abraham WT, Gilbert EM *et al.* Combined oral positive inotropic and beta-blocker therapy for treatment of refractory class IV heart failure. *J Am Coll Cardiol* 1998;**31**:1336–1340.

105 Lewis EF, Johnson PA, Johnson W *et al.* Preferences for quality of life or survival expressed by patients with heart failure. *J Heart Lung Transpl* 2001;**20**: 1016–1024.

106 Pimobendan in Congestive Heart Failure (PICO) Investigators. Effect of pimobendan on exercise capacity in patients with heart failure: Main results from the Pimobendan in congestive heart failure (PICO) Trial. *Heart* 1996;**76**:223–231.

107 Xamoterol in Severe Heart Failure Study Group. Xamoterol in severe heart failure. *Lancet* 1990;**336**: 1–6.

108 Marius-Nunez AL, Heaney L, Fernandez RN *et al.* Intermittent inotropic therapy in an outpatient setting: A cost-effective therapeutic modality in patients with refractory heart failure. *Am Heart J* 1996;**132**: 805–808.

109 Cesario D, Clark J, Maisel A. Beneficial effects of intermittent home administration of the inotrope/vasodilator milrinone in patients with end-stage congestive heart failure: a preliminary study. *Am Heart J* 1998;**135**:121–129.

110 Stevenson LW, Dracup KA, Tillisch JH. Efficacy of medical therapy tailored for severe congestive heart failure in patients transferred for urgent cardiac transplantation. *Am J Cardiol* 1989;**63**:461–464.

111  Feldman AM. Oral enoximone in intravenous inotrope-dependent subjects (EMOTE): a phase III, randomized double-blind, placebo-controlled parallel study. Late-Breaking and Recent Clinical Trials. Presented at the 8th Annual Scientific Meeting of the Heart Failure Society of America; 12–15 September 2004 Toronto, Ontario, Canada.

112  Kishore HJ, Mandeep MR, Ventura HO *et al.* Home inotropic Therapy in Advanced Heart Failure: Cost Analysis and Clinical Outcomes. *Chest* 1997;**112**:1298–1303.

**CHAPTER 8**

# Antiarrhythmic therapy in heart failure

*Igino Contrafatto,* MD *& Leslie A. Saxon,* MD

## Introduction

Patients with cardiac dilatation and systolic dysfunction commonly present with ventricular arrhythmias or with supraventricular tachyarrhythmias. The former are associated with an increase in mortality while the latter may result in cardiac decompensation or worsening symptoms. While sudden death, a common feature of heart failure, is most often thought to be due to a ventricular tachyarrhythmia the event may also be caused by ischemic events, electrolyte disturbances, vascular events or bradyarrhythmias, and other pulseless supraventricular rhythms. The recent demonstration that implantable-cardiac defibrillators (ICD) can prolong survival in patients with compromised left ventricular function due to either coronary artery disease or idiopathic dilated cardiomyopathy has provided the first definitive therapy for treating ventricular arrhythmias occurring in the setting of heart failure. However, clinical trial data still suggests that a substantial number of patients are treated with antiarrhythmic agents even if an ICD is in place. Furthermore, while ICD's can effect benefit in patients with ventricular tachyarrhythmias, other important forms of rhythm disturbances including atrial fibrillation and other supra-ventricular arrhythmias may require pharmacologic treatment. Finally, pharmacologic therapy may be effective in decreasing the firing rate and prolonging battery life in patients with ICD's. Therefore, this chapter will discuss the relationship between arrhythmias and outcomes in patients with heart failure and present data regarding the effectiveness of antiarrhythmic therapy in the treatment of patients with left ventricular dysfunction.

## Premature ventricular beats and nonsustained ventricular tachycardia: prevalence and implications

The prevalence of both symptomatic and asymptomatic ventricular arrhythmias is very high in patients with the clinical syndrome of heart failure (HF). Early studies, using ambulatory ECG monitoring, revealed the presence of ventricular couplets, multiform premature ventricular contractions (PVCs), or both in up to 87% of patients with HF. The occurrence of nonsustained ventricular tachycardia (NSVT) was observed in 54% of patients. Interestingly, the prevalence of asymptomatic nonsustained ventricular arrhythmias was not correlated with the severity of heart failure [1]. In more recent studies performed in HF patients, treated with background medical therapy consisting of angiotensin-converting enzyme (ACE) inhibitor in association with beta-receptor blockade, the prevalence of ventricular arrhythmias is very similar to that observed prior to adoption of these therapies. Ventricular couplets are present in 85% of patients and NSVT in 61% of patients with NYHA class III/IV HF, detected on ambulatory ECG screening [2].

In the majority of patients, the occurrence of PVCs or NSVT is asymptomatic so that the clinical significance and treatment implications rest on the potential for the ventricular arrhythmias to predict adverse clinical events. Whether the presence of ventricular arrhythmias observed represent a marker of disease severity or an independent predictor of increased risk of events is unknown. The relationship between the presence of asymptomatic ventricular arrhythmias and subsequent risk of sudden death have been extensively explored, but studies have reached conflicting conclusions regarding the role of ventricular arrhythmias and mortality risk in patients with HF [1–9].

In the 1980s, several studies showed a direct relationship between complex arrhythmias (PVCs, couplets, and NSVT) and subsequent mortality risk in patients with left ventricular dysfunction, and this association was established for both sudden and nonsudden modes of cardiac death and for both ischemic and nonischemic etiologies of left ventricular dysfunction [3–7]. In these early studies, the standard medical treatments for HF did not include ACE inhibitor and beta-receptor blockade therapy, and the primary etiology of HF was mostly due to nonischemic factors, such as arterial hypertension [8]; while contemporary HF patients are more likely to have ischemic left ventricular dysfunction [9]. Conversely, many subsequent studies did not identify asymptomatic ventricular arrhythmias as independent predictor of mortality in HF patients. These data also suggested that as HF severity increased, the predominant mode of death was due to pump dysfunction rather than sudden death, which was more prevalent in less severe symptom class HF [10].

In a recent study, involving 1080 patients with advanced heart failure (NYHA class III–IV), 290 deaths were observed over a 21-month follow-up period and 139 (48%) of these were classified as sudden death. Multivariate analysis did not identify the presence of asymptomatic ventricular arrhythmias as an independent predictor of sudden death and the detection of ventricular arrhythmias did not provide other significant incremental prognostic information [2]. The mechanism of sudden death in patients with HF may not be solely due to ventricular tachyarrhythmias. In a group of 216 patients with advanced HF hospitalized for evaluation for cardiac transplantation (mean LVEF 18% ± 8%), Luu et al. reviewed the causes of 20 inhospital cardiac arrests and found that bradycardia or electromechanical dissociation was the cause of death in 13 patients (62%) and ventricular tachycardia or fibrillation (VT/VF) in the other (38%). Interestingly, the patients who suffered a bradycardia/electromechanical

dissociation arrest were similar to those who had a VT/VF arrest with respect to age, ventricular arrhythmia history, ventricular function, and serum potassium levels. Only the serum sodium levels were significantly lower in patients with bradycardia/electromechanical dissociation arrests [11]. Similarly, the characteristics of an observed NSVT event such as rapid rate and prolonged duration did not appear to independently identify an increased risk of death. In the CHF-STAT study of low-dose amiodarone versus placebo in patients with mild to severe NYHA symptom class HF, there was an 80% incidence of NSVT on 24-h ambulatory Holter among 674 patients. The incidence of NSVT was similar in NYHA class II, III, and IV patients. Those patients with short duration of NSVT (3–14 beats) versus those with longer duration (≥15 beats) of NSVT did not differ by risk. Similarly, the rate of the NSVT did not predict risk (slow NSVT at 100–120 bpm versus NSVT >120 bpm). In this study only left ventricular ejection fraction was identified as an independent predictor of sudden death [12].

As mentioned above, the mode of cardiac death appears to differ according to the severity of the symptoms' class in heart failure populations studied. The risk of sudden death is relatively higher in NYHA functional class I and II, and accounts for 50–60% of all deaths. The primary mode of death in more advanced symptom class HF is pump failure, and sudden death accounts for only 20–40% of deaths, although the yearly mortality is much higher [10,13].

## Antiarrhythmic agents classification

Antiarrhythmic agents have traditionally been grouped according to their mechanism of action. A classification system proposed by Vaughan–Williams, and widely used, subdivides drugs into four broad classes according to their effects on the myocardium, particularly the myocardial cell action potential [14] (Table 8.1). A more modern view is that all antiarrhythmic agents exercise their effects by interacting with specific membrane cell's targets. The most important target of these agents is the ion channel, the pore-forming protein structure that controls the ionic currents flowing

**Table 8.1** Vaughan–Williams classification of antiarrhythmic drugs.

| Class | Effect on myocardial cell | Electrophysiologic effect | Drug |
|---|---|---|---|
| I | Blockade of $Na^+$ channels | Slow conduction velocity | A: Quinidine, Procainamide, Disopyramide |
| | | | B: Lidocaine, Mexiletine, Tocainide, Phenytoin |
| | | | C: Flecainide, Encainide, Propafenone, Moricizine |
| II | Blockade of $\beta$-receptors | Antiadrenergic effect | Metoprolol, Atenolol, Carvedilol, Bisoprolol, Propranolol |
| III | Blockade of $K^+$ channels | Prolong repolarization phase | Amiodarone, Bretylium, Sotalol, Dofetilide, Ibutilide, Azimilide |
| IV | Blockade of $Ca^{++}$ channels | Slow heart rate and AV nodal conduction | Diltiazem, Verapamil |

during the action potential and drug specificity is a property of drugs that are able to target a single population of ion channels. The Vaughan–Williams classification has been useful for clinicians to the extent that it has allowed prediction of patient's response to a given antiarrhythmic agent that can often be measured by changes on the surface ECG. However, it has received criticism because many drugs have been found to have more than one effect, or, like digoxin, have an antiarrhythmic effect not included in the classification. For example, quinidine has both class I and III effects, while amiodarone has multiple class actions. In addition, some drugs, like amiodarone, exert other important pharmacological actions such as inhibition of specific metabolic pathways, alteration of hemodynamic status, and interaction with thyroid hormone receptors. A strength of the Vaughan–Williams classification is that drugs of a common class frequently exhibit similar toxicities, most notably proarrhythmia. Proarrhythmia is defined as the potential for an antiarrhythmic agent to cause a new arrhythmia or worsened arrhythmia.

Class I agents are associated with increased mortality, when compared to placebo in patients with HF or ischemic ventricular dysfunction, when used to prevent or treat ventricular or supraventricular arrhythmias. Patients receiving class I antiarrhythmic agents for atrial fibrillation (AF) and who had a history of HF have been shown to have a threefold risk of cardiac death and a sixfold risk of arrhythmic death presumably attributed to ventricular proarrhythmia [15]. An extensive discussion of these agents used in HF patients is given in later sections.

Class II antiarrhythmic agents, the beta-receptor blocking agents, reduce all-cause and sudden mortality and improve the functional class and LV systolic function [10,16]. At present, only three beta-receptor blocking agents, carvedilol, metoprolol, and bisoprolol have demonstrated a mortality benefit in patients with HF in well-conducted placebo-controlled trials [10,17–20] (Table 8.2). Other $\beta$-receptor blocking agents may have no beneficial or even an adverse effect on mortality. This may be particularly true in $\beta$-blockers with a sympathomimetic effect, such as xamoterol and possibly bucindolol [24,37,38].

The class III antiarrhythmic agents are currently the most valuable treatment option for achieving both efficacy and safety in patients with HF. The main effects of class III antiarrhythmic agents are exerted through action on the potassium-channel in the myocardial cell membrane, and most of the antiarrhythmic agents of this class block the rapid component of the delayed potassium-channel rectifier ($IK_r$) thereby prolonging the action potential duration through a prolongation of the repolarization period. This action results in prolongation of the QT interval on the ECG [39]. Prolongation of repolarization leads to an increase in the refractory period and limits the time in which the myocytes can be stimulated. Excessive prolongation of ventricular repolarization period may induce early afterdepolarizations, which are the primary trigger for *torsade de pointes* or polymorphic VT.

Among the class III antiarrhythmic agents, amiodarone has the best efficacy profile for treating both atrial and ventricular arrhythmias in HF, and decreases heart failure hospitalization risk [29,30]. A meta-analysis of 13 trials of low-dose

**Table 8.2** Clinical trials of antiarrhythmic drugs (class I–IV) and digoxin in patients with CHF and/or LV dysfunction.

| Trial | Number of patients | Drug tested | Entry criteria | Primary endpoint | Results |
|---|---|---|---|---|---|
| **Class I sodium-channel blockers** | | | | | |
| CAST I [21] | 1498 | Encainide/ flecainide/placebo | MI, PVCs, EF $\leq$ 55% ($\leq$40% if MI $\geq$90 days) | Arrhythmic death | Premature termination (increased mortality in encanide and flecainide groups) |
| CAST II [22] | 1325 | Moricizine/placebo | MI, PVCs, EF $\leq$ 55% ($\leq$40% if MI $\geq$90 days) | Total mortality | Premature termination (increased mortality in moricizine group) |
| CASH [23] | 153 | Propafenone/ICD | Survivors of cardiac arrest (mean EF 43%) | Total mortality or recurrence cardiac arrest | Premature termination (increased mortality in propafenone group) |
| **Class II $\beta$-blockers** | | | | | |
| US Carvedilol [17] | 1094 | Carvedilol/placebo | Mild, moderate, or severe heart failure, EF $\leq$ 35% | Death or hospitalization for card reasons | Premature termination due to reduction mortality in the carvedilol group |
| MERIT-HF [10] | 3991 | Metoprolol/placebo | NYHA II–IV and EF $\leq$ 40% | Total mortality | Premature termination due to reduction mortality in the metoprolol group |
| CIBIS-II [20] | 2647 | Bisoprolol/placebo | NYHA III/IV and EF $\leq$ 35% | Total mortality | Premature termination due to reduction mortality in the bisoprolol group |
| CAPRICORN [18] | 1959 | Carvedilol/placebo | MI with EF $\leq$ 40% | Total mortality or hospitalization for card reasons | Primary end point neutral but all-cause mortality alone reduced in carvedilol treated patients |
| BEST [24] | 2708 | Bucindolol/placebo | NYHA III/IV and EF $\leq$ 35% | Total mortality | Premature termination because no difference in mortality was found |
| COPERNICUS [19] | 2289 | Carvedilol/placebo | NYHA III/IV and EF $\leq$ 25% | | Mortality reduction on carvedilol |
| **Class III potassium-channel blockers** | | | | | |
| SWORD [25] | 3121 | d-sotalol/placebo | MI and EF$\leq$40% (if remote MI: history of heart failure) | Total mortality | Premature termination because of increased mortality in the d-sotalol group |
| EMIAT [26] | 1486 | Amiodarone/ placebo | MI with EF$\leq$40% | Total mortality | No effect on total mortality |

*Continued*

**Table 8.2** Continued.

| Trial | Number of patients | Drug tested | Entry criteria | Primary end point | Results |
|---|---|---|---|---|---|
| DIAMOND-MI [27] | 1510 | Dofetilide/placebo | Recent MI with EF≤40% | Total mortality | No effect on total mortality |
| ALIVE [28] | 3717 | Azimilide/placebo | MI and EF≤15% and low heart rate variability | Total mortality | No effect on total mortality |
| GESICA [29] | 516 | Amiodarone/ controls (no placebo) | NYHA II–IV and EF≤35% | Total mortality | Mortality reduction on amiodarone |
| STAT-CHF [30] | 674 | Amiodarone/ placebo | NYHA I–IV and EF≤40% | Total mortality | No effect on total mortality |
| DIAMOND-CHF [31] | 1518 | Dofetilide/ placebo | NYHA III–IV and EF≤35% within1month | Total mortality | No effect on total mortality |
| SCD-HeFT [32] | 1692 | Amiodarone/ placebo/ICD | NYHA II–III and EF≤35% | Total mortality | No benefit of Amiodarone on mortality |
| **Class IV calcium-channel blockers** | | | | | |
| MDPIT [33] | 2466 | Diltiazem/placebo | Previous MI | Total mortality and reinfarction | Overall neutral, but more cardiac events in patients with anterior-lateral Q MI and EF ≤ 40% |
| DAVIT II [34] | 1775 | Verapamil/placebo | Acute MI | Total mortality and reinfarction | Neutral in subgroup with heart failure |
| **Digoxin** | | | | | |
| DIG [35] | 6800 | Digoxin/placebo | HF and EF≤45% | Total mortality or hospitalization | Neutral on mortality, but reduced rate of hospitalization in digoxin treatment |

*Source:* Adapted from [36].

amiodarone found that amiodarone therapy results in a decreased mortality risk in patients with HF (4% per year versus 5.7% per year in controls [40]). However, most of these trials did not have a placebo control group and were performed in the late 1980s early 90s when the use of $\beta$-receptor blockers was still uncommon. While amiodarone is a class III antiarrhythmic agent, it also has additional effects on the fast sodium and slow calcium channels as well as a noncompetitive $\beta$-blocker effect [41]. Experimentally, amiodarone has been shown to abolish calcium-dependant early afterdepolarization and this may explain the lower incidence of proarrhythmia associated with its use [42,43]. The antiadrenergic effects of amiodarone can be used to slow heart rate in severely decompensated HF patients deemed to be unsuitable for $\beta$-blocker therapy [44]. The direct effects of amiodarone to decrease sympathetic nerve activity to a similar extent to that of $\beta$-blockers has been demonstrated using nuclear MIBG scanning ($I^{123}$-metaiodobenzylguanidine) in patients with dilated cardiomyopathy [45]. Amiodarone use also decreases serum levels of brain natriuretic peptide (BNP), reduces heart rate as well as the frequency of PVCs [46].

Chronic amiodarone use does have several adverse effects and the most serious of them is pulmonary toxicity, which occurs most commonly at moderately high doses. Low-dose amiodarone is better tolerated but it is not free of adverse effects. In a meta-analysis involving 1465 patients on chronic maintenance amiodarone dose $\leq$400 mg/day (mean daily dose range 152–330 mg), a mean follow-up of 12 months, the odds of developing adverse effects was significant for thyroid (odds ratio, OR 4.2), neurologic (OR 2.0), skin (OR 2.5), ocular (OR 3.4), and bradycardic (OR 2.2) events. A trend toward increased odds of pulmonary toxicity was also noted (OR 2.0), but this did not reach statistical significance ($p = 0.07$). The incidence of amiodarone discontinuation was 22.9% (OR 1.52, $p = 0.003$ [47]).

Dofetilide is a novel, class III antiarrhythmic drug that selectively inhibits the rapid component of the delayed rectifier potassium current and prolongs the refractory period. As a pure class III agent, it has no negative inotropic effects even in patients with markedly reduced left ventricular function and does not affect cardiac conduction or sinus-node function [48]. In patients with AF/flutter, dofetilide has been shown to restore and chronically maintain sinus rhythm in 31–54% of treated patients, with higher efficacy among patients with atrial flutter [48,49]. In patients with advanced cardiac HF, dofetilide does not appear to increase mortality. In the DIAMOND study, dofetilide significantly reduced the overall risk of hospitalization for worsening HF regardless of whether AF was present or absent at baseline. Among patients with AF at baseline, after 1 month of therapy with dofetilide, 12% had conversion to sinus rhythm (versus 1% with placebo). Among patients in sinus rhythm at baseline, AF developed less frequently with dofetilide than with placebo (11 of 556 patients versus 35 of 534 patients, $p < 0.001$) over a follow-up of 18 months [31]. The main adverse effect of dofetilide is a proarrhythmic effect. In the DIAMOND study, 3.3% of patients developed *torsade de pointes* and in 76% of these patients the arrhythmia occurred within 3 days following the initiation of therapy. This is consistent with the observation that the peak increase in the corrected QT interval occurs within the first days of treatment with dofetilide.

Sotalol in its *d*-enantiomeric form (*d*-sotalol) is a pure, class III antiarrhythmic agent, whic blocks

only the rapid component of the delayed IK$_r$. Unlike the commercially available *dl*-sotalol, *d*-sotalol has no $\beta$-receptor blocking effect. Unfortunately, the slow component of the delayed potassium rectifier (IK$_s$), which is not blocked by dofetilide and *d*-sotalol, is activated more at increased heart rate and increased levels of catecholamines. Thus, these drugs may inadequately protect patients at risk of arrhythmias provoked by ischemia and/or sympathetic stimulation. *d*-Sotalol is not approved for use as it has been shown to increase mortality, compared to placebo, in patients with left ventricular dysfunction [25].

Other class III agents such as azimilide and ambasilide block both the slow and rapid components of the delayed potassium rectifier (IK$_r$ + IK$_s$), therefore theoretically have additional protective potential against arrhythmias provoked by sympathetic stimulation and/or increased heart rate. Azimilide has shown a neutral effect on mortality in patients with depressed LV function [50] and is effective in AF prevention or treatment in these patients [28] (Table 8.2). Dronedarone is a noniodinated amiodarone derivative with little effect on thyroid receptors but may have adverse effects in HF patients [51].

The class IV antiarrhythmic drugs encompass two cardioselective calcium antagonists, diltiazem and verapamil. These agents have never found a place in the treatment of patients with HF, due to their negative inotropic effects. The testing of these two agents has been performed primarily in post-MI patients with or without reduced LV systolic function because of the drugs' vasodilatory properties. While the Multicenter Diltiazem Post-Infarction Trial (MDPIT) showed a direct harmful effect of diltiazem in post-MI patients with HF, the Danish Verapamil Infarction Trial II (DAVIT II) showed a neutral effect of verapamil in similar population [33,34].

## Other drugs used in HF with antiarrhythmic properties

Digoxin is used extensively in the treatment of HF for its positive inotropic and AV nodal blocking effects (see Chapter 2). The mechanism of action of digoxin is due to the inhibition of sodium–potassium (Na$^+$–K$^+$) ATPase, which in myocardial cells leads to slowing of A–V conduction and an increase in contractility. The ATPase inhibitory effects of digoxin are also present in other organs. These effects include the inhibition of ATPase in vagal afferent fibers and the kidneys. These effects may benefit the HF patients by attenuating activation of the neurohormonal system [52]. Proarrhythmic risks associated with *Digitalis* use, primarily observed at excessive serum levels, include both sino-atrial and A–V block as well as ventricular tachyarrhythmias. The only large survival study of digoxin versus placebo in HF showed no beneficial effect on total mortality [35] (Table 8.2). Digoxin use was compared to placebo in 6800 patients; death from worsening HF was reduced by 12%, but was offset by a similar increase in presumed arrhythmic death. Based on this study, digoxin should not be used with the aim of increasing survival in HF but may play a role in patients who are receiving optimal medical therapy yet are still symptomatic [53].

## Use of antiarrhythmic drug therapy and relation to outcomes

The relationship between PVC's or NSVT as a marker of risk for total and sudden death mortality was an established observation for post-MI patients with ventricular dysfunction, prior to the emergence of thrombolytic therapy for acute MI [3]. In the 1990s, studies were performed in this patient population, utilizing antiarrhythmic drug therapy, to determine if arrhythmia suppression would reduce the risk. This strategy of PVC suppression

to reduce mortality risk was referred to as the 'PVC Hypothesis' [21,22,25,30] (Table 8.2). The initial trials enrolled patients with depressed LVEF, without specifically targeting those with HF. Two well-conducted blinded, randomized, and controlled trials of prophylactic antiarrhythmic drug therapy were the Cardiac Arrhythmia Suppression Trials I and II (CAST). In the initial open-label phase of these studies, the class I antiarrhythmic drugs Encainide, Flecainide, and Moricizine had to be effective in suppressing ventricular arrhythmias in post-MI patients with mild to moderate reduction of LV function. Patients were subsequently randomized to the effective drug versus placebo. These studies were prematurely terminated due to excess mortality in the drug treatment arms [21,22]. The etiology of the increased risk of death was thought to be due to drug-induced proarrhythmia occurring in the setting of infarct scar and recurrent ischemia. These studies were critical to dispensing the PVC hypothesis and lead to a tendency toward not treating asymptomatic NSVT in patients with ischemic LV dysfunction.

Figure 8.1 summarizes the results of trials studying the effects of antiarrhythmic drugs to reduce mortality after MI. Only $\beta$-receptor blocking agents, amiodarone and dofetilide are associated with improved outcome. Propafenone, a class I antiarrhythmic agent, was tested in the CASH study against Amiodarone and the ICD in cardiac arrest survivors. All patients had a reduced LVEF at randomization. The propafenone arm was terminated after 11 months because the total mortality

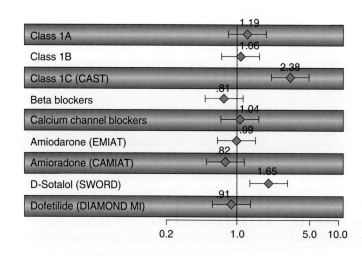

**Figure 8.1** Summary of the effects of antiarrhythmic agent on mortality in post-MI patients. (Adapted from Echt [21], Waldo 1996, Julian 1997, Kober 2000 [25–27], Cairns 1997 [54].)

and recurrence of cardiac arrest were significantly higher than in ICD-treated patients (23% and 12% versus 0%); and at 2 years mortality was significantly reduced in the ICD group compared also to the amiodarone treatment group (12.6% versus 19.6%) [23].

Four large-scale clinical trials have evaluated class III antiarrhythmic agents for primary prevention of death in HF patients [25,29–31]. In the STAT-CHF study low-dose amiodarone versus placebo was tested in 674 patients with HF and asymptomatic ventricular arrhythmias [30]. There was no significant difference in overall mortality between the two treatment groups, despite amiodarone's effectiveness in suppressing ventricular arrhythmias. Amiodarone also significantly increased the LVEF by 42% at 2 years. However, there was a trend towards combined reduction in hospitalizations and cardiac death, which was significant in patients with nonischemic cardiomyopathy in the amiodarone treated group (relative risk 0.56, $p = 0.01$). In the GESICA study, amiodarone was tested in an open label, randomized protocol, in 516 patients with advanced HF [29]. There were 87 deaths in the amiodarone group (33.5%) compared to 106 in the control group (41.4%) (risk reduction 28%, $p = 0.024$). There was a nonsignificant reduction in sudden death (risk reduction 27%, $p = 0.16$). The decrease in mortality was independent of the presence of NSVT. Side effects of amiodarone were reported in 17 patients (6.1%), and it was withdrawn in 12 patients. The majority of patients randomized to the STAT-CHF trial had an ischemic etiology of HF. This is in contrast to the GESICA trial where the majority of patients had nonischemic cardiomyopathy.

In the SWORD study, the class III agent $d$-sotalol, was tested in survivors of MI with left ventricular dysfunction (EF $\leq$ 40%) and a history of overt HF. The study was prematurely terminated because of the higher mortality in the $d$-sotalol group (5% versus 3.1%) [25]. In the DIAMOND-CHF study, the effect of dofetilide on survival was compared to placebo. No overall effect was seen on mortality. However, significant beneficial effects of dofetilide on morbidity were observed – the overall risk of hospitalization for worsening heart failure was reduced – regardless of whether AF was present or absent at baseline. In patients in AF at randomization, conversion to sinus rhythm after 1 month of treatment was 12% with dofetilide versus 1% with placebo. The recurrence or new onset of AF was also significantly reduced in the dofetilide group (11 of 556 patients versus 35 of 534 placebo treated patients, $p < 0.001$) [31].

Until the recent Sudden Cardiac Death Heart failure Trial (SCD-HeFT) [32], it appeared that low-dose amiodarone had a role in the treatment of patients with nonischemic cardiomyopathy for primary prevention indications. However, the SCD-HeFT investigators found no mortality benefit to low-dose amiodarone versus placebo therapy in patients with moderate HF due to both ischemic and nonischemic etiologies. The ICD demonstrated a 23% reduction in mortality risk compared to placebo over a 48 months follow-up [32].

There are many large studies evaluating the use of $\beta$-receptor blocking therapy that have demonstrated its efficacy for mortality and sudden death reduction in HF patients, most likely due to the favorable effects of $\beta$-blockade on attenuating neurohormonal activation rather than arrhythmia suppression (Table 8.2). Beta-receptors blocker therapies, along with the use of ACE inhibitors and aldosterone antagonists, have resulted in a significant improvement in HF survival over the past two decades with a 5-year-adjusted survival of 52% in 1996–2000 versus 43% in 1979–84 [55]. However, in HF patients with a history of VT/VF or a positive electrophysiologic study after MI, the ICD is superior therapy compared to amiodarone, sotalol, or propafenone [23,56–58]. The clinical trials of primary prevention with ICD or CRT–D (cardiac resynchronization therapy defibrillator therapy) when added to established medical therapy for HF show a further improvement in survival [32,59–61].

## Other indications for antiarrhythmic agent therapy

With the increase in the number of patients eligible for a primary prevention ICD, the number of patients that may require additional antiarrhythmic drug treatment for arrhythmia suppression may also increase. Since the goal of arrhythmia management is to provide symptomatic arrhythmia control, the use of combined therapy for patients

**Table 8.3** Trials of antiarrhythmics in reducing ICD therapies.

| Trial | Drug | Result |
|---|---|---|
| AVID [56] | Amiodarone 42%<br>Others 58$ | Reduction in number of shocks (↓ 1.4)<br>Increase time to shock (3.9→11 months) |
| CASCADE [64] | Amiodarone | Reduction shocks and syncopal shocks |
| Pacifico 1999 [65] | Sotalolo | Reduction shock (48% RR)<br>Reduction inappropriate shocks |
| Singer 2004 [67] | Azimilide/placebo | Reduction shock/year (36→9) |

with persistent sustained VT is between 40% and 70% of ICD patients [62]. There are other several reasons to consider adding an antiarrhythmic agent in patients with an ICD. These include prevention of recurrences of arrhythmias, hence reduction in the frequency of ICD discharge, reduction in the spontaneous ventricular tachycardia rate to permit an effective antitachycardia pacing from the ICD, and reduction of AF or other supraventricular tachycardias that may induce inappropriate shocks. Additionally, antiarrhythmic agent drug therapy may render some VT more amenable to ablative therapy. However, antiarrhythmic drug use in ICD patients can also have deleterious effects. They include proarrhythmia, slowing of the spontaneous VT rate below the rate of detection of the ICD, rendering previously effective antitachycardia pacing ineffective, elevating defibrillation thresholds, altering the sensing capability of the device by altering native QRS morphology, slowing the heart rate, and deterioration of quality of life [63]. Thus, antiarrhythmic therapy even in the presence of an ICD must be used with great caution.

The potential of an antiarrhythmic agent to increase ventricular defibrillation thresholds is present with the use of amiodarone and this may require retesting the ICD after initiating this agent. However, studies have still shown potential benefit in patients with an ICD. For example, in the AVID trial, the addition of antiarrhythmic drug to ICD therapy was associated with a significant increase in the time to the next arrhythmic event (3.9 months before drug to 11.2 months after drug) and a reduction in the number of ICD shocks (1.4 fewer shocks, $p = 0.05$). In 42% of cases the added antiarrhythmic agent was amiodarone [52] (Table 8.3). Similarly, in the CASCADE study, patients treated with amiodarone were less likely

to receive a shock from the ICD and also syncopal shocks were less common in these patients [64]. In addition, in a randomized placebo-controlled study, *dl*-sotalol was used in 302 patients with a previously implanted ICD. The group receiving sotalol had a lower risk of the combined endpoint of death or delivery of a shock for any reason (48% risk reduction). There was also a significant reduction in the occurrence of inappropriate shocks in the sotalol group [65]. The reduction of shock events from an ICD appears also to have a positive prognostic value. In patients with LVEF ≤35%, the occurrence of shock versus no shock more than doubles the risk of death at 2 years follow-up [66]. Finally, it should be noted that the development of new pharmacologic agents may provide new opportunities to decrease the firing rate of an ICD. For example, another new class III antiarrhythmic drug, azimilide, in a preliminary study in 172 patients was shown to reduce the incidence of ICD therapies and appears well-tolerated without adverse effects on LV function or defibrillation threshold, in patients with a history of HF and remote MI [67].

## Atrial fibrillation

### Incidence and prognosis

Supraventricular arrhythmias (SVA) are commonly observed in patients with HF. Indeed, patients with HF have a 5% yearly incidence of SVA requiring hospitalization or drug treatment [68]. Longer duration of HF, older age, and LV size are the most significant predictors of developing SVA. Thus, as the population ages and as patients with HF live longer the incidence and prevalence of SVA can be expected to increase. The presence of SVA has an important impact on this patient population as morbidity and mortality associated with the development of SVA in HF patients is significantly higher than in those that maintain sinus rhythm. In a large population of patients with HF, after adjustment for other clinical variables including LVEF, the occurrence of SVA resulted an independent risk of death (RR, 2.45), stroke (RR, 2.35), and hospitalization due to worsening of HF (RR, 3.00) [68].

Atrial fibrillation is the most common SVA that complicates HF and along with HF have been described as the 'two new epidemics of cardiovascular disease' [69]. In one report, the incidence of AF and HF doubles for every decade of increase in age [70,71]. However, it should be noted that these data are not universally accepted as a recent population-based cohort study showed that the rate of new HF cases has been stable over the past two decades and that the increased HF prevalence is a consequence of improved survival and aging of the population [55]. The prevalence of AF also increases with severity of HF, from 10% in patients in NYHA functional class II to 40% in patients in functional class IV HF symptoms. The propensity of AF and HF to coexist is explained partially because the syndrome of HF creates the milieu for the development of AF [72,73].

The combination of AF and HF also carries an adverse prognosis the cause of which is most likely multifactorial. The development of AF may be a marker of deterioration of ventricular function or increased neurohormonal activation. Alternatively, AF may play a causal role in HF exacerbation by causing loss of atrial transport, rapid ventricular rate response, or thromboembolism [74,75]. An experimental study showed that the irregular sequence of ventricular cycle length (R–R intervals) resulting from AF was associated with adverse hemodynamic consequences independent of heart rate that may have particularly adverse effects in HF [76]. In addition, the presence of AF impacts mortality in patients with HF. Despite some controversy, most studies found AF to be a risk factor for mortality [77,78]. In patients with advanced HF, the presence of AF is also associated with reduced survival (52% versus 79% survival), over a mean follow-up of 236 days [79]. In the same study, the sudden death-free survival was significantly worse for AF patients than for sinus rhythm patients (69% versus 82%).

The goals of treatment of AF in HF patients are to relieve symptoms, to improve functional capacity, and to reduce the risk of associated morbidities including embolic risk [80]. Anticoagulation is critical in HF patients with either chronic or paroxysmal atrial fibrillation, in order to reduce embolic episodes [81], while the role of chronic anticoagulation is less certain in patients with HF without AF or history of embolic episodes (see Chapter 9). A retrospective analysis of 6797 patients enrolled in the SOLVD study, found that warfarin use was associated with a significant reduction in all-cause mortality (hazard ratio HR 0.76, $p = 0.0002$) [82,83].

The first treatment strategy for AF aims at restoring and maintaining sinus rhythm (rhythm control) whereas the second focuses exclusively on optimizing the ventricular rate (rate control). Rhythm control strategies include electrical cardioversion and antiarrhythmic treatment. As previously stated, amiodarone is the preferred agent in HF. In the Canadian trial of atrial fibrillation, low-dose amiodarone was effective at maintaining sinus rhythm in 65% of patients after cardioversion, at 16 months of follow-up, versus only 37% of patients maintaining sinus rhythm when treated with sotalol or propafenone [84] (Table 8.4).

In addition to the use of antiarrhythmic agents, other therapies have been used in HF in an effort to restore or maintain sinus rhythm. The surgical procedure, known as the 'maze procedure' is effective in curing medically refractory AF and can be performed as an adjunct to any major cardiac surgical procedure [87]. The evolution of this technique has lead to less invasive surgical approaches (maze-III) and epicardial procedures with use of various sources of ablative energy, such as radiofrequency, cryo-energy, and microwaves to create conduction block to cure AF [88]. Another nonpharmacological strategy for restoration and maintenance of sinus rhythm is transvenous radiofrequency catheter ablation of the left atrium with isolation of the four pulmonary veins [89]. This technique has promisingly been applied in patients with HF and evidence of extensive atrial remodeling [90,91].

For rate-control, the spectrum of available antiarrhythmic agents free of adverse effects in HF is rather narrow. Digoxin, calcium antagonists, and

**Table 8.4** Low-dose amiodarone and dofetilide trials in AF and LV dysfunction patients.

| Trial | Patients | Drug | LVEF | AF free | Follow up | Dose |
|---|---|---|---|---|---|---|
| Canadian trial AF [84] | 403 | Amiodarone/ sotalolo/ propafenone + DC shock | ≤ 50% in 20% of patients | Amiodarone 65% Sotalol 37% Propafenone 37% | 16 months | Loading then 200 mg |
| Gosselink 1992 [85] | 89 | Amiodarone + DC shock (no controls) | ≤ 35% and HF | Amiodarone 93% | 6 months | Loading then 200 mg |
| CHF-STAT [86] | 103 | Amiodarone/ Placebo No DC shock | 25% ±8 and HF | Amiodarone 32% Placebo 8% | 12 months | Loading then 200 mg |
| DIAMOND 1999 [25] | 391 | Dofetilide/ Placebo No DC shock | ≤ 35% and HF | Dofetilide 12% Placebo 1% | 1 month | 250–500 μg/day |

$\beta$-receptor blockers, either alone or combined, have been widely used with variable success. Low-dose amiodarone (200 mg/daily) can be used for rate control safely and effectively. The CHF-STAT study data showed that amiodarone has a significant efficacy in reducing the mean and maximal ventricular response in AF patients [86]. A nonpharmacologic treatment modality for ventricular rate control is ablation of the atrioventricular node and insertion of a rate-responsive ventricular pacemaker. This has been demonstrated to improve ventricular function in patients with AF and rapid ventricular rate [92]. In one-third of patients, after AV nodal ablation LVEF is reported nearly to normalize, suggesting that atrial fibrillation-induced EF reduction is reversible in many patients [93].

The effect on mortality of the two strategies, rhythm control versus rate control, has not yet been tested solely in patients with HF. A recent large trial (AFFIRM) [94] found a nonsignificant increase in mortality risk in the rhythm control group compared with the rate-control group (HR 1.15, $p = 0.08$), in patients over 65 years of age or having at least one risk factor for stroke. In the study only 939 (23%) patients had a history of HF and for this subgroup there was a trend toward a better prognosis for the rhythm-control group. In addition, a further follow-up analysis of the same population showed that the presence of sinus rhythm was associated with lower risk of death, but the use of antiarrhythmic drugs was not associated with improved survival, suggesting that any beneficial antiarrhythmic effect of drugs could be offset by their adverse effects [95]. Interestingly, however, among the drugs used in the rhythm-control group, amiodarone was used for initial therapy in only 37% of patients and sotalol in 31% of patients. This relatively large use of sotalol versus amiodarone concurs with the SWORD study results of sotalol in HF patients, and confirms its deleterious effects [25].

Other forms of nonpharmacological therapy of AF have also been investigated for both rate and rhythm control. For example, a stand-alone implantable atrial defibrillator was found to be of limited practical value because of patient discomfort during shocks. In patients with indications for pacemaker implantation, the use of a physiologic modality of stimulation (atrial pacing or dual chamber) reduces AF occurrence compared to ventricular pacing [96]. A new device capable of providing biventricular pacing, ventricular and atrial shock therapy separately is under investigation (Renewal 3 AVT, Guidant Corp).

## Conclusion

Ventricular arrhythmias are very frequent in patients with HF and, unless they are sustained and symptomatic, their presence does not appear to worsen the prognosis. While a variety of antiarrhythmic agents are effective at suppressing these arrhythmias, all but amiodarone are associated with worsened outcome. However, the increasing number of HF patients indicated for an ICD will likely create the need for increased use of antiarrhythmic agents in order to decrease the number of shocks and preserve, and amiodarone is the agent of choice, although in the presence of an ICD Sotalol or Dofetilide can be considered.

Atrial fibrillation is very frequent in patients with HF, and some studies indicate that it carries a worse prognosis. In contrast to ventricular arrhythmias, antiarrhythmic drugs in AF patients with HF are still the mainstay of therapy. However, the long-term efficacy of antiarrhythmic drugs for preventing AF recurrence is far from ideal. In addition, it is not yet clear whether aggressive attempts to maintain sinus rhythm with drugs, electrical cardioversion, or ablation procedures, offer a better prognosis than heart rate control strategy and prevention of thrombo-embolism. By contrast, $\beta$-blockers, another form of antiarrhythmia therapy is effective in improving LV function and reducing sudden death and total mortality in HF patients; however, it remains unclear whether these salutary benefits are due to its 'antiarrhythmic' properties or to the profound effects it has on cardiac remodeling and myocyte biology. Ideally, new antiarrhythmic agents will become available in the future that will fill the unmet needs of these pharmacologic agents.

## References

1 Francis GS. Development of arrhythmias in the patient with congestive heart failure: pathophysiology, prevalence and prognosis. Am J Cardiol 1986;**57**:3B–7B.

2 Teerlink JR, Jalaluddin M, Anderson S et al. Ambulatory ventricular arrhythmias in patients with heart failure do not specifically predict an increased risk of sudden death. PROMISE (Prospective Randomized Milrinone Survival Evaluation) Investigators. Circulation 2000;**101**:40–46.

3 Bigger JT Jr, Fleiss J, Kleiger R et al. The relationships among ventricular arrhythmias, left ventricular dysfunction, and mortality in the 2 years after myocardial infarction. Circulation 1984;**69**:250–258.

4 Meinertz T, Hofmann T, Kasper W et al. Significance of ventricular arrhythmias in idiopathic dilated cardiomyopathy. Am J Cardiol 1984;**53**:902–907.

5 Holmes J, Kubo SH, Cody RJ et al. Arrhythmias in ischemic and nonischemic dilated cardiomyopathy: prediction of mortality by ambulatory electrocardiography. Am J Cardiol 1985;**55**:146–151.

6 Von Olshausen K, Schafer A, Mehmel HC et al. Ventricular arrhythmias in idiopathic dilated cardiomyopathy. Br Heart J 1984;**51**:195–201.

7 Unverferth DV, Magorien RD, Moeschberger ML et al. Factors influencing the one-year mortality of dilated cardiomyopathy. Am J Cardiol 1984;**54**:147–152.

8 McKee PA, Castelli WP, McNamara PM et al. The natural history of congestive heart failure: the Framingham study. N Engl J Med 1971;**285**:1441–1446.

9 Andersson B, Wantiarrhythmic agent gstein F. Spectrum and outcome of congestive heart failure in a hospitalized population. Am Heart J 1993;**126**:632–640.

10 Effect of metoprolol CR/XL in chronic heart failure: Metoprolol CR/XL Randomised Intervention Trial in Congestive Heart Failure (MERIT-HF). Lancet 1999;**353**:2001–2007.

11 Luu M, Stevenson WG, Stevenson LW et al. Diverse mechanisms of unexpected cardiac arrest in advanced heart failure. Circulation 1989;**80**:1675–1680.

12 Singh SN, Fisher SG, Carson PE et al. Prevalence and significance of nonsustained ventricular tachycardia in patients with premature ventricular contractions and heart failure treated with vasodilator therapy. Department of Veterans Affairs CHF STAT Investigators. J Am Coll Cardiol 1998;**32**:942–947.

13 Kjekshus J. Arrhythmias and mortality in congestive heart failure. Am J Cardiol 1990;**65**:42I–48I.

14 Vaughan Williams EM. A classification of antiarrhythmic actions reassessed after a decade of new drugs. J Clin Pharmacol 1984;**24**:129–147.

15 Flaker GC, Blackshear JL, McBride R et al. Antiarrhythmic drug therapy and cardiac mortality in atrial fibrillation. The Stroke Prevention in Atrial Fibrillation Investigators. J Am Coll Cardiol 1992;**20**:527–532.

16 Metra M, Giubbini R, Nodari S et al. Differential effects of beta-blockers in patients with heart failure: A prospective, randomized, double-blind comparison of the long-term effects of metoprolol versus carvedilol. Circulation 2000;**102**:546–551.

17 Packer M, Bristow MR, Cohn JN et al. The effect of carvedilol on morbidity and mortality in patients with chronic heart failure. U.S. Carvedilol Heart Failure Study Group. N Engl J Med 1996;**334**:1349–1355.

18 Dargie HJ. Effect of carvedilol on outcome after myocardial infarction in patients with left-ventricular dysfunction: the CAPRICORN randomised trial. Lancet 2001;**357**:1385–1390.

19 Packer M, Coats AJ, Fowler MB et al. Effect of carvedilol on survival in severe chronic heart failure (COPERNICUS). N Engl J Med 2001;**344**:1651–1658.

20 The Cardiac Insufficiency Bisoprolol Study II (CIBIS-II): a randomised trial. Lancet 1999;**353**:9–13.

21 Echt DS, Liebson PR, Mitchell LB *et al*. Mortality and morbidity in patients receiving encainide, flecainide, or placebo. The Cardiac Arrhythmia Suppression Trial. *N Engl J Med* 1991;**324**:781–788.

22 The Cardiac Arrhythmia Suppression Trial II Investigators. Effect of the antiarrhythmic agent moricizine on survival after myocardial infarction. *N Engl J Med* 1992;**327**:227–233.

23 Siebels J, Kuck KH. Implantable cardioverter defibrillator compared with antiarrhythmic drug treatment in cardiac arrest survivors (the Cardiac Arrest Study Hamburg). *Am Heart J* 1994;**127**:1139–1144.

24 Beta-Blocker Evaluation of Survival Trial Investigators (BEST). A trial of the beta-blocker bucindolol in patients with advanced chronic heart failure. *N Engl J Med* 2001;**344**:1659–1667.

25 Waldo AL, Camm AJ, deRuyter H *et al*. Effect of *d*-sotalol on mortality in patients with left ventricular dysfunction after recent and remote myocardial infarction. The SWORD Investigators. Survival With Oral *d*-Sotalol. *Lancet* 1996;**348**:7–12.

26 Julian DG, Camm AJ, Frangin G *et al*. Randomised trial of effect of amiodarone on mortality in patients with left-ventricular dysfunction after recent myocardial infarction: EMIAT. European Myocardial Infarct Amiodarone Trial Investigators. *Lancet* 1997;**349**:667–674.

27 Kober L, Bloch Thomsen PE, Moller M *et al*. Effect of dofetilide in patients with recent myocardial infarction and left-ventricular dysfunction: a randomised trial. *Lancet* 2000;**356**:2052–2058.

28 Pratt CM, Singh SN, Al-Khalidi HR *et al*. The efficacy of azimilide in the treatment of atrial fibrillation in the presence of left ventricular systolic dysfunction: results from the Azimilide Postinfarct Survival Evaluation (ALIVE) trial. *J Am Coll Cardiol* 2004;**43**:1211–1216.

29 Doval HC, Nul DR, Grancelli HO *et al*. Randomized trial of low-dose amiodarone in severe congestive heart failure. Grupo de Estudio de la Sobrevida en la Insuficiencia Cardiaca en Argentina (GESICA). *Lancet* 1994;**344**:493–498.

30 Singh SN, Fletcher RD, Fisher SG *et al*. Amiodarone in patients with congestive heart failure and asymptomatic ventricular arrhythmia. Survival Trial of Antiarrhythmic Therapy in Congestive Heart Failure. *N Engl J Med* 1995;**333**:77–82.

31 Torp-Pedersen C, Moller M, Bloch-Thomsen PE *et al*. Dofetilide in patients with congestive heart failure and left ventricular dysfunction. Danish Investigations of Arrhythmia and Mortality on Dofetilide Study Group. *N Engl J Med* 1999;**341**:857–865.

32 Bardy G. SCD-HeFT: The Sudden Cardiac Death in Heart Failure Trial. American College of Cardiology. 8 March 2004. New Orleans. http://sicr.org/scdheft_results_acc_lbcc.pdf

33 The effect of diltiazem on mortality and reinfarction after myocardial infarction. The Multicenter Diltiazem Postinfarction Trial Research Group. *N Engl J Med* 1988;**319**:385–392.

34 Effect of verapamil on mortality and major events after acute myocardial infarction (the Danish Verapamil Infarction Trial II–DAVIT II) *Am J Cardiol* 1990;**66**:779–785.

35 The Digitalis Investigation Group. The effect of digoxin on mortality and morbidity in patients with heart failure. *N Engl J Med* 1997;**336**:525–533.

36 Brendorp B, Pedersen OD, Elming H *et al*. Can antiarrhythmic drugs save lives in patients with congestive heart failure? *Expert Rev Cardiovasc Ther* 2003;**1**:191–202.

37 The Xamoterol in Severe Heart Failure Study Group. Xamoterol in severe heart failure. *Lancet* 1990;**336**:1–6.

38 Andreka P, Aiyar N, Olson LC *et al*. Bucindolol displays intrinsic sympathomimetic activity in human myocardium. *Circulation* 2002;**105**:2429–2434.

39 The Sicilian gambit. A new approach to the classification of antiarrhythmic drugs based on their actions on arrhythmogenic mechanisms. Task Force of the Working Group on Arrhythmias of the European Society of Cardiology. *Circulation* 1991;**84**:1831–1851.

40 Connolly SJ. Meta-analysis of antiarrhythmic drug trials. *Am J Cardiol* 1999;**84**:90R–93R.

41 Kodama I, Kamiya K, Toyama J. Amiodarone: ionic and cellular mechanisms of action of the most promising class III agent. *Am J Cardiol* 1999;**84**:20R–28R.

42 Middlekauff HR, Wiener I, Saxon LA *et al*. Low-dose amiodarone for atrial fibrillation: time for a prospective study? *Ann Intern Med* 1992;**116**:1017–1020.

43 Hohnloser SH, Singh BN. Proarrhythmia with class III antiarrhythmic drugs: definition, electrophysiologic mechanisms, incidence, predisposing factors, and clinical implications. *J Cardiovasc Electrophysiol* 1995;**6**:920–936.

44 Choo DC, Huiskes B, Jones J *et al*. Amiodarone rescue therapy for severe decompensated heart failure initially unsuitable for beta-blockers. *J Cardiovasc Pharmacol Ther* 2003;**8**:187–192.

45 Toyama T, Hoshizaki H, Seki R *et al*. Efficacy of amiodarone treatment on cardiac symptom, function, and sympathetic nerve activity in patients with dilated cardiomyopathy: comparison with beta-blocker therapy. *J Nucl Cardiol* 2004;**11**:134–141.

46 Shiga T, Hosaka F, Wakaumi M *et al*. Amiodarone decreases plasma brain natriuretic peptide level in patients with heart failure and ventricular tachyarrhythmia. *Cardiovasc Drugs Ther* 2003;**17**:325–333.

47 Vorperian VR, Havighurst TC, Miller S *et al.* Adverse effects of low dose amiodarone: a meta-analysis. *J Am Coll Cardiol* 1997;**30**:791–798.

48 Singh SN, Berk MR, Yellen LG *et al.* Efficacy and safety of oral dofetilide in maintaining normal sinus rhythm in patients with atrial fibrillation/flutter: a multicenter study. *Circulation* 1997;**96**:I-383 (abstr).

49 Greenbaum R, Campbell TJ, Channer KS *et al.* Conversion of AF and maintainance of sinus rhythm by dofetilide. *Eur Heart J* 1998;**19**:Suppl:661 (abstr).

50 Camm AJ, Pratt CM, Schwartz PJ *et al.* Mortality in patients after a recent myocardial infarction: a randomized, placebo-controlled trial of azimilide using heart rate variability for risk stratification. *Circulation* 2004;**109**:990–996.

51 Doggrell SA, Hancox JC. Dronedarone: an amiodarone analogue. *Expert Opin Investig Drugs* 2004;**13**: 415–426.

52 Gheorghiade M, Ferguson D. Digoxin. A neurohormonal modulator in heart failure? *Circulation* 1991;**84**:2181–2186.

53 Packer M, Gheorghiade M, Young JB *et al.* Withdrawal of digoxin from patients with chronic heart failure treated with angiotensin-converting-enzyme inhibitors. RADIANCE Study. *N Engl J Med* 1993;**329**:1–7.

54 Cairns JA, Connolly SJ, Roberts R *et al.* Randomised trial of outcome after myocardial infarction in patients with frequent or repetitive ventricular premature depolarisations: CAMIAT. Canadian Amiodarone Myocardial Infarction Arrhythmia Trial Investigators. *Lancet* 1997;**349**:675–682.

55 Roger VL, Weston SA, Redfield MM *et al.* Trends in heart failure incidence and survival in a community-based population. *JAMA* 2004;**292**:344–350.

56 The Antiarrhythmics versus Implantable Defibrillators (AVID) Investigators. A comparison of antiarrhythmic-drug therapy with implantable defibrillators in patients resuscitated from near-fatal ventricular arrhythmias. *N Engl J Med.* 1997;**337**:1576–1583.

57 Moss AJ, Hall WJ, Cannom DS *et al.* Improved survival with an implanted defibrillator in patients with coronary disease at high risk for ventricular arrhythmia. Multicenter Automatic Defibrillator Implantation Trial Investigators. *N Engl J Med* 1996;**335**:1933–1940.

58 Buxton AE, Lee KL, Fisher JD *et al.* A randomized study of the prevention of sudden death in patients with coronary artery disease. Multicenter Unsustained Tachycardia Trial Investigators. *N Engl J Med* 1999;**341**:1882–1890.

59 Moss AJ, Zareba W, Hall WJ *et al.* Prophylactic implantation of a defibrillator in patients with myocardial infarction and reduced ejection fraction. *N Engl J Med* 2002;**346**:877–883.

60 Bristow MR, Saxon LA, Boehmer J *et al.* Cardiac-resynchronization therapy with or without an implantable defibrillator in advanced chronic heart failure. *N Engl J Med* 2004;**350**:2140–2150.

61 Kadish A, Dyer A, Daubert JP *et al.* Prophylactic defibrillator implantation in patients with nonischemic dilated cardiomyopathy. *N Engl J Med* 2004;**350**: 2151–2158.

62 Dougherty AH. Interactions between antiarrhythmic drugs and implantable cardioverter-defibrillators. *Curr Opin Cardiol* 1996;**11**:2–8.

63 Page RL. Effects of antiarrhythmic medication on implantable cardioverter-defibrillator function. *Am J Cardiol* 2000;**85**:1481–1485.

64 Greene HL. The CASCADE Study: randomized antiarrhythmic drug therapy in survivors of cardiac arrest in Seattle. CASCADE Investigators. *Am J Cardiol* 1993;**72**:70F–74F.

65 Pacifico A, Hohnloser SH, Williams JH *et al.* Prevention of implantable-defibrillator shocks by treatment with sotalol. d, l-Sotalol Implantable Cardioverter-Defibrillator Study Group. *N Engl J Med* 1999;**340**:1855–1862.

66 Pacifico A, Ferlic LL, Cedillo-Salazar FR *et al.* Shocks as predictors of survival in patients with implantable cardioverter-defibrillators. *J Am Coll Cardiol* 1999;**34**:204–210.

67 Singer I, Al-Khalidi H, Niazi I *et al.* Azimilide decreases recurrent ventricular tachyarrhythmias in patients with implantable cardioverter defibrillators. *J Am Coll Cardiol* 2004;**43**:39–43.

68 Mathew J, Hunsberger S, Fleg J *et al.* Incidence, predictive factors, and prognostic significance of supraventricular tachyarrhythmias in congestive heart failure. *Chest* 2000;**118**:914–922.

69 Braunwald E. Shattuck lecture – cardiovascular medicine at the turn of the millennium: triumphs, concerns, and opportunities. *N Engl J Med* 1997;**337**:1360–1369.

70 Kannel WB, Belanger AJ. Epidemiology of heart failure. *Am Heart J* 1991;**121**:951–957.

71 Benjamin EJ, Levy D, Vaziri SM *et al.* Independent risk factors for atrial fibrillation in a population-based cohort. The Framingham Heart Study. *JAMA* 1994;**271**: 840–844.

72 Li D, Fareh S, Leung TK *et al.* Promotion of atrial fibrillation by heart failure in dogs: atrial remodeling of a different sort. *Circulation* 1999;**100**:87–95.

73 Shinbane JS, Wood MA, Jensen DN *et al.* Tachycardia-induced cardiomyopathy: a review of animal models and clinical studies. *J Am Coll Cardiol* 1997;**29**: 709–715.

74 Pozzoli M, Cioffi G, Traversi E *et al.* Predictors of primary atrial fibrillation and concomitant clinical and hemodynamic changes in patients with chronic heart failure:

a prospective study in 344 patients with baseline sinus rhythm. *J Am Coll Cardiol* 1998;**32**:197–204.

75 Alam M, Thorstrand C. Left ventricular function in patients with atrial fibrillation before and after cardioversion. *Am J Cardiol* 1992;**69**:694–696.

76 Clark DM, Plumb VJ, Epstein AE *et al.* Hemodynamic effects of an irregular sequence of ventricular cycle lengths during atrial fibrillation. *J Am Coll Cardiol* 1997;**30**:1039–1045.

77 Dries DL, Exner DV, Gersh BJ *et al.* Atrial fibrillation is associated with an increased risk for mortality and heart failure progression in patients with asymptomatic and symptomatic left ventricular systolic dysfunction: a retrospective analysis of the SOLVD trials. Studies of Left Ventricular Dysfunction. *J Am Coll Cardiol* 1998;**32**:695–703.

78 Wang TJ, Larson MG, Levy D *et al.* Temporal relations of atrial fibrillation and congestive heart failure and their joint influence on mortality: the Framingham Heart Study. *Circulation* 2003;**107**:2920–2925.

79 Middlekauff HR, Stevenson WG, Stevenson LW. Prognostic significance of atrial fibrillation in advanced heart failure. A study of 390 patients. *Circulation* 1991;**84**:40–48.

80 Saxon LA. Atrial fibrillation and dilated cardiomyopathy: therapeutic strategies when sinus rhythm cannot be maintained. *Pacing Clin Electrophysiol* 1997;**20**: 720–725.

81 Fuster V, Ryden LE, Asinger RW *et al.* ACC/AHA/ESC guidelines for the management of patients with atrial fibrillation: executive summary. *J Am Coll Cardiol* 2001;**38**:1231–1266.

82 Al-Khadra AS, Salem DN, Rand WM *et al.* Warfarin anticoagulation and survival: a cohort analysis from the Studies of Left Ventricular Dysfunction. *J Am Coll Cardiol* 1998;**31**:749–753.

83 Dries DL, Domanski MJ, Waclawiw MA *et al.* Effect of antithrombotic therapy on risk of sudden coronary death in patients with congestive heart failure. *Am J Cardiol* 1997;**79**:909–913.

84 Roy D, Talajic M, Dorian P *et al.* Amiodarone to prevent recurrence of atrial fibrillation. Canadian Trial of Atrial Fibrillation Investigators. *N Engl J Med* 2000;**342**:913–920.

85 Gosselink AT, Crijns HJ, Van Gelder IC *et al.* Low-dose amiodarone for maintenance of sinus rhythm after cardioversion of atrial fibrillation or flutter. *JAMA* 1992;**267**:3289–3293.

86 Deedwania PC, Singh BN, Ellenbogen K *et al.* Spontaneous conversion and maintenance of sinus rhythm by amiodarone in patients with heart failure and atrial fibrillation: observations from the veterans affairs congestive heart failure survival trial of antiarrhythmic therapy (CHF-STAT). The Department of Veterans Affairs CHF-STAT Investigators. *Circulation* 1998;**98**:2574–2579.

87 Cox JL, Ad N, Palazzo T *et al.* Current status of the Maze procedure for the treatment of atrial fibrillation. *Semin Thorac Cardiovasc Surg* 2000;**12**:15–19.

88 Manasse E, Barbone A, Ghiselli S *et al.* Surgical treatment of atrial fibrillation in the beating heart: a novel approach. *Ital Heart J* 2003;**4**:872–874.

89 Haissaguerre M, Jais P, Shah DC *et al.* Spontaneous initiation of atrial fibrillation by ectopic beats originating in the pulmonary veins. *N Engl J Med* 1998;**339**:659–666.

90 Pappone C, Oreto G, Rosanio S *et al.* Atrial electroanatomic remodeling after circumferential radiofrequency pulmonary vein ablation: efficacy of an anatomic approach in a large cohort of patients with atrial fibrillation. *Circulation* 2001;**104**:2539–2544.

91 Li-Fern H, Pierre J, Prashantan S *et al.* Catheter Ablation for atrial fibrillation in congestive heart Failure. *N Engl J Med* 2004;**351**:2373–2383

92 Edner M, Caidahl K, Bergfeldt L *et al.* Prospective study of left ventricular function after radiofrequency ablation of atrioventricular junction in patients with atrial fibrillation. *Br Heart J* 1995;**74**:261–267.

93 Ozcan C, Jahangir A, Friedman PA *et al.* Significant effects of atrioventricular node ablation and pacemaker implantation on left ventricular function and long-term survival in patients with atrial fibrillation and left ventricular dysfunction. *Am J Cardiol* 2003;**92**: 33–37.

94 Wyse DG, Waldo AL, DiMarco JP *et al.* A comparison of rate control and rhythm control in patients with atrial fibrillation. Atrial Fibrillation Follow-up Investigation of Rhythm Management (AFFIRM) Investigators. *N Engl J Med* 2002;**347**:1825–1833.

95 Corley SD, Epstein AE, DiMarco JP *et al.* Relationships between sinus rhythm, treatment, and survival in the Atrial Fibrillation Follow-Up Investigation of Rhythm Management (AFFIRM) Study. *Circulation* 2004;**109**:1509–1513.

96 Skanes AC, Krahn AD, Yee R *et al.* Progression to chronic atrial fibrillation after pacing: the Canadian Trial of Physiologic Pacing. CTOPP Investigators. *J Am Coll Cardiol* 2001;**38**:167–172.

## CHAPTER 9

# Treating the hypercoagulable state of heart failure: modifying the risk of arterial and venous thromboembolism

*Geno J. Merli,* MD, FACP *& Howard H. Weitz,* MD, FACC, FACP

## Introduction

Heart failure affects nearly five million people in the United States with more than 500 000 new cases diagnosed annually [1]. In patients older than 65 years, heart failure is the most frequent indication for hospitalization and the most frequent discharge diagnosis submitted for Medicare reimbursement [2]. Currently, the mortality of heart failure is related to its severity ranging from 5% to 10% in patients with mild symptoms to 30% to 40% in severe cases [3]. There are two major areas of risk for thromboembolic disease in patients with heart failure. Arterial thromboembolism has been reported to occur with an incidence of 0.9 to 42.4 events per 100 patient years [4]. The incidence of lower extremity deep vein thrombosis in hospitalized heart failure patients is 16% [5]. In this chapter the mechanism for the development of a hypercoagulable state in heart failure, the incidence of arterial and venous thromboembolic events, and management strategies to prevent these complications are presented.

## Coagulation pathophysiology in heart failure

Stasis, intimal injury, and hypercoagulability all contribute to the development of thrombosis. Their presence in heart failure contributes to the development of arterial or venous thromboembolic events

(Table 9.1). In order to better appreciate the impact of the pathophysiologic changes that heart failure has on the coagulation process, studies using surrogate markers for activation of the clotting system must be reviewed.

Stasis, secondary to heart failure, has an effect on the venous and arterial circulation.

**Table 9.1** Prothrombotic features of heart failure.

*Stasis*
  Dilated cardiac chambers
  Decreased cardiac output
  Slowed circulatory time
  Immobility secondary to worsening ejection fraction

*Endothelial dysfunction*
  Increased level of von Willebrand factor
  Increased plasminogen activator inhibitor 1 (PAI – 1)
    Related to increased angiotensin II levels with HF
  Decreased tissue plasminogen activator (tPA)
    Related to increased angiotensin II levels with HF

*Hypercoagulability*
  Markers of thrombin formation
    Thrombin antithrombin thrombin (TAT)
    Fibrinopeptide A
    D-Dimer
  Markers of platelet activation
    Beta thromboglobulin
    P – selectin
  Increased plasma viscosity
  Increased fibrinogen

With the reduction in left ventricular ejection fraction (LVEF), the patient's functional capacity is decreased as documented by the New York Heart Association classification. Reduced functional capacity translates to immobility that is an independent risk factor for the development of DVT/PE. Intracardiac stasis secondary to left ventricular dilatation is also a stimulus for thrombus formation. Sbarouni et al. demonstrated the plasma and blood flow viscosity in patients with moderate to severe heart failure in sinus rhythm was increased when compared to controls and these changes may increase the risk for thromboembolic events [6]. In addition, an abnormal reduction or absence of blood flow by Doppler studies was demonstrated in heart failure patients with intracardiac thrombi. The degree of reduction in ejection fraction has also been shown to increase the risk of stroke as demonstrated in the SAVE trial with a relative risk of stroke by 1.86 when the LVEF was $\leq 28\%$ [7].

Intimal injury in heart failure is manifested by endothelial dysfunction. This process can be best demonstrated by von Willebrand factor (vWF), nitric oxide (NO), and angiotensin II. von Willebrand factor is a marker of endothelial damage or dysfunction [8]. An increase in vWF enhances platelet aggregation and platelet adhesion to the endothelium resulting in an increased risk for thrombosis. Gibbs et al. demonstrated a significant increase in the levels of vWF in class III and IV heart failure patients [9]. In the control group, vWF levels of $106 \pm 31$ IU were documented while the levels in the heart failure cohort were $136 \pm 27$ IU ($p \leq 0.0001$). In this study there was a trend toward high vWF levels in patients with more severe symptoms of heart failure (NYHA class III and IV) but this difference did not reach statistical significance. Elevated levels of vWF have been associated with an increased risk of reinfarction and mortality in post-myocardial infarction patients as shown by Jansson et al. [10].

In vivo studies have shown that heart failure patients have impaired production of endothelium-derived NO. Low levels of NO causes endothelial dysfunction that promotes platelet and monocyte adhesion to endothelial surfaces, which permit the release of prothrombotic mediators from activated platelets [11,12]. Heart failure increases the level

of angiotensin II and norepinephrine. The former substance stimulates the release of endothelium-derived endothelin that increases the expression from endothelial and smooth muscle cells of plasminogen activator inhibitor-1 (PAI-1), which inhibits the release of tissue plasminogen activator (tPA) [13]. In addition angiotensin II degrades bradykinin, which is a potent stimulus of vascular release of tPA [14]. These three effects on the endothelium in patients with heart failure increase the risk for thrombus formation.

Hypercoagulablity in heart failure can best be demonstrated by assessing surrogate markers that reflect activation of the clotting process as well as platelet function. Activation of the clotting process can be measured by evaluating the formation of prothrombin fragment $1 + 2$ (F $1 + 2$), thrombin–antithrombin III complex (TAT), fibrinopeptide A (FPA), and D-dimers. Prothrombin fragment $1 + 2$ forms from prothrombin when factor Xa cleaves the C-terminal half of the molecule. Elevated plasma levels of F $1 + 2$ indicate an increase in factor Xa generation due to activation of the clotting system. When thrombin is generated from prothrombin its biological activity is neutralized by antithrombin III forming equimolar complexes of TAT in the circulating plasma. Elevated levels of TAT suggest increased in vivo thrombin generation. Thrombin specifically cleaves FPA from the amino terminal of fibrinogen's alpha chain and initiates fibrin generation. D-dimers are fibrin degradation products formed when thrombin generates fibrin from fibrinogen, which is subsequently lysed by plasmin. Elevated levels of D-dimers indicate not only thrombin generation but also activation of the fibrinolytic system for clot dissolution. These four markers have all been shown to be elevated in patients with heart failure [15–17].

The final segment of hypercoagulability is the activation of platelets secondary to heart failure. Platelet factor IV (PF4) and beta-thromboglobulin (BTG) are measures of platelet activation. Jafri et al. demonstrated that in patients with heart failure levels of BTG were significantly elevated to $89 \pm 62$ IU versus $50 \pm 59$ IU in normal individuals [11]. The same author also reported platelet activation using surface activation as detected by electron microscopy in patients with severe heart failure [18]. Mehta et al. also demonstrated increased platelet activation by measuring platelet aggregates, which were elevated in patients with heart failure [19].

All of the above evidence supports the prothrombotic state created by heart failure. The question is whether this hypercoagulable state translates to the development of an increased incidence of arterial and venous thromboembolic events.

## Clinical manifestations of the prothrombotic state of heart failure

Stroke is a major complication of heart failure with a reported annual risk of approximately 1.5% as compared to <0.5% in the general population [20]. In patients with NYHA class III or IV heart failure with a concomitant ejection fraction of <20% the incidence of stroke has been reported to be as high as 4% [20]. In fact, the SAVE study reported an inverse relationship between stroke risk and LVEF, with an 18% increase in stroke for every 5% reduction in ejection fraction [21]. In order to better understand the risk for stroke in heart failure with sinus rhythm, a review of the literature will shed more light on this thromboembolic complication as well as approaches to preventing these complications.

Fuster et al. evaluated 104 non-anticoagulated patients with idiopathic dilated cardiomyopathy and reported an incidence of 3.5 arterial embolic events per 100 patient years [22]. Approximately 50% of the patients died within the first year of follow up, which may have been an indication of a more complicated heart failure population. In a study by Ciaccheri et al. in 126 patients with dilated cardiomyopathy, arterial thromboemboli were reported at 1.4 events per 100 patient years [23]. The incidence of atrial fibrillation was 12% in this latter study versus the 23% in the Fuster et al. series. The CONSENSUS study enrolled patients with NYHA class IV heart failure patients with and without atrial fibrillation [24]. Three of 253 patients suffered a fatal stroke during a 6-month follow-up period for an estimated incidence of 2.3 fatal strokes per 100 patient years.

Another physiologic aspect that must be considered is the correlation between the degree of left ventricular dysfunction and the incidence of stroke. In a study by Kyrle et al. the association between arterial embolism and the severity of left ventricular dysfunction demonstrated an embolization risk of 67% for severe, 47% in moderate, and 20% in mild left ventricular dysfunction [25]. The V-HeFT study demonstrated that heart failure patients with a stroke had a lower ejection fraction (29.6% versus 26.3%) and peak oxygen consumption (14.2 mL/kg/min versus 12.6 mL/kg/min) than heart failure patients without stroke [26]. Along with the above, another aspect that has been assessed is the correlation between left ventricular function and left ventricular mural thrombi. In a small study Yokota et al. demonstrated that patients with cardiac thrombus had a lower ejection fraction (25%) than patients without thrombus (39%) [27]. In a subgroup analysis it was shown that 9 of 11 patients with thrombi had severe apical dyskinesis or akinesis compared to 12 of 29 patient without thrombi. Maze et al. studied 20 patients with mural thrombi and 20 with dilated cardiomyopathy and no mural thrombi and found that the inflow and systolic flow velocity at the ventricular apex was markedly lower in those with thrombi [28]. The study concluded that mural thrombi result from segmental wall motion abnormalities or aberrant flow through the left ventricle rather than a globally depressed ejection fraction. Despite these findings two other studies found no relationship between left ventricular thrombus and ejection fraction, NYHA class, or fractional shortening [29,30].

## Preventing thromboembolism in the patient with heart failure

Most of the information regarding the effects of anticoagulation on the risk of thromboembolism in patients with heart failure comes from retrospective analysis of large multicenter clinical trials. The SOLVD trials (Studies of Left Ventricular Dysfunction) included patients with symptomatic (LVEF <35%) and asymptomatic heart failure [31–36] (Table 9.2). The administration of aspirin or warfarin was not randomized and was at the discretion of the investigator. Analysis of these studies suggested that patients receiving aspirin had a lower incidence of sudden cardiac death and thromboembolism than the controls. Thromboembolism was only significantly reduced in women (RR 0.47,

**Table 9.2** Post hoc analysis of heart failure trials.

| Study | Type | Number of patients | Intervention | Outcome (Sroke) |
|-------|------|--------------------|--------------|-----------------|
| SOLVD [31–36] | Retrospective cohort analysis EF <35% | 6767 | ASA and Warfarin investigator's choice | Women RR 0.47 Men RR 0.77 |
| V-HeFT I [26] | Retrospective cohort analysis EF <40% | 642 I | ASA and Warfarin investigator's choice | 0.5 events/100pt-yrs ASA 2.7 events/100pt-yrs No Rx 2.9 events/100pt-yr Warf |
| V-HeFT II [37] | Retrospective cohort analysis EF <40% | 804 | ASA and Warfarin | 1.6 events/100pt-yrs ASA 2.1 events/100pt-yrs No Rx 4.9 events/100pt-yrs Warf |
| SAVE [21] | Cohort analysis Post-MI, asymptomatic heart failure | 2231 | Warfarin, ASA | ASA RR 0.44 Warfarin RR 0.19 |
| PROMISE [38] | Retrospective cohort analysis NYHA III or IV | 1088 | ASA and Warfarin investigator's choice | Warfarin 0.6% stroke ASA 3.3% stroke |

RR= Relative risk; Pt-yrs = Patient-years
*Source*: Adapted from [4].

95% CI 0.24–0.92, $p = 0.03$) and borderline in men (RR 0.77, 95% CI 0.59–1.00, $p = 0.06$). A further analysis showed that antiplatelet therapy use was associated with a reduced all-cause mortality (adjusted hazard ratio HR 0.12, 95% CI 0.73–0.92, $p = 0.005$) and reduced risk of death or hospitalization for heart failure (HR 0.81, 95% CI 0.74–0.89, $p < 0.0001$). This effect was substantially reduced in those patients receiving enalapril therapy. In the patients receiving warfarin, there was also a reduction in the risk of sudden cardiac death. There was no direct comparison between Aspirin and warfarin therapy in these studies.

The V-HeFT trials (Vasodilator Heart Failure Trial) included patients with symptomatic heart failure with radiologic, electrocardiographic, or radionuclide evidence of left ventricular dysfunction [26,37] (Table 9.2). In V-HeFT I, 12.6% of the patient-years follow up and in V-HeFT II, 27.3% of patient-years follow up included antiplatelet therapy with aspirin, dipyridamole, or both [26,37]. In V-HeFT I there was 184 patient years of treatment with antiplatelet agents and the incidence of thromboembolism was 0.5 events per 100 patient years compared to 2.7 events per 100 patient years ($p = 0.07$) in those not receiving treatment. This trend was not reproduced in V-HeFT II with thromboembolic events occurring at 1.6 events per 100 patient years in the antiplatelet group versus

2.1 events per 100 patient years in the untreated group. For those patients treated with warfarin the incidence of thrombosis in the V-HeFT I was 2.9 events per 100 patient years and in V-HeFT II 4.9 events per 100 patient years. There was no significant difference compared to the control group. These two studies did not compare aspirin and warfarin.

The SAVE study (Survival and Ventricular Enlargement) included patients post myocardial infarction with LVEF of <40% and asymptomatic for heart failure [21] (Table 9.2). In those patients treated with antiplatelet therapy there was a 56% reduction in total stroke risk (RR 0.44, 95% CI 0.29–0.65). On the other hand in those patients that received warfarin there was an associated 81% reduction in stroke risk (RR 0.19, 95% CI 0.13–0.27). Again as in the SOLVD and V-HeFT I, II studies there was no direct comparisons of the treatments.

Data from the PROMISE trial (Prospective Randomized Milrinone Survival Evaluation) was retrospectively reviewed to assess the incidence of stroke in those patients receiving warfarin or aspirin [38] (Table 9.2). The warfarin treated patients had a 0.6% (1 of 181 patients) stroke rate while the aspirin group had a 3.3% (12 of 361 patients) incidence ($p \leq 0.05$). The authors concluded that warfarin was more effective than aspirin in a select population of heart failure patients with NYHA class III or IV and an ejection fraction of less than 20%.

The WASH study (Warfarin/Aspirin Study in Heart Failure), which was a prospective, open-labeled, blinded endpoint design trial, randomized 279 patients to warfarin (INR 2–3), aspirin (300 mg, Q 24 h), or no treatment [39]. The follow up was $27 \pm 1$ month for the composite endpoints of death, nonfatal myocardial infarction, and nonfatal stroke. There were no significant differences between the three groups with respect to these endpoints (26% warfarin versus 33% aspirin versus 26% no treatment respectively). However, there were five major bleeding events one in the aspirin group and four in those receiving warfarin. The authors concluded that because of insufficient power from the planned sample size, the efficacy of aspirin or warfarin could not be determined and a more appropriately powered study was needed. The WATCH trial (Warfarin Antiplatelet Trial and Chronic Heart Failure) had planned to enroll 4500 patients but entered only 1587 patients with NYHA class III–IV symptoms and an LVEF <35% who were receiving angiotensin converting enzyme inhibitors and diuretics. Subjects were randomized to receive warfarin (INR 2–3) or blinded antiplatelet therapy with aspirin (162 mg) or clopidogrel (75 mg) [40]. The primary outcome was death from all causes, nonfatal myocardial infarction, and nonfatal stroke. This trial was terminated early because of inadequate enrollment. The currently ongoing WARCEF trial (Warfarin versus Aspirin in Reduced Cardiac Ejection Fraction) is a prospective trial evaluating warfarin (INR 2–3) against aspirin (325 mg, Q 24 h) with the composite endpoint of all-cause mortality, stroke, and hemorrhage over a 5-year period [41].

## Guideline recommendations for anticoagulation in ambulatory heart failure patients

Having reviewed all the above data what conclusions and recommendations can be derived based on the evidence provided. The ACC/AHA guidelines for the evaluation and management of chronic heart failure recommends that antiplatelet or warfarin therapy not be used for the prevention of stroke in those heart failure patients with normal sinus rhythm [42]. Warfarin anticoagulation (INR 2–3) is recommended for patients with heart failure who have paroxysmal or chronic atrial fibrillation or a previous thromboembolic event (level of evidence A) [42]. The Heart Failure Society of America supports this statement but recommends that warfarin be considered for patients with LVEF of 35% or less but this be done with careful consideration of risks and benefits of anticoagulation (level of evidence B) [43]. The Cochrane Review by Lip and Gibbs concluded that there is no evidence from long-term randomized controlled trials to recommend the use of aspirin to prevent thromboembolic events in patients with heart failure in sinus rhythm [20]. In addition, they found no evidence that warfarin is superior to aspirin in patients with heart failure and sinus rhythm. The American College of Chest Physicians guidelines on antithrombotic therapy recommends that patients with nonischemic heart failure should not receive routine aspirin or warfarin therapy (Grade 1B evidence) and all other heart failure patients should receive aspirin whether or not they are receiving angiotensin converting enzyme inhibitors (Grade 1C+evidence) [44]

## Heart failure and the incidence and treatment of venous thrombosis

As discussed in the earlier section on arterial thromboembolic events in heart failure, there are no studies solely devoted to assessing the incidence of venous thrombosis in patients with heart failure. Therefore, we will focus our attention on large prospective randomized placebo-controlled trials in heterogeneous populations of hospitalized medically ill patients as well as a few retrospective post hoc analyses.

Samama et al. randomized 1102 hospitalized patients older than 40 years of age to receive placebo, enoxaparin 20 mg, or enoxaparin 40 mg once daily for 6 to 14 days [5]. The primary outcome was venous thromboembolism (VTE) diagnosed by bilateral leg venography on day 6 through 14 or earlier, if indicated by symptoms and

**Table 9.3** Incidence of venous thromboembolism (day 1–14) in heart failure.

| Heart failure | Number of patients | Placebo | Enoxaparin | RR | P |
|---|---|---|---|---|---|
| Class III | 151 | 9/73 (12.3%) | 4/78 (5.1%) | 0.42 (0.13–1.29) | 0.2 |
| Class IV | 44 | 5/23 (21.7%) | 0/21 (0%) | – | 0.05 |
| Total HF | 195 | 14/96 (14.6%) | 4/99 (4%) | 0.29 (0.10–0.84) | 0.02 |

*Source*: Data from [46].

signs. The overall incidence of deep vein thrombosis (DVT) was 5.5% in the enoxaparin 40 mg group while the placebo and enoxaparin 20 mg group had respectively 14.9% and 15% thrombotic events. The overall incidence of VTE can be further defined with respect to proximal DVT. The enoxaparin 40 mg had a 1.7% incidence compared to 4.9% with the placebo and 4.5% in the enoxaparin 20 mg groups. At the completion of the fourteenth day of prophylaxis, symptomatic nonfatal pulmonary emboli occurred in four patients, three in the placebo group and one with enoxaparin 20 mg. Subgroup analysis of patients in this trial with NYHA class III or IV heart failure demonstrated that VTE occurred in 14.6% (14 of 96) of patients receiving placebo and 4% in those randomized to enoxaparin (40 mg, SC, Q 24 h). This was a 72% relative risk reduction with a $p < 0.02$ [45,46] (Table 9.3).

Kleber *et al.* randomized 451 medically ill hospitalized patients to either enoxaparin 40 mg once daily or unfractionated heparin 5000 units, subcutaneous, every 8 h for $10 \pm 2$ days [47]. The primary efficacy measure was confirmed VTE up to 1 day after completion of prophylaxis. Deep vein thrombosis was documented by bilateral venography or at autopsy. Suspected pulmonary embolism was verified by a ventilation perfusion scan, pulmonary angiography, or autopsy. Thromboembolic events were confirmed in 8.4% (20 of 239) of patients in the enoxaparin group and 10.4% (22 of 212) of patients in the unfractionated heparin group. Major bleeding occurred in one patient in the enoxaparin group and one patient in the unfractionated heparin group. In this study, patients with heart failure (class III and IV) were evaluated with respect to the two pharmacologic interventions. The enoxaparin group had a 9.7% incidence of DVT and the unfractionated heparin patients were documented to have a 16.1% thrombotic event rate.

Emerson *et al.* evaluated the efficacy of unfractionated low-dose heparin in the prevention of VTE in 78 acute myocardial infarction patients [48]. In this trial radiolabeled fibrinogen scanning was use as the DVT endpoint. Of the 37 unfractionated heparin-treated patients two (5%) developed DVT while 14 (34%) of the 41 control group had thrombosis. Five patients in the control group had pulmonary emboli. In the control group of 41 patients, 14 had concomitant congestive heart failure. Deep vein thrombosis was documented in 8 of these 14 (57%) patients. Although this study was not designed to evaluated congestive heart failure as a risk factor, it did define a trend toward thrombosis in patients with acute myocardial infarction and concomitant congestive heart failure.

In order to further delineate the risk of congestive heart failure for the development of VTE, Howell *et al.* completed a retrospective, case control study that examined whether congestive heart failure due to left ventricular dysfunction was an independent risk factor for acute VTE in an outpatient population and that this risk would correlate with diminishing LVEFs [49]. A logistic regression model, which took into account other risk factors such as previous VTE, recent surgery, and obesity for developing VTE, demonstrated that congestive heart failure patients were more likely to develop VTE than patients without this state with an adjusted odds ratio of 2.6 (95% CI, 1.4–4.7) (Table 9.4). A second logistic regression model demonstrated that the risk of VTE increased as the LVEF decreased. Patients with an LVEF of <20% had an odds ratio of 38.3 (95% CI 9.6) compared with study patients having no available LVEF measurement (Table 9.5). This second model also identified previous VTE as a very powerful predictor of VTE as well as other

Table 9.4 Logistic regression model evaluating CHF and Odds of VTE.

| Risk factor | Odds ratio (95% CI) |
| --- | --- |
| CHF | 2.61 (1.44, 4.73) |
| Prior VTE | 35.50 (14.48, 87.04) |
| Surgical state | 9.86 (4.34, 22.38) |
| Obesity | 3.66 (1.85, 7.23) |

Source: With permission from [49].

Table 9.5 Logistic regression model evaluating LVEF and VTE.

| Risk factor | Odds ratio (95% CI) |
| --- | --- |
| LVEF <20% | 38.3 (9.6, 152.5) |
| LVEF 20–44% | 2.8 (1.4, 5.7) |
| LVEF >45% | 1.7 (1.03, 2.9) |
| Prior VTE | 43.4 (17.0, 111.1) |
| Surgical state | 10.6 (4.6, 24.6) |
| Obesity | 3.9 (1.9, 7.6) |

Source: With permission from [49].

predictors such as surgical state and obesity. This study supports the clinical-pathologic concept that as LVEF decreases, venous stasis worsens, exercise tolerance decreases, and immobility increases. The sequelae all contribute to the development of VTE.

## Recommendations for the prevention of thrombosis in hospitalized patients

The data given earlier does support the increased risk that heart failure affords the hospitalized medically ill patients. The Seventh American College of Chest Physicians Guidelines on antithrombotic therapy recommends that in acutely ill medical patients who have been admitted to the hospital with congestive heart failure or severe respiratory disease, or who are confined to bed and have one or more additional risk factors, including active cancer, previous VTE, sepsis, acute neurologic disease, or inflammatory bowel disease receive VTE prophylaxis with either unfractionated heparin (UFH) (5000 units, SC, Q 8 h) or low molecular weight heparin (LMWH, enoxaparin 40 mg, SC, Q 24 h or dalteparin 5,000 IU, SC, Q 24 h) for the duration of their hospital confinement

(Grade IA recommendation) [50]. The remaining unanswered questions are the post-hospitalization incidence of VTE and the need for extended prophylaxis. This will be answered by the soon to be completed EXCLAIM trial.

## Conclusion

There is no question that heart failure activates the clotting process, increases platelet aggregation, and disrupts endothelial function. All of these factors could increase the risk for the development of arterial or venous thromboembolic events. The data reviewed at best had a number of short comings but a snap shot of arterial and venous thrombotic events were provided. There needs to be large randomized prospective trials to answer the question of incidence as well as preventive measures that are safe and efficacious for long-term use especially as there are currently five million Americans with heart failure and 500 000 new cases each year.

## References

1 Benatar D, Bondmass M, Ghitelman J, Avitall B. Outcomes of chronic heart failure. *Arch Intern Med* 2003;**163**:347–352.

2 Jessup M, Brozena S. Medical progress: heart failure. *N Engl J Med* 2003;**348**:2007–2018.

3 Massie B, Shah NB. Evolving trends in the epidemiologic factors of heart failure: rationale for preventive strategies and comprehensive disease management. *Am Heart J* 1997;**133**:703–712.

4 Baker DW, Wright RF. Management of heart failure: IV anticoagulation for patients with heart failure due to left ventricular systolic dysfunction. *JAMA* 1994;**272**:1614–1618.

5 Samama M, Cohen A, Darmon J *et al.* A comparison of enoxaparin with placebo for the prevention of venous thromboembolism in acutely ill medical patients. *N Engl J Med* 1999;**341**:793–800.

6 Sbarouni E, Bradshaw A, Andreotti F *et al.* Relationship between hemostatic abnormalities and neuroendocrine activity in heart failure. *Am Heart J* 1994;**127**:607–612.

7 Loh E, Sutton MS, Wun CC *et al.* Ventricular dysfunction and the risk of stroke after myocardial infarction. *N Engl J Med* 1997;**336**:251–257.

8 Lip G, Blann A. von Willebrand factor and its relevance to cardiovascular disorders. *Br Heart J* 1995;**74**:580–583.

9  Gibbs CR, Blann AD, Watson RDS, Lip GYH. Abnormalities of hemorheological, endothelial, and platelet function in patients with chronic heart failure in sinus rhythm: effects of angiotensin-converting enzyme inhibitor and beta blocker therapy. *Circulation* 2001;**103**: 1746–1751.

10 Jansson J, Nilsson T, Johnson O. von Willebrand factor in plasma: a novel risk factor for recurrent myocardial infarction and death. *Br Heart J* 1991;**66**:351–355.

11 Jafri SM, Ozawa T, Mammen E *et al.* Platelet function, thrombin and fibrinolytic activity in patients with heart failure. *Eur Heart J* 1993;**14**:205–212.

12 Kubo S, Rect-or T, Bank A *et al.* Endothelium-dependent vasodilatation is attenuated in patients with heart failure. *Circulation* 1991;**84**:1589–1596.

13 Vaughan DE, Rouleau JL, Ridker PM *et al.* Effects of ramipril on plasma fibrinolytic balance in patients with acute anterior myocardial infarction. *Circulation* 1997;**96**:442–447.

14 Brown NJ, Vaughan DE. Role of angiotensin II in coagulation and fibrinolysis. *Heart Fail Rev* 1999;**3**: 193–198.

15 Gibbs C, Blann A, Watson R, Lip G. Abnormalities of hemorheological, endothelial, and platelet function in patients with chronic heart failure in sinus rhythm: effects of angiotensin-converting enzyme inhibitor and beta blocker therapy. *Circulation* 2001;**103**:1746–1751.

16 Yamamoto K, Ikeda U, Furuhashi K *et al.* The coagulation system is activated in idiopathic cardiomyopathy. *J Am Coll Cardiol* 1995;**25**:1634–1640.

17 Jafri S, Mammen E, Masura J, Goldstein S. Effects of warfarin on markers of hypercoagulability in patients with heart failure. *Am Heart J* 1997;**134**:27–36.

18 Jafri S, Riddle J, Raman S *et al.* Altered platelet function in patients with severe congestive heart failure. *Henry Ford Hosp J* 1986;**34**:156–159.

19 Mehta J, Mehta P. Platelet function studies in heart disease. Enhanced platelet aggregate formation in congestive heart failure. *Circulation* 1979;**60**:497–503.

20 Lip GYH, Gibbs CR. Antiplatelet agents versus control or anticoagulation for heart failure in sinus rhythm: a Cochrane systematic review. *Q J Med* 2002;**95**:461–468.

21 Loh E, Sutton MS, Wun CC *et al.* Ventricular dysfunction and the risk of stroke after myocardial infarction. *N Engl J Med* 1997;**336**:251–257.

22 Fuster V, Gersh B, Giuliani E *et al.* The natural history of idiopathic dilated cardiomyopathy. *Am J Cardiol* 1981;**47**:525–530.

23 Ciaccheri M, Castelli Q, Cecchi F *et al.* Lack of correlation between intracavitary thrombosis detected by cross-sectional echocardiography and systemic emboli in patients with dilated cardiomyopathy. *Br Heart J* 1989;**62**:26–29.

24 CONSENSUS Trial Study Group. Effects of enalapril on mortality in severe congestive heart failure. *N Engl J Med* 1987;**316**:1429–1435.

25 Kyrle P, korninger C, Gossinger H *et al.* Prevention of arterial and pulmonary embolism by oral anticoagulants in patients with dilated cardiomyopathy. *Thromb Haemost* 1985;**54**:521–523.

26 Dunkman WB, Johnson GR, Carson PE, Bhat G, Farrell L, Cohn JN, for the V-HeFT VA Cooperative Studies Group. Incidence of thromboembolic events in congestive heart failure. *Circulation* 1993;**87**:V194-101.

27 Yokota Y, Kawanishi H, Hayakawa M *et al.* Cardiac thrombus in dilated cardiomyopathy: relationship between left ventricular pathophysiology and left ventricular thrombus. *Jpn Heart J* 1989;**30**:1–11.

28 Maze SS, Kotler MN, Parry WR. Flow characteristics in the dilated left ventricle with thrombus. *J Am Coll Cardiol* 1989;**13**:873–881.

29 Katz SD, Marnatz PR, Biasucci L *et al.* Low incidence of stroke in ambulatory patients with heart failure: a prospective study. *Am Heart J* 1993;**126**: 141–146.

30 Stratton JR, Resnick AD. Increased embolic risk in patient with left ventricular thrombi. *Circulation* 1987;**75**: 1004–1011.

31 The SOLVD Investigators. Effect of enalapril on survival in patients with reduced left ventricular ejection fractions and congestive heart failure. *N Engl J Med* 1991;**325**:293–302.

32 The SOLVD Investigators. Effect of enalapril on mortality and the development of heart failure in asymptomatic patients with reduced left ventricular ejection fractions. *N Engl J Med* 1992;**327**:685–691.

33 Al-Khadra AS, Salem DN, Rand WM *et al.* Antiplatelet agents and survival: a cohort anlaysis from the Studies of Left Ventricular Dysfunction (SOLVD) trial. *J Am Coll Cardiol* 1998;**31**:419–425.

34 Al-Khadra AS, Salem DN, Rand WM *et al.* Warfarin anticoagulation and survival: a cohort analysis from the Studies of Left Ventricular Dysfunction. *J Am Coll Cardiol* 1998;**31**:749–753.

35 Dries DL, Domanski MJ, Waclawiw AA, Gersh BJ. Effect of antithrombotic therapy on risk of sudden coronary death in patient with congestive heart failure. *Am J Cardiol* 1997;**79**:909–913.

36 Dries DL, Rosenberg YD, Waclawiw MA, Domanski MJ. Ejection fraction and risk of thromboembolic events in patients with systolic dysfunction and sinus rhythm: evidence for gender differences in the studies of left ventricular dysfunction trials. *J Am Coll Cardiol* 1997;**29**:1074–1080.

37 Cohn JN, Archibald DG, Ziesche S, Franciosa JA *et al.* Effect of vasodilator therapy on mortality in

chronic congestive heart failure: results of a Veterans Administration Cooperative Study. *N Engl J Med* 1986;**314**:1547–1552.

38 Falk RH, Pollak A, Tandon PK, Packer M. The effect of warfarin on prevalence of stroke in patients with severe heart failure. *J Am Coll Cardiol* 1993;**21**:218A.

39 Cleland JGF, Findlay I, Jafri S *et al*. The Warfarin/Aspirin Study in Heart Failure (WASH): a randomized trial comparing antithrombotic strategies for patients with heart failure. *Am Heart J* 2004;**148**:157–164.

40 Massie BM, Krol WF, Ammon SE *et al*. The Warfarin and Antiplatelet Therapy in Heart Failure Trial (WATCH): rationale, design, and baseline patient characteristics. *J Card Fail* 2004;**10**:101–112.

41 Pulerwitz T, Rabbani LE, Pinney SP. A rationale for the use of anticoagulation in heart failure management. *J Thromb Thrombolysis* 2004;**17**(2):87–93.

42 Hunt SA, Baker DW, Chin MH *et al*. ACC/AHA guidelines for the evaluation and management of chronic heart failure in adults: Executive summary. *J Am Coll Cardiol* 2001;**38**:2101–2113.

43 Heart Failure Society of America. HFSA guidelines for management of patients with heart failure caused by left ventricular systolic dysfunction: pharmacologic approaches. *J Card Fail* 1999;**5**:357–382.

44 Harrington RA, Becker RC, Ezekowitz M *et al*. Antithrombotic therapy for coronary artery disease. *Chest* 2004;**126**:513S–548S.

45 Alikhan R, Cohen A, Combe S *et al*. Risk factors for venous thromboembolism in hospitalized patients with acute medical illness: analysis of the MEDENOX Study. *Arch Intern Med* 2004;**164**:963–968.

46 Alikahan R, Cohen A, Combe S *et al*. Prevention of venous thromboembolism in medical patients with enoxaparin: a subgroup analysis of the MEDENOX study. *Blood Coagul Fibrinolysis* 2003;**14**:341–346.

47 Kleber F, Witt C, Vogel G *et al*. Randomized comparison of enoxaparin with unfractionated heparin for the prevention of venous thromboembolism in medical patients with heart failure or severe respiratory disease. *Am Heart J* 2003;**145**:614–621.

48 Emerson P, Marks P. Preventing thromboembolism after myocardial infarction: effect of low dose heparin or smoking. *Br Med J* 1977;**1**:18–20.

49 Howell MD, Geraci JM, Knowelton AA. Congestive heart failure and outpatient risk of venous thromboembolism: a retrospective, case-control study. *J Clin Epidemiol* 2001;**54**:810–816.

50 Geerts WH, Pineo GF, Heit JA *et al*. Prevention of venous thromboembolism. *Chest* 2004;**126**:338S–400S.

## CHAPTER 10

# Vasodilator and nitrates

*Abdul Al-Hesayen,* MD, FRCPC *& John D. Parker,* MD, FRCP(C), FACC

## Introduction: the rationale for vasodilator therapy in chronic congestive heart failure

Ventricular afterload is elevated in patients with chronic heart failure (HF) secondary to left ventricular systolic dysfunction. This elevation in afterload is multifactorial in origin, driven primarily by increases in ventricular dimensions, and exacerbated by increased peripheral vascular resistance, abnormalities in aortic impedance, and a relative decrease in ventricular wall thickness (eccentric hypertrophy).

Preload is also elevated in the setting of chronic HF caused by left ventricular systolic dysfunction. Once again, the etiology is multifactorial. Ventricular diastolic dimensions are increased driven by adverse ventricular remodeling. Diastolic properties of the ventricle are abnormal with a decrease in chamber distensibility. The chronic heart failure syndrome is characterized by salt and water retention and a subsequent increase in circulating blood volume. This increase in preload is associated with an increase in diastolic ventricular pressures at rest and/or with exercise and is responsible for the congestive symptoms that are present in a significant proportion of patients with HF.

More than 30 years ago, it was recognized that the chronic increases in preload and afterload that are associated with chronic HF secondary to dilated cardiomyopathy, played an important role in the pathophysiology, symptomatic status, and progression of chronic HF. This recognition was followed by experimentation that documented the ability of vasodilator therapy to have favorable effects on the hemodynamic status of patients with chronic HF. As such, vasodilator therapy was shown to be

associated with a reduction in filling pressures, an increase in cardiac output in response to afterload reduction, and a reduction in functional mitral insufficiency with a paradoxical maintenance of systemic blood pressure despite the vasodilator-induced reduction in systemic arterial resistance.

Vasodilator-induced reductions in afterload and preload are translated into an improvement in ventricular efficiency (Figure 10.1). The reductions in preload and afterload lower myocardial oxygen consumption in the face of unchanged or increased ventricular work [1,2]. This increase in ventricular efficiency may have an important impact on disease progression as HF secondary to systolic dysfunction represents a situation of increased myocardial oxygen demand in the face of limited energy substrate supply. These beneficial effects on preload,

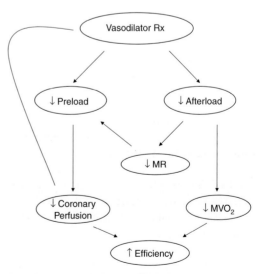

**Figure 10.1** Rationale for vasodilator therapy in HF.

afterload, and myocardial oxygen consumption provide the rationale for vasodilator therapy in chronic HF.

## Nitroprusside

Nitroprusside is the sodium or potassium salt of the ferric cyanide and nitric acid molecule. It has been available since the 1850s. It is a nitrovasodilator relaxing both arterial and venous smooth muscle. It produces its effects through the nonenzymatic release of nitric oxide. This in turn activates soluble guanylate cyclase thereby increasing intracellular concentration of cGMP, which reduces calcium influx across the plasma membrane and its release from the sarcoplasmic reticulum. The release of nitric oxide is accompanied by cyanide release, which is converted in the liver into thiocynate by mitochondrial rhodanase. Thiocynate is excreted by the kidney [3,4]. In 1929, Johnson provided the first description of the hypotensive effects of nitroprusside in humans, however concern that this hypotensive effect was related to the release of cyanide prevented its wide spread use [5]. It was not until 1955, that Page et al. demonstrated its efficacy and safety in treating hypertensive crisis [6]. Broader application was prompted by reports in the early 1970s of improvement in cardiac function in patients with depressed left ventricular function in response to nitroprusside infusion [7].

Nitroprusside is a balanced arterial and venous vasodilator. As such, it has beneficial effects on both preload and afterload (Figure 10.2). Nitroprusside infusion is associated with a reduction in ventricular filling pressures. This preload reduction is multifactorial in origin. Nitroprusside-induced venodilation results in an increase in venous capacitance with attendant shift of blood from the central to the peripheral circulation [8]. Nitroprusside infusion is associated with an increase in cardiac output and a reduction in mitral regurgitation. Both effects are related to a reduction of afterload. Unlike nitrates, this increase in cardiac output is associated with a reduction in renal vascular resistance and an increase or preservation of renal blood flow [9].

In addition, it has been suggested that nitroprusside has primary myocardial effects with a positive impact on left ventricular relaxation and diastolic distensibility [10]. As such, some have suggested that nitroprusside can decrease the slope of the diastolic pressure–volume relationship reflecting an increase in diastolic distensibility [11]. It has been argued that part of the downward shift of the left ventricular pressure–volume relationship is related to diminished pericardial constraint in response to a reduction in ventricular volumes. To address this question Paulus et al. using an elegant bilateral intracoronary infusion technique, documented that nitroprusside hastened LV relaxation and improved diastolic distensibility in the absence of systemic hemodynamic effects [12]. This observation has been made both in normal ventricles and in patients with severe pressure overload hypertrophy [12,13].

These hemodynamic changes are associated with a neutral or beneficial neurohormonal profile. Acutely, nitroprusside is associated with a reduction or no change in cardiac sympathetic activity [14,15]. This observation speaks about the impairment of baroreceptor control of cardiac sympathetic activity, an observation that has been recently extended to the kidney [16]. Furthermore, nitroprusside reduced endothelin levels by 50% and abolished pulmonary release of both ET-1 and big ET-1 that is characteristic of severe heart failure [17,18]. In addition, brain natriuretic peptide (BNP) levels are reduced by 25% after 1 day of therapy with nitroprusside [18].

Nitroprusside is used extensively in the treatment of decompensated heart failure of multiple etiologies. In the setting of an acute coronary syndrome complicated by LV failure, nitroprusside is effective in reducing filling pressures and increasing cardiac output. Although intravenous nitroglycerin is now used more commonly in this setting, nitroprusside can still be useful in certain patients with ongoing ischemia and severe systemic hypertension. A randomized study of nitroprusside was conducted in patients with LV failure in the context of acute myocardial infarction. The study showed no mortality benefit from a 48-h infusion of nitroprusside given routinely to patients with a pulmonary capillary wedge pressure >12 mmHg [19]. Importantly, this study was limited by an extremely small sample size. Recently, Khot et al. reported on the safety and efficacy of nitroprusside infusion in the patients with decompensated HF

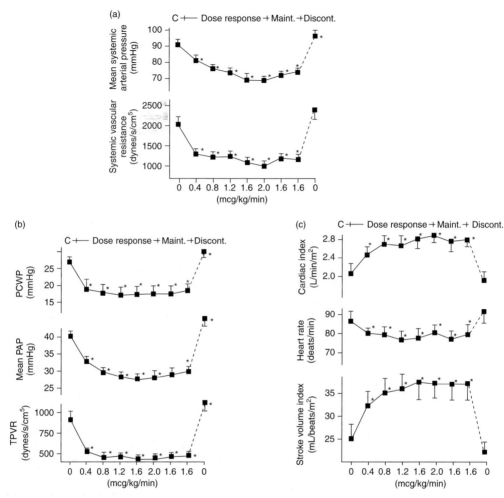

**Figure 10.2** Hemodynamic effects of nitroprusside.

and aortic stenosis (Figure 10.3) [20]. Today, nitroprusside continues to be used in the management and tailored therapy of advanced HF although the recent introduction of intravenous BNP may reduce its utilization in this setting [18]. Finally, nitroprusside continues to be used in the testing of pulmonary vascular reactivity in patients being considered for cardiac transplantation.

## Hydralazine

Hydralazine is a potent arterial vasodilator. It appears to be an endothelium-independent vasodilator although its exact mechanism of action remains unclear. Hydralazine is quite selective as an arterial vasodilator. Its primary hemodynamic

effect is to lower peripheral vascular resistance. Although hydralazine does lower left ventricular filling pressures in patients with CHF, this effect is less prominent when compared to that observed with nitroprusside or the organic nitrates. This relative lack of preload reduction provided the rationale for combining hyrdalazine with organic nitrates, a combination that yields a balanced vasodilatory effect. The combination of nitrates and hydralazine has been shown to result in additive hemodynamic effects compared to each drug on its own [21,22].

The systemic and pulmonary hemodynamic effects of hydralazine have been well-documented in patients with HF. Acutely, hydralazine causes a reduction in both systemic and pulmonary vascular

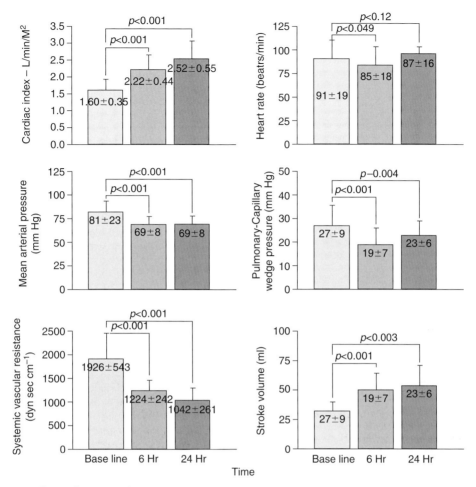

**Figure 10.3** Efficacy of nitroprusside in patients with decompensated HF due to aortic stenosis.

resistance. This afterload reduction is accompanied by a 60–70% increase in stroke volume and cardiac output leading to a minimal reduction in systemic arterial pressure (5%) (Figure 10.4) [23]. These beneficial acute hemodynamic changes are maintained during exercise although they have not been shown to translate into an increase in exercise capacity for hydralazine therapy on its own. The response to hydralazine appears to be dependent on LV chamber size. Patients with an LVEDD >60 mm show a greater increase in cardiac output and improvement in renal function compared to patients with an LVEDD <60 mm [24]. Chronic hydralazine administration has been shown to be associated with sustained beneficial hemodynamic effects for up to 8 months [25]. However, a subset of patients develop tolerance to these

therapeutic effects despite preserved responses to other vasodilators [24].

Hydralazine therapy reduces renal vascular resistance and causes an increase in renal blood flow. Although this increase in renal blood flow is not accompanied by an increase in glomerular filtration rate acutely, it resulted in an increase in creatinine clearance after 3 days of therapy [26]. Hydralazine can have sympathoexcitatory effects mediated by arterial baroreceptor responses secondary to reductions in arterial blood pressure. Increases in coronary sinus norepinephrine concentrations have been reported in some patients following administration of hydralazine, an observation that suggests cardiac sympathetic activation [27]. Other authors have documented a positive inotropic response to hydralazine suggesting that this pharmacodynamic

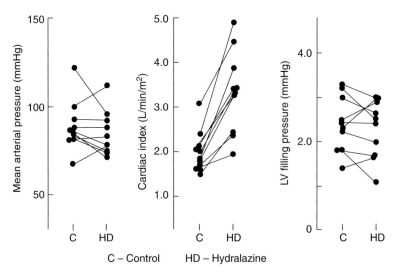

**Figure 10.4** Hemodynamic effects of Hydralazine.

effect might be secondary to stimulation of the sympathetic nervous system [28]. Finally, hydralazine has been reported to increase myocardial oxygen consumption by increasing heart rate and minute ventricular stroke work. Although this effect could be deleterious in patients with ischemic heart disease, this effect is offset by an increase in coronary blood flow [29].

Interestingly, it is now recognized that hydralazine has antioxidant effects, something which is of relevance to the observation that the combination of nitrates and hydralazine has beneficial effects on clinical outcome in chronic heart failure. This antioxidant effect has been documented in *in vitro* studies where hydralazine has been shown to inhibit the generation of reactive oxygen species by blocking the actions of NADH and NADPH oxidases [30].

The combination of hydralazine and isosorbide dinitrate was the first vasodilator regiment that was shown to have a mortality benefit in patients with moderate heart failure [31]. The hemodynamic effects of these two vasodilators are complementary to each other. Furthermore, hydralazine has been shown to prevent the development of tolerance to nitrates [30]. This combination was superseded by angiotensin converting enzyme inhibitor (ACEI) therapy with the publication of the V-HeFT II trial [32]. However, there has been a recent interest in the potential role of adding the combination

therapy to ACEI therapy. The interest stems from a subgroup analysis of V-HeFT I and II showing a race-based difference in the response to hydralazine and isosorbide dinitrate therapy [33]. Recently, this was confirmed with the publication of the A-HeFT protocol. This study reported a 43% reduction in mortality in black patients treated with hydralazine and isosorbide dinitrate in addition to standard therapy including ACEI and beta-blockers (Figure 10.5) [34].

### The organic nitrates

Nitrates are prodrugs that require intracellular metabolic biotransformation to liberate nitric oxide (NO) prior to producing their known myriad of pharmacological effects. NO activates guanylate cyclase causing the conversion of guanosine triphosphate to cGMP, with subsequent smooth muscle cell relaxant effects. The exact mechanism of the denitration process leading to the liberation of NO remains controversial, although recent development points to a central role of mitochondrial aldehyde dehydrogenase in the biotransformation of nitroglycerine [35].

Nitrates exert their hemodynamic effects through vasodilatation of the capacitance veins and conductive arteries with a preferential effect on the venous side of the circulation [36]. Most of the beneficial effects of nitrate therapy in the setting of heart failure are mediated through

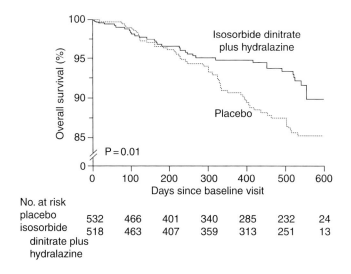

No. at risk

| | | | | | | | |
|---|---|---|---|---|---|---|---|
| placebo | 532 | 466 | 401 | 340 | 285 | 232 | 24 |
| isosorbide dinitrate plus hydralazine | 518 | 463 | 407 | 359 | 313 | 251 | 13 |

**Figure 10.5** Effects of isosorbide dinitrate plus hydralazine on mortality in black patients with heart failure.

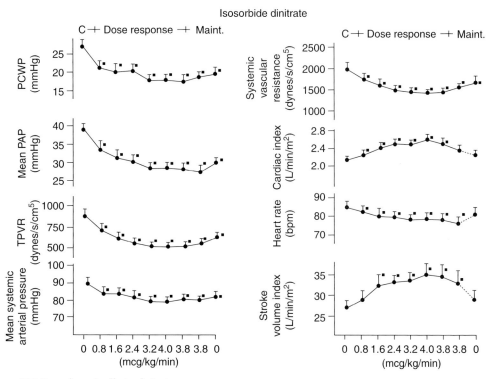

**Figure 10.6** Hemodynamic effects of nitrates.

preload reduction (Figure 10.6). Nitrate therapy lowers ventricular filling pressures via venodilatation, which leads to a shift of intracardiac and central blood volume to the peripheral circulation causing a reduction in ventricular volumes and diastolic wall stress [37–39]. Through their effects on conductive arteries they reduce systemic blood pressure and ventricular afterload with a resultant increase in cardiac output [38,39]. However, this increase in cardiac output is not uniformly distributed among all cardiovascular beds. Nitrates increase limb blood flow and reduce renal blood flow with no alteration in splanchnic and hepatic blood flow [39]. This observation is of potential importance when managing patients with decompensated heart failure and reduced renal function although no clear adverse impact on clinical outcome has ever been documented. Mitral regurgitation is common in patients with heart failure and nitrate therapy reduces the regurgitant fraction through its effects on both ventricular volume and afterload [40,41].

Despite their beneficial hemodynamic effects when given acutely, it has been documented that a significant portion of this acute effect is lost during sustained therapy, a phenomenon known as nitrate tolerance. Tolerance to the hemodynamic effects of the organic nitrates has been documented in a number of studies [42,43]. Interpretation of the clinical impact of sustained nitrate therapy on clinical outcomes in patients with chronic CHF requires an understanding of this phenomenon. In this setting, almost all studies have used hemodynamic markers to document tolerance (this is defined as loss of hemodynamic effectiveness). The mechanism(s) of tolerance appear to be multifactorial and has recently been reviewed in detail [44,45]. Importantly, the presence of tolerance is dependent upon the type of long-acting nitrate applied, the pharmacokinetic characteristics of the formulation and, to some extent, the vascular bed which is studied. Indeed, early studies done with isosorbide dinitrate suggested that tolerance to the effect of this medication on the pulmonary vasculature was less apparent than that observed in the systemic arterial bed. The loss of hemodynamic effects during sustained nitrate administration in congestive heart failure is usually not total. For example, when one examines the impact of nitrates on filling pressures, it is clear that during sustained therapy with most formulations there is significant loss of the acute effects of these drugs on filling pressures. Nevertheless, in most studies filling pressures do not return completely to baseline but remain somewhat lower than it was prior to the initiation of nitrate therapy. This is important because there is evidence that minor reductions in filling pressures may be associated with beneficial effects on, for example, cardiac sympathetic activity [46]. Furthermore, these subtle reductions in filling pressures may be associated with beneficial effects on

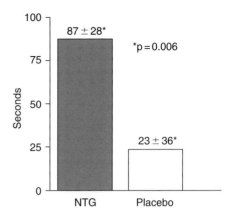

**Figure 10.7** Effects of nitrates on exercise tolerance.

myocardial oxygen consumption and thus improve the energetics of LV chamber function over time. Importantly, even the acute hemodynamic effects of nitrates are not observed in all patients. It has been documented that patients with elevated right atrial pressure or peripheral edema are resistant to the hemodynamic effects of nitrates [47]. This resistance is reversed with diuretic therapy [47].

Nitrates improve exercise tolerance in heart failure patients. They progressively increase exercise duration in the setting of heart failure over a 3-month period (Figure 10.7) [48]. Although prior studies had documented a beneficial effect of nitrates on exercise capacity in chronic HF, the more recent results confirm that they are beneficial in patients already treated with ACEI. The mechanism of this improvement is multifactorial. The reduction in filling pressures and mitral regurgitation during activity with nitrates may be partly responsible [40].

Chronic heart failure is a state of energy deprivation and nitrates may help in correcting this imbalance [1]. First, preload and afterload are important determinants of myocardial oxygen consumption and both are reduced by nitrate therapy. Second, nitrates by reducing LV diastolic pressure help in averting subendocardial ischemia [49]. Although nitrates do not increase coronary blood flow, this observation in not surprising given its close correlation with myocardial oxygen requirements that is reduced commensurate with the reduction in preload and afterload. Indeed, nitrate therapy has been shown to reduce myocardial oxygen consumption in heart failure patients [50]. Importantly, unlike sodium nitroprusside, the risk of myocardial ischemia due to coronary steal is reduced due to the lack of an effect of nitrates on resistance vessels.

Nitrates have the capacity to relieve angina in patients with dilated cardiomyopathy by a number of mechanisms. They have been shown to improve collateral blood flow in patients with severe epicardial coronary disease. Their primary mechanism of reducing angina appears to be preload reduction. This has certainly been the long accepted mechanism through which nitrates improve angina when given acutely. Importantly, in patients with an ischemic cardiomyopathy, the presence of epicardial coronary disease can be aggravated by the presence of elevated cardiac filling pressures. Therefore, the use of nitrates in patients with elevated filling pressures can lead to quite dramatic improvements in angina. Indeed, in this era of ACE inhibition and angiotension II receptor antagonist, the primary role for nitrates in the therapy of angina may be in the relief of ischemia.

No hard outcome data exist for nitrates on their own in the treatment of HF. However, nitrates in combination with hydralazine improved survival in the V-HeFT trial when added to a combination of digoxin and diuretics [31]. As such, the independent beneficial effects of nitrates on long-term outcome in chronic heart failure remain uncertain. Furthermore, during the past decade, multiple studies in both animal models and humans have documented that sustained nitrate therapy is associated with increased free radical production, increased sensitivity of the vasculature to vasoconstriction, as well as the development of endothelial dysfunction in multiple vascular beds [51]. Although these findings have not been shown to have adverse effects on clinical outcome, they do cast a shadow over the benefit of widespread use of organic nitrates in chronic congestive heart failure.

## Summary

In summary, intravenous vasodilators can play an important role in the management of patients with acutely decompensated HF. In particular, nitroprusside and more frequently nitroglycerin can provide salutary benefits in patients with high peripheral vascular resistance and low cardiac output. The role of oral vasodilators has undergone change over the past few years as new agents have replaced the combination of hydralazine and isosorbide dinitrate in the pharmacologic regimen for treatment of chronic heart failure. Indeed, the Guidelines of the ACC/AHA note that the combination of hydralazine and isosorbide dinitrate 'should not be used for the treatment of heart failure patients who have no prior use of an ACE inhibitor and should not be substituted for ACE inhibitors in patients who are tolerating ACE inhibitors without difficulty [52]'. However, the combination of hydralazine and isosorbide dinitrate may be considered in patients who are intolerant of an ACEI; however, there are no trials that support the use of this combination in patients with persistent symptoms and intolerance of renin–angiotensin system inhibitors. Perhaps the most exciting information regarding the use of vasodilators comes from the recent A-HeFT trial that demonstrated a significant survival benefit of the combination of hydralazine and isosorbide dinitrate when added to routine therapy with an ACEI or a beta-blocker in African American patients with HF. Whether or not these results are relevant to some proportion of the non-African American population will require further study.

## References

1 De Marco T, Chatterjee K, Rouleau JL, Parmley WW. Abnormal coronary hemodynamics and myocardial energetics in patients with chronic heart failure caused by ischemic heart disease and dilated cardiomyopathy. *Am Heart J* 1988;**115**:809–815.

2 Miller RR, Vismara LA, Zelis R, Amsterdam EA, Mason DT. Clinical use of sodium nitroprusside in chronic ischemic heart disease. Effects on peripheral vascular resistance and venous tone and on ventricular volume, pump and mechanical performance. *Circulation* 1975;**51**:328–336.

3 Palmer RF, Lasseter KC. Drug therapy. Sodium nitroprusside. *N Engl J Med* 1975;**292**:294–297.

4 Schulz V. Clinical pharmacokinetics of nitroprusside, cyanide, thiosulphate and thiocyanate. *Clin Pharmacokinet* 1984;**9**:239–251.

5 Cohn JN, Burke LP. Nitroprusside. *Ann Intern Med* 1979;**91**:752–757.

6 Page IH, Corcoran AC, Dustan HP, Koppanyi T. Cardiovascular actions of sodium nitroprusside in animals and hypertensive patients. *Circulation* 1955;**11**:188–198.

7  Franciosa JA, Limas CJ, Guiha NH, Rodriguera E, Cohn JN. Improved left ventricular function during nitroprusside infusion in acute myocardial infarction. *Lancet* 1972;**1**:650–654.

8  Pouleur H, Covell JW, Ross J, Jr. Effects of nitroprusside on venous return and central blood volume in the absence and presence of acute heart failure. *Circulation* 1980;**61**:328–337.

9  Leier CV. Regional blood flow responses to vasodilators and inotropes in congestive heart failure. *Am J Cardiol* 1988;**62**:86E–93E.

10  Kelly RA, Balligand JL, Smith TW. Nitric oxide and cardiac function. *Circ Res* 1996;**79**:363–380.

11  Herrmann HC, Ruddy TD, Dec GW, Strauss HW, Boucher CA, Fifer MA. Diastolic function in patients with severe heart failure: comparison of the effects of enoximone and nitroprusside. *Circulation* 1987;**75**: 1214–1221.

12  Paulus WJ, Vantrimpont PJ, Shah AM. Acute effects of nitric oxide on left ventricular relaxation and diastolic distensibility in humans. Assessment by bicoronary sodium nitroprusside infusion. *Circulation* 1994;**89**:2070–2078.

13  Matter CM, Mandinov L, Kaufmann PA, Vassalli G, Jiang Z, Hess OM. Effect of NO donors on LV diastolic function in patients with severe pressure-overload hypertrophy. *Circulation* 1999;**99**:2396–2401.

14  Newton GE, Parker JD. Cardiac sympathetic responses to acute vasodilation. Normal ventricular function versus congestive heart failure. *Circulation* 1996;**94**:3161–3167.

15  Kaye DM, Jennings GL, Dart AM, Esler MD. Differential effect of acute baroreceptor unloading on cardiac and systemic sympathetic tone in congestive heart failure. *J Am Coll Cardiol* 1998;**31**:583–587.

16  Al Hesayen A, Parker JD. Impaired baroreceptor control of renal sympathetic activity in human chronic heart failure. *Circulation* 2004;**109**:2862–2865.

17  Stangl K, Dschietzig T, Richter C *et al*. Pulmonary release and coronary and peripheral consumption of big endothelin and endothelin-1 in severe heart failure: acute effects of vasodilator therapy. *Circulation* 2000;**102**:1132–1138.

18  Johnson W, Omland T, Hall C *et al*. Neurohormonal activation rapidly decreases after intravenous therapy with diuretics and vasodilators for class IV heart failure. *J Am Coll Cardiol* 2002;**39**:1623–1629.

19  Cohn JN, Franciosa JA, Francis GS *et al*. Effect of short-term infusion of sodium nitroprusside on mortality rate in acute myocardial infarction complicated by left ventricular failure: results of a Veterans Administration cooperative study. *N Engl J Med* 1982;**306**:1129–1135.

20  Khot UN, Novaro GM, Popovic ZB *et al*. Nitroprusside in critically ill patients with left ventricular dysfunction and aortic stenosis. *N Engl J Med* 2003;**348**:1756–1763.

21  Massie B, Chatterjee K, Werner J, Greenberg B, Hart R, Parmley WW. Hemodynamic advantage of combined administration of hydralazine orally and nitrates non-parenterally in the vasodilator therapy of chronic heart failure. *Am J Cardiol* 1977;**40**:794–801.

22  Massie BM, Kramer B, Shen E, Haughom F. Vasodilator treatment with isosorbide dinitrate and hydralazine in chronic heart failure. *Br Heart J* 1981;**45**:376–384.

23  Chatterjee K, Parmley WW, Massie B *et al*. Oral hydralazine therapy for chronic refractory heart failure. *Circulation* 1976;**54**:879–883.

24  Packer M, Meller J, Medina N, Yushak M, Gorlin R. Hemodynamic characterization of tolerance to long-term hydralazine therapy in severe chronic heart failure. *N Engl J Med* 1982;**306**:57–62.

25  Chatterjee K, Ports TA, Brundage BH, Massie B, Holly AN, Parmley WW. Oral hydralazine in chronic heart failure: sustained beneficial hemodynamic effects. *Ann Intern Med* 1980;**92**:600–604.

26  Cogan JJ, Humphreys MH, Carlson CJ, Rapaport E. Renal effects of nitroprusside and hydralazine in patients with congestive heart failure. *Circulation* 1980;**61**:316–323.

27  Daly P, Rouleau JL, Cousineau D, Burgess JH, Chatterjee K. Effects of captopril and a combination of hydralazine and isosorbide dinitrate on myocardial sympathetic tone in patients with severe congestive heart failure. *Br Heart J* 1986;**56**:152–157.

28  Elkayam U, Roth A, Hsueh W, Weber L, Freidenberger L, Rahimtoola SH. Neurohumoral consequences of vasodilator therapy with hydralazine and nifedipine in severe congestive heart failure. *Am Heart J* 1986;**111**: 1130–1138.

29  Magorien RD, Brown GP, Unverferth DV *et al*. Effects of hydralazine on coronary blood flow and myocardial energetics in congestive heart failure. *Circulation* 1982;**65**:528–533.

30  Munzel T, Kurz S, Rajagopalan S *et al*. Hydralazine prevents nitroglycerin tolerance by inhibiting activation of a membrane-bound NADH oxidase. A new action for an old drug. *J Clin Invest* 1996;**98**:1465–1470.

31  Cohn JN, Archibald DG, Ziesche S *et al*. Effect of vasodilator therapy on mortality in chronic congestive heart failure. Results of a Veterans Administration Cooperative Study. *N Engl J Med* 1986;**314**:1547–1552.

32  Cohn JN, Johnson G, Ziesche S *et al*. A comparison of enalapril with hydralazine-isosorbide dinitrate in the treatment of chronic congestive heart failure. *N Engl J Med* 1991;**325**:303–310.

33  Exner DV, Dries DL, Domanski MJ, Cohn JN. Lesser response to angiotensin-converting-enzyme inhibitor therapy in black as compared with white patients with left ventricular dysfunction. *N Engl J Med* 2001;**344**: 1351–1357.

34 Taylor AL, Ziesche S, Yancy C et al. Combination of isosorbide dinitrate and hydralazine in blacks with heart failure. N Engl J Med 2004;**351**:2049–2057.

35 Chen Z, Zhang J, Stamler JS. Identification of the enzymatic mechanism of nitroglycerin bioactivation. Proc Natl Acad Sci USA 2002;**99**:8306-8311.

36 Parker JD, Parker JO. Nitrate therapy for stable angina pectoris. N Engl J Med 1998;**338**:520–531.

37 Gold HK, Leinbach RC, Sanders CA. Use of sublingual nitroglycerin in congestive failure following acute myocardial infarction. Circulation 1972;**46**:839–845.

38 Bussmann WD, Schofer H, Kaltenbach M. Effects of intravenous nitroglycerin on hemodynamics and ischemic injury in patients with acute myocardial infarction. Eur J Cardiol 1978;**8**:61–74.

39 Leier CV, Bambach D, Thompson MJ, Cattaneo SM, Goldberg RJ, Unverferth DV. Central and regional hemodynamic effects of intravenous isosorbide dinitrate, nitroglycerin and nitroprusside in patients with congestive heart failure. Am J Cardiol 1981;**48**: 1115–1123.

40 Stevenson LW, Brunken RC, Belil D et al. Afterload reduction with vasodilators and diuretics decreases mitral regurgitation during upright exercise in advanced heart failure. J Am Coll Cardiol 1990;**15**:174–180.

41 Gibbs JS, Keegan J, Wright C, Fox KM, Poole-Wilson PA. Pulmonary artery pressure changes during exercise and daily activities in chronic heart failure. J Am Coll Cardiol 1990;**15**:52–61.

42 Bogaert MG, Rosseel MT, Deschaepdryver AF. Cardiovascular effects of glyceryldinitrates as compared to glyceryltrinitrate. Arch Int Pharmacodyn Ther 1968;**176**: 458–460.

43 Bogaert MG, De Schaepdryver AF. Tolerance towards glyceryl trinitrate (trinitrin) in dogs. Arch Int Pharmacodyn Ther 1968;**171**:221–224.

44 Gori T, Parker JD. Nitrate tolerance: a unifying hypothesis. Circulation 2002;**106**:2510–2513.

45 Gori T, Parker JD. The puzzle of nitrate tolerance: pieces smaller than we thought? Circulation 2002;**106**: 2404–2408.

46 Azevedo ER, Newton GE, Floras JS, Parker JD. Reducing cardiac filling pressure lowers norepinephrine spillover in patients with chronic heart failure. Circulation 2000;**101**:2053–2059.

47 Kulick D, Roth A, McIntosh N, Rahimtoola SH, Elkayam U. Resistance to isosorbide dinitrate in patients with severe chronic heart failure: incidence and attempt at hemodynamic prediction. J Am Coll Cardiol 1988;**12**:1023–1028.

48 Elkayam U, Johnson JV, Shotan A et al. Double-blind, placebo-controlled study to evaluate the effect of organic nitrates in patients with chronic heart failure treated with angiotensin-converting enzyme inhibition. Circulation 1999;**99**:2652–2657.

49 Unverferth DV, Magorien RD, Lewis RP, Leier CV. The role of subendocardial ischemia in perpetuating myocardial failure in patients with nonischemic congestive cardiomyopathy. Am Heart J 1983;**105**:176–179.

50 Gray R, Chatterjee K, Vyden JK, Ganz W, Forrester JS, Swan HJ. Hemodynamic and metabolic effects of isosorbide dinitrate in chronic congestive heart failure. Am Heart J 1975;**90**:346–352.

51 Munzel T, Sayegh H, Freeman BA, Tarpey MM, Harrison DG. Evidence for enhanced vascular superoxide anion production in nitrate tolerance. A novel mechanism underlying tolerance and cross-tolerance. J Clin Invest 1995;**95**:187–194.

52 Hunt SA, Abraham WT, Chin MH et al. ACC-AHA 2005 Guideline update for the diagnosis and management of chronic heart failure in the adult. Summary Article A Report of the American College of Cardiology/American Heart Association Task Force on Practice Guidelines (Writing Committee to Update the 2001 Guidelines for the Evaluation and Management of Heart Failure). J Am Coll Cardiol 2005;**46**:1116–1143.

## CHAPTER 11

# Natriuretic peptides for the treatment of heart failure

*Jonathan D. Sackner-Bernstein,* MD, *Hal Skopicki,* MD, PHD *&*
*Keith D. Aaronson,* MD, MSC

## Introduction

Dyspnea and fatigue may profoundly limit the quality of life experienced by patients with left ventricular dysfunction, and are reflected by clinical signs of volume overload, elevated cardiac filling pressures and diminished end-organ perfusion. Treatments must balance between the opposing targets of relieving organ congestion, a reflection of increased risk of hospitalization and cardiovascular events [1] and antagonizing mediators of left ventricular remodelling [2]. Thus standard therapies include neurohormonal antagonists [2] and agents to optimize hemodynamic status and volume control [3].

However, much like the mythological Scylla and Charybdis, navigating between the symptoms of dyspnea and fatigue is not simply a matter of reversing volume overload. While diuretics are potent means of relieving congestion they are associated with activation of the renin–angiotensin system [4] and can exacerbate electrolyte abnormalities [5] and glucose intolerance [6]. Despite these concerns, no prospective, randomized placebo-controlled study has established the net clinical effects of diuretics in acutely decompensated heart failure. Alternative treatments, such as the vasodilators nitroglycerin and nitroprusside, can reduce preload and afterload acutely but are associated with tachyphylaxis, by-product toxicity, and/or ineffective dosing regimens [7,8]. And while inotropic agents are useful for enhancing renal perfusion and augmenting diuresis, clinical studies

have demonstrated that their use is associated with increased risks of tachyarrhythmias and mortality [9,10].

Natriuretic peptides have been advocated as potential front-line agents for the treatment of acutely decompensated heart failure [11]. Similar to catecholamines and angiotensin II, they have multiple effects on the cardiovascular system. Preliminary studies suggested natriuretic, diuretic, and vasodilatory actions, clinical trials in acutely decompensated heart failure patients have not consistently demonstrated these effects. Recent evidence has emerged suggesting the need for caution with their clinical use.

This chapter will attempt to synthesize the pathophysiologic and clinical roles of natriuretic peptides and critically evaluate their potential role as therapy for patients with decompensated heart failure. In so doing, the extent of investigation, limitations of the literature, research are also presented, all with the perspective that the utility of any therapy can only be defined based on the net effects on clinical outcomes.

## Mechanisms of action

Natriuretic peptides were named, in part, based on the natriuresis accompanying diuresis precipitated by the injection of an extract of atrial tissue in rats [12–14]. Further study demonstrated that the heart secretes two peptides with natriuretic properties, atrial natriuretic peptide (ANP) from the atria and b-type natriuretic peptide (BNP) from the ventricles [15–17]. Synthesized within the kidney, the natriuretic peptide urodilatin is most closely related to ANP, with the exception the addition of an NH$_2$ terminal extension [127] is primarily synthesized in the brain, but is also produced by vascular endothelial cells [18–20]. All four share in common a 17-amino acid ring structure and exert their actions via second messenger activation, after binding to natriuretic peptide receptors (NPR-A and NPR-B), to generate cyclic guanosine monophosphate (cGMP) [21]. The type-A receptor, present in larger blood vessels, adrenal glands, and kidneys, binds ANP and BNP albeit with a lower affinity for BNP. The type-B receptor, expressed in the adrenal glands, kidneys, and brain is specific for CNP [22]. Type-C receptors are believed to be involved in receptor-mediated endocytotic degradation of the natriuretic peptides [23]. While ANP, BNP and urodilatin exert their vascular effects by increasing intracellular cGMP levels, GNP activity appears at least partly cGMP-independent, acting via a tyrosine kinase dependent pathway [128].

The secretion of ANP is elicited by atrial stretch [24]. Early studies of this 28-amino acid peptide demonstrated vasodilatory, natriuretic, and neurohormonal inhibitory properties, seemingly ideal responses for atria contending with a volume challenge. ANP was found to produce natriuresis by inhibiting sodium reabsorption in the collecting duct, increasing glomerular filtration rate, and sodium filtration; vasodilation via direct relaxation of vascular smooth muscle; and inhibition of the release or action of renin, angiotensin II, aldosterone, and vasopressin [25,26]. However, the exceedingly short serum half-life of ANP (2–5 min in humans with a metabolic clearance rate of 14–25 mL/min/kg) [26] and the development of pharmacogenic tolerance made its clinical application challenging.

B-type natriuretic peptide is synthesized and released by ventricular myocytes and fibroblasts in response to myocardial stretch [27,28]. A multitude of studies have shown that increased serum BNP concentrations are highly predictive of major cardiovascular events in patients with either acutely decompensated or chronic heart failure and the magnitude of BNP release is in direct proportion to ventricular wall stretch [29–36]. It is endogenously synthesized as a propeptide (proBNP), which is proteolytically cleaved and then secreted into the blood as C-terminal BNP (a 32 amino acid peptide) and an N-terminal-proBNP fragment. Only the C-terminal BNP is biologically active. BNP shares nearly identical physiological actions with ANP [37]. Endogenous BNP has a half-life of 18–22 min and (similar to ANP) its clearance is affected by two major mechanisms, binding to the NPR-C receptor on cell surfaces followed by endocytosis and lysosomal degradation and direct proteolysis by neutral endopeptidase [38]. Urodilatin is a paracrine peptide secreted by renal distal tubular cells. The addition of the terminal NH$_2$ appears to provide a longer half life than ANP [129]. Its physiologic effects appear similar to other natriuretic peptides, though its secretion within the kidney and its inhibition of sodium reabsorption via amiloride sensitive channels suggests greater relevance than the other peptides to the control of salt and water balance [130].

Therefore, identification of neutral endopeptidase inhibitors, which would prolong the action of natriuretic peptides, became a therapeutic goal [39]. While initial investigations demonstrated rapid natriuresis, diuresis, and vasodilation in response to neutral endopeptidase inhibition by candoxatrilat and candoxatril [40,41], these effects were not maintained with chronic use. Ecadotril produced desirable physiologic effects acutely, but a phase II trial of 279 patients treated for 3–4 months showed no improvement in clinical status. Alarmingly, a numerically greater number of patients died on active therapy (0 versus 3%, $p$ = ns) [42]. The IMPRESS trial reported that omapatrilat, which blocks both neutral endopeptidase and angiotensin converting enzyme, reduced the risk of mortality or major morbidity compared to enalapril [43]. However, the larger OVERTURE trial demonstrated that omapatrilat could only be considered noninferior to enalapril, not superior [44]. More ominous to the fate of omapatrilat was the increased risk of angioedema [45,46]. Therefore, the search for a synthetic analog of BNP became a primary therapeutic focus.

## Clinical effects of natriuretic peptides

Administration of ANP to normal volunteers was found to induce significant natriuresis and diuresis

[47,48]. However, while confirming that ANP produced a marked natriuretic effect in normal controls, Cody *et al.* noted that the effect was more modest in patients with heart failure [49]. Similarly, initial studies of recombinant BNP (nesiritide) in normal volunteers showing its diuretic effect at doses of 0.007–0.014 µg/kg/min [50] and the report of increased natriuresis, diuresis, glomerular filtration rate, filtration fraction, and filtered load of sodium compared with placebo in the absence of changes in renal blood flow [51]. Thus began the investigation of natriuretic peptides for human use including the ANP analogs anaritide [131] and carperitide (the later marketed for the treatment of acutely decompensated heart failure in Japan) and recombinant BNP (nesiritide).

In animal studies, compared to ANP, BNP has been shown to have greater natriuretic actions, decreased susceptibility for degradation by neutral endopeptidase, and an enhanced ability to augment intracellular cGMP [52,53]. Urodilatin has greater potency than BNP as a venodilator in human heart failure [132].

Preclinical investigations of recombinant BNP confirmed its similar physiological activities to endogenous BNP [54,55]. After intravenous bolus administration, BNP achieves 90% of its peak effects within 30 min and has a mean terminal elimination half-life of 18–20 min. Even though BNP is partly eliminated via renal filtration, dosage adjustment is not required for patients with renal insufficiency.

Nesiritide induces formation of cGMP in smooth muscle cells, which should result in balanced arterial and venous vasodilation [11,56]. It also can stimulate renal excretion of sodium while blunting the activation of the renin–angiotensin–aldosterone and sympathetic nervous systems [57–61]. Importantly, the dose response for each of these physiologic effects was different.

## Effect of nesiritide on clinical symptoms in acutely decompensated heart failure

### Comparison to placebo

The lack of meaningful impact of nesiritide on clinical status is an underappreciated aspect of the clinical trial results to date. In VMAC, through

nesiritide treated patients had better dyspnea scores at 3 hours after initiation of therapy, there were no differences between nesiritide and placebo on the severity of dyspnea at any other time point. In parallel, there were no points in time when patients felt better overall. These observations suggest that the difference at the 3 hour time point may be a statistical fluke [69].

Improvement in clinical status by nesiritide relative to placebo was first demonstrated in patients with severely decompensated heart failure undergoing invasive hemodynamic monitoring [62]. Subsequently, the VMAC study demonstrated nesiritide's ability to improve symptoms of dyspnea relative to placebo in a broader population of patients admitted to the hospital with acutely decompensated heart failure whether or not invasive monitoring was indicated [63]. Both trials demonstrated rapid symptomatic relief of dyspnea and a reduction in pulmonary capillary wedge pressure [62,63].

While the effects were consistent and statistically significant, the nature of the effects may cast some doubt on the clinical relevance of these statistical advantages. For example, the Nesiritide Study Group Efficacy Trial (NSGET) administered placebo or one of two doses of nesiritide (0.3 µg bolus with an infusion of 0.015 or 0.6 µg followed by an infusion at 0.03 µg/kg/min) in double-blind fashion for 6 h [62]. At the end of 6 h, dyspnea improved significantly more frequently for nesiritide treated patients (12%, 56%, 50% improved on placebo, nesiritide 0.015 or 0.03 µg/kg/min infusions respectively, $p < 0.001$). However, the results were not as robust in the VMAC trial which used the standard dosing regimen of 2 µg/kg bolus followed by an infusion of 0.01 µg/kg/min. While dyspnea was affected more favorably during nesiritide treatment ($p = 0.034$), the frequency that patients reporting that their dyspnea improved moderately or markedly was less striking (35% versus 44%, for placebo and any dose of nesiritide, respectively) as was the frequency of any improvement noted, even if only mild, according to the patient (64% versus 76%, for placebo and any dose of nesiritide) [63]. Similar findings were reported by these two trials when assessing patient rated impact on overall well-being. While NSGET demonstrated greater improvement in global clinical status in patients receiving nesiritide after 6 h of higher dose infusions (0.015 or 0.03 µg/kg/min) [62], there were no statistical differences between the effects of nesiritide and placebo after 3 h of the standard dosing regimen (0.01 µg/kg/min infusion) [63].

### Comparison to nitroglycerin

While VMAC confirmed nesiritide's effectiveness at relieving dyspnea compared to placebo at 3 hours after initiation of therapy, superiority over nitroglycerin was not established at any point of time within the first 24 h [63]. After 3 h of therapy, 44% of nesiritide and 47% of nitroglycerin treated patients reported moderate or marked improvement in dyspnea, while 73% and 76% reported any improvement ($p = 0.6$). There were no significant differences in the patient's global assessment between the two drugs, with 45% versus 41% reporting moderate or marked improvement and 66% and 75% any improvement for nitroglycerin and nesiritide therapy ($p = 0.3$).

This lack of superiority for effectiveness is particularly relevant when coupled with an analysis of the safety of nesiritide, relative to nitrates or placebo. While ease of administration, tolerability (Table 11.1), and consistency of the reduction in pulmonary capillary wedge pressure are relevant benefits to nesiritide use, its association with worsening renal function and overall safety concerns mitigate its theoretical advantages. The hemodynamic advantages of nesiritide, as well as these safety issues, are addressed in sections that follow.

### Nesiritide as a diuretic and natriuretic

Nesiritide has not been proven to promote diuresis or natriuresis in patients with acutely decompensated heart failure at its approved doses and should not be used for such purposes [64]. While a preliminary study in patients with heart failure reported a trend towards greater net urine output during a 24 h infusion with high dose nesiritide (infused at doses of 0.015, 0.03, or 0.05 µg/kg/min) [65], a larger study showed a trend towards *less* net urine output with nesiritide than placebo, although nesiritide treated patients received diuretics less frequently than the control group patients [66].

A diuretic sparing effect was also suggested by Colucci *et al.* who controlled for diuretic administration during a 6 h comparison between nesiritide and placebo in patients hospitalized with severely decompensated heart failure. Nesiritide treatment at doses of 0.015 and 0.03 µg/kg/min resulted in 560 and 659 mL urine output over the 6 h observation period compared to 380 mL during placebo therapy ($p = 0.004$) [62]. Moreover, after the 6 h blinded phase, it was the more frequent diuretic use in placebo-treated patients that led to similar urine output between groups by 24 h [67]. The VMAC trial reported similar urine output over 24 h for patients treated with nitroglycerin or nesiritide (2959 ±1543 versus 2969 ± 1838 mL, respectively) [67], with diuretics administered most frequently in the nitroglycerin group (94% versus 85% respectively, $p = 0.001$) [63]. Considering the adverse neurohormonal effects of diuretics [4], if this diuretic sparing effect by nesiritide were to be proven it would likely prove to be clinically advantageous.

**Table 11.1** Adverse events associated with nitroglycerin and nesiritide where the frequency was greater in nitroglycerin or there appeared to be a dose-related incidence with nesiritide [88].

| Adverse event | Nitroglycerin | Nesiritide infusion rate (µg/kg/min) | | |
| | | 0.01 | 0.015 | 0.03 |
|---|---|---|---|---|
| Asymptomatic hypotension | 17 (8%) | 17 (8%) | 31 (12%) | 49 (20%) |
| Symptomatic hypotension | 10 (5%) | 10 (5%) | 2 (11%) | 42 (17%) |
| Bradycardia | 1 (<1%) | 2 (1%) | 8 (3%) | 13 (5%) |
| Headache | 44 (20%) | 19 (9%) | 23 (9%) | 17 (7%) |
| Nausea | 13 (6%) | 7 (3%) | 24 (9%) | 33 (13%) |

Despite the perception that nesiritide is diuretic sparing [68], this effect of nesiritide remains an unproven hypothesis. However while more patients in the notroglycerin group were treated with concomitant diuretics, the average doses of diuretics administered to each group were similar (range: 153–173 mg/day of furosemide) [69] accounting for the Braunwald committee's recommendation not to view nesiritide as a diuretic [64].

## Effect of nesiritide on hemodynamics

Studies indicate variable, dose-dependent effects of nesiritide on venodilation, afterload reduction, improvement in cardiac index, and coronary vasodilation.

### Effect as venodilator

Nesiritide is an effective venodilator and has been demonstrated to be superior to low-dose nitroglycerin [63]. The mechanism of venodilation is incompletely defined, but data suggests that inhibition of venous tone results in recruitment of venous capacitance vessels with little or no effect on conduit veins [132]. In patients with or without decompensated heart failure, nesiritide produces prompt reduction in cardiac filling pressures at doses as low as 0.01 µg/kg/min [63,65,70]. When administered following a bolus of 2 mg at an infusion rate of 0.01 µg/kg/min, pulmonary capillary wedge pressure decreases significantly within 15 min when compared to placebo or intravenous low-dose nitroglycerin (starting at 5 µg/min with a median dose of 13 µg/min) ($-3.5 \pm 5.3$ versus $-1.2 \pm 3.8$ and $-1.2 \pm 3.6$ mmHg for nesiritide, nitroglycerin, and placebo, respectively, $p < 0.05$ for nesiritide versus nitroglycerin and nesiritide versus placebo). After 3 h, these differences persist ($-5.8 \pm 6.5$ versus $-3.8 \pm 5.3$ versus $-1 \pm 4.2$ mmHg for nesiritide, nitroglycerin and placebo, respectively, $p < 0.05$ for nesiritide versus nitroglycerin and nesiritide versus placebo). There were no differences on the change in wedge pressure between fixed dose nesiritide and titrated nitroglycerin infusions after 12 or 24 h of therapy, although adjustable dose nesiritide was associated with statistically significant reductions in wedge pressure than nitroglycerin therapy [63]. There were no statistically significant differences between the effects of nesiritide and nitroglycerin

on right atrial pressure after 3 h ($-3.1 \pm 4.6$ versus $-2.6 \pm 3.5$ mmHg, respectively) [63].

### Effect on afterload

Compared to placebo in either stable or acutely decompensated heart failure patients, nesiritide at doses of 0.015 or 0.03 µg/kg/min lowers systolic blood pressure approximately 5–8 mmHg within 3 h [66] and up to 5–10 mmHg after 6 h [62].

When used at currently recommended doses, nesiritide lowered systemic vascular resistance within 1 h relative to placebo therapy. However, there were no differences between nesiritide and placebo-treated patients after 3 h of therapy. Nesiritide did lower pulmonary vascular resistance relative to placebo within one hour, an effect that lasted through 3 h, the final time measurements were made relative to placebo in the VMAC trial [63].

Compared to nitroglycerin there were no statistical differences between nesiritide and nitroglycerin on systemic or pulmonary vascular resistances at any time point over the first 24 h of blinded medication administration [63]. This suggests that at the recommended dose, nesiritide is predominantly a venodilator without significant arteriolar vasodilation.

### Cardiac index

In patients without heart failure, cardiac output was not increased after an infusion of nesiritide that included a bolus of 2 mg followed by a 0.01 µg/kg/min infusion [70]. In parallel, when assessed in patients with acute decompensation of heart failure (ADHF), the effects of nesiritide on cardiac index were not as robust as its effects on cardiac filling pressures.

In patients with heart failure, nesiritide infused at doses of 0.015, 0.03, and 0.06 µg/kg/min significantly increased cardiac index after 3 h. When compared to placebo, the magnitude of the effect was less after a 24 hours of nesiritide relative to placebo [66]. The study with the second largest population studied (NSGET: 127 patients) reported that cardiac index increased significantly at doses of 0.015 and 0.03 µg/kg/min (by 18% and 28%, respectively) after a 6 h infusion of nesiritide relative to placebo but was not designed to provide data beyond that 6 hour time point [54,62].

However, the VMAC study reported little effect on cardiac index when starting with current recommended dosing, 2 μg/kg bolus followed by an infusion of 0.01 μg/kg/min. In the subgroup of 246 patients who underwent measurement of cardiac hemodynamics in VMAC relative to both nitroglycerin and placebo therapies, nesiritide administration resulted in a significant increase in cardiac index by the first hour that was no longer significantly greater than placebo or low-dose nitroglycerin by the third hour of therapy, consistent with the pharmacodynamic effect of the bolus administration and little effect from the ongoing infusion [63].

### Coronary vasodilation

Nesiritide may be an effective coronary vasodilator. In patients without heart failure treated with a bolus of 2 mg followed by a 0.01 μg/kg/min infusion, nesiritide increased epicardial coronary diameter from $2.6 \pm 0.8$ mm at baseline to $3.0 \pm 0.8$ mm at 15 min and then $3.0 \pm 0.9$ mm at 30 min ($p = 0.007$ compared with baseline). Coronary resistance decreased from $4.4 \pm 5.0$ mmHg/min/mL at baseline to $3.4 \pm 4.7$ at 15 min ($p = 0.019$) and $3.3 \pm 3.7$ at 30 min ($p < 0.046$) [70]. In conjunction with the preliminary observations on the effects of natriuretic peptides as adjuncts to coronary interventions and in patients with recent myocardial infarction [61,71], these data support further investigation in coronary disease [72].

The lack of effect of nesiritide on systemic vascular resistance coupled with the lack of a consistent or sustained increase in cardiac index supports the hypothesis that nesiritide is a more potent venodilator than arterial vasodilator when administered at the dose of 0.01 μg/kg/min. Therefore, when nesiritide is administered at its approved doses, lowering of pulmonary capillary wedge pressure should be expected while changes in cardiac index may be less consistent and pulmonary vascular resistance is likely to remain unaffected, particularly when comparing the effects of nesiritide to the vasodilator nitroglycerin.

### Effect of natriuretic peptides on remodeling

In patients with systolic dysfunction, therapies that favorably affect ventricular remodeling tend to improve the natural history of the disease [73]. If natriuretic peptides were to blunt the activation of both renin–angiotensin–aldosterone and sympathetic nervous systems and lower ventricular filling pressures in patients with systolic dysfunction [57–61,63], it is plausible that they would therefore favorably affect ventricular remodeling [61,71].

Mechanistic studies are available to support an important role for natriuretic peptides in the development of deleterious remodeling and the potential for reverse remodeling. BNP is produced rapidly after experimental myocardial infarction and its serum level in heart failure is correlated with the severity of myocardial wall stress. More recent investigations underscore the complex role of BNP in myocardial healing. Mice that lack the *BNP* gene still develop similarly to animals with the *BNP* gene [74]. However, in the presence of pressure overload from aortic banding, marked myocardial fibrosis appeared in those mice lacking BNP. Experimental infarction in normal mice is also associated with a gradient of BNP expression (with greater production and release in the periinfarct zone) suggesting a prominent role for BNP in regulating myocardial remodeling [75].

The net effects of BNP may be modulated by its temporal relationship to an event. Mice that overexpress BNP appear to be at higher risk of myocardial rupture in the early days after infarction [74], associated with increased infiltration of neutrophils and release of local MMP-9. The increased activity of this gelatinase was associated with enhanced collagen breakdown without parallel increase in collagen synthesis. Ventricular geometry was improved in animals that survived without rupture of 6 weeks, supporting the view that BNP plays a central role in regulating the balance between mitigating ventricular remodeling and predisposing to myocardial rupture [76]. The Burnett laboratory recently reported that canine fibroblasts secrete BNP in abundance when stimulated by TNF-α and, in parallel, degradative collagenase production is increased [28]. Together, these data suggests that continued local production of BNP in the myocardium may regulate fibroblast-induced wound healing.

While there are no clinical data evaluating the remodeling and scarring effects of nesiritide in humans, investigation of the effects of the ANP analog carperitide is ongoing. An open label pilot study has demonstrated that carperitide significantly reduced left ventricular filling pressure in patients who suffered an acute infarction and had heart failure with documented left ventricular dysfunction [77]. A randomized pilot trial has also assessed the effects of carperitide in patients undergoing angioplasty. Relative to placebo therapy, the 20 patients randomized to carperitide had smaller left ventricular and diastolic volume index (LVEDVI) at 1 and 6 months and a higher ejection fraction after 6 months [71]. In 60 patients randomized to ANP or nitroglycerin after an anterior infarction, left ventricular remodeling appeared to be attenuated by ANP [61]. Additional studies are underway to investigate the role of carperitide as an adjunct to coronary interventions [72].

## Effect of natriuretic peptides on neurohormones

Natriuretic peptides can antagonize the release and effects of several neurohormones that are known to contribute to the progression of heart failure [2]. These include members of the renin–angiotensin–aldosterone system [57–61], the sympathetic nervous system [60], and the endothelin pathway [61,78]. Each of these three systems produces adverse effects when activated long term, particularly vasoconstriction and sodium and water retention, which can be opposed by the pharmacologic effects of natriuretic peptides.

Non-hypotensive doses of ANP [79] and BNP [80] are sympathoinhibitory in patients with heart failure. Even doses that produce mild hypotension (approximately 5 mmHg change) are not associated with any evidence of sympathoexcitation. As nesiritide is used as an infusion during clinical decompensation for a period of hours or days, it remains unclear whether the neurohormonal antagonism reported acutely with high dose therapy will be relevant to standard dosing regimens administered either briefly or as prolonged infusions. The potential for long-term effects on neurohormonal activation remains an untested hypothesis.

## Effect of natriuretic peptides on circulating blood volume

Natriuretic peptides may also reduce ventricular filling pressure by affecting body water distribution. Administration of ANP results in shifts of intravascular volume to the extravascular space along with protein extravasation, as reflected by hemoconcentration in excess of that predicted by the degree of diuresis [81,82]. Similarly, nesiritide tends to increase hematocrit slightly within the first 2 days of therapy with resolution by day 5 and has been associated with trends towards a greater incidence of hypoalbuminemia in phase II trials [67]. Although likely less important than the vasodilatory effects of nesiritide, a reduction in circulating blood volume could contribute to the lowering of pulmonary capillary wedge and right atrial pressures. This finding may also explain the prolonged hypotension during nesiritide infusion that persisted beyond the time predicted based on the pharmacologic half-life of the drug [63], although this effect of nesiritide seems more likely to be related to delayed clearance of cGMP. Further studies will be required to determine whether this is a clinically relevant effect and if so identify those patients at risk. There is no suggestion in the literature that such a phenomenon, if present, would have any prognostic relevance.

## Safety of recombinant BNP

At the time of initial FDA approval, the clinical trials database for nesiritide in acutely decompensated heart failure included 755 patients with heart failure treated with nesiritide infused at the currently approved doses (0.01–0.03 µg/kg/min) but only 273 treated at the approved starting dose (2 µg/kg bolus and 0.01 µg/kg/min infusion). Of these patients, a smaller number suffered from acutely decompensated heart failure, defined as those patients requiring therapy within the first 24 h of a heart failure hospitalization. Presumably, owing to the *perception* of a low risk of adverse events relative to other standard therapies for this clinical setting, nesiritide was approved for the acute lowering of pulmonary capillary wedge pressure and relief of dyspnea due to volume overload [67]. However, no randomized clinical trial defined the long-term safety associated with nesiritide administration, even when used as therapy for acutely decompensated heart failure [64,83]. Moreover, despite preliminary evidence suggesting safety in the outpatient setting (FUSION), no long term, adequately powered safety or efficacy studies have been performed for treatment of outpatients with chronic heart failure.

In addition to these limitations, the clinical trials database with nesiritide offers particularly little guidance for three specific patient populations, those with concomitant ischemia, those with preserved ejection fraction, and those with baseline creatinine above 2.0 mg/dL prior to the initiation of therapy. First, the clinical trial database included only 27 patients who had been admitted for an acute coronary syndrome within 7 days prior to nesiritide infusion. Second, while VMAC permitted study enrolment whether or not ventricular systolic function was impaired, ejection fraction was not measured in this study. Only 9% (35 of 373) of patients enrolled in trials who received nesiritide had ejection fraction documented to be above 40%. Third, while nesiritide has been purported to be nephroprotective [11,51], only 19% (147 of 755) of patients who received nesiritide in clinical trials had an initial creatinine above 2.0 mg/dL prior to therapy. The association between worsening renal function and nesiritide use underscores the caution necessary when considering nesiritide for patients with preexisting chronic kidney disease.

## Effect of nesiritide on ventricular arrhythmias

The theoretical advantages of nesiritide in acutely decompensated heart failure patients appear most striking in comparison to positive inotropes. While dobutamine and milrinone can improve cardiac output and renal blood flow, positive inotropic agents are proarrhythmic and their use in heart failure patients has been associated with an increased risk of death [9,10,84–87]. In contrast, proarrhythmia has not been associated with nesiritide therapy [88,89]. Similar to nitroglycerin and nitroprusside and unlike the inotropes, nesiritide does not affect intracellular calcium [90]. The lack of proarrhythmic risk may prove relevant to the outpatient setting, as the presence of ventricular

arrhythmias in FUSION-1 was no greater for the nesiritide treated group than the control group, although positive inotropes were administered to 58% of the patients in the control group but only 1.4% in the nesiritide group, perhaps biasing an assessment of proarrhythmic risk in favor of nesiritide. The lower proarrhythmic risk may indicate that nesiritide can be administered in the absence of continuous ECG monitoring, providing additional logistical and economic advantages.

However, the lack of proarrhythmic effect does not necessarily preclude risk. Silver and colleagues compared survival between groups of patients treated with dobutamine or nesiritide within 180 days of treatment in a post hoc subset analysis from a trial where patients were randomized, open-label, to standard care or nesiritide, where the dose of nesiritide was blinded [113]. The analysis selected the subset of patients in the standard care group who were treated with dobutamine at the discretion of the investigators (58% of the standard care group). Dobutamine treated patients appeared to be at higher risk of death than those treated with nesiritide infused at 0.015 µg/kg/min, whereas those patients randomized to an infusion of 0.03 µg/kg/min appeared to be at similar risk of death as the dobutamine treated patients. While the apparent benefit at lower doses may be cited as evidence that vasodilator therapy is preferable to positive inotropic agents, there can be no escaping the suggestion that nesiritide may have a narrow therapeutic window (Figure 11.1). This finding is one that parallels prior experience with vesnarinone [133] and tezosentan [134], drugs developed for heart failure that proved to be associated with significant and relevant risks.

## Effect on renal function

Both baseline renal dysfunction and acute transient worsening of renal function are associated with increased morbidity and mortality in patients with cardiovascular disease [91–95]. Moreover, renal dysfunction, whether measured by serum creatinine [92,96,97], glomerular filtration rate [98,99], or calculated creatinine clearance [100–102], can predict outcome in patients with chronic heart failure [98–102] and in those hospitalized for acutely decompensated heart failure [103–106].

Even minimal increases in serum creatinine of just 0.1 mg/dL were predictive of worsened outcome, independent of baseline creatinine [106]. The relationship between transient increases in creatinine and worse outcome has been demonstrated at levels of 0.3 up to 0.5 mg/dL [103–107]. Although worsening renal function is a surrogate suggesting risk and not proof of harm, the data supporting its relevance are as strong as any other in patients with acutey decompensated heart failure, including wedge pressure, cardiac output, and neurohormonal activity.

It is important to consider the evolution of the beliefs of the effects of nesiritide on renal function. Preliminary mechanistic studies suggested that nesiritide might improve renal blood flow and

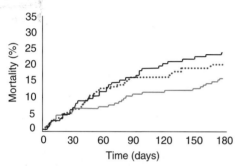

Log Rank test:
Dobutamine versus Nesiritide 0.03 *p*=0.45
Dobutamine versus Nesiritide 0.015 *p*=0.04
Nesiritide 0.015 versus 0.03 *p*=0.19

— Dobutamine 5 μg/kg/min (*n*=141)
···· Nesiritide 0.03 μg/kg/min (*n*=179)
— Nesiritide 0.015 μg/kg/min (*n*=187)

**Figure 11.1** Risk of death after treatment with nesiritide (0.015 or 0.03 μg/kg/min) or dobutamine (5 μg/kg/min) [113].

enhance the glomerular filtration rate [56]. Several review papers reinforced this perspective, as was summarized by the report from the BNP Consensus Panel, a panel supported by an educational grant from the manufacturers of nesiritide [11]. In addition, a retrospective analysis of the VMAC trial reported that patients with or without preexistent chronic kidney disease responded equally well to nesiritide treatment without increased risk of renal dysfunction [63,108].

Yet the effects of nesiritide used at recommended dose on renal function in the VMAC trial, based on prospectively defined parameters, were not reported [11]. For each of these three definitions, nesiritide was associated with numerically more patients with worsened renal function than was nitroglycerin therapy [69] (Table 11.2).

The clinical relevance was demonstrated by Gottlieb and colleagues who investigated the effects of nesiritide on renal function in fifteen patients with chronic renal insufficiency (serum creatinine rose from a baseline of $1.5 \pm 0.4$ to $1.8 \pm 0.8$ mg/dL at time of trial initiation) and chronic heart failure associated with volume overload [109]. No benefits on renal function were associated with a 24 h infusion of nesiritide relative to placebo, despite careful measurement of glomerular filtration rate (by iothalamate clearance), effective renal plasma flow (by para-amino hippurate clearance), urinary sodium excretion, and urine output. Of note, their was a trend suggesting nesiritide reduced effective renal plasma flow relative to placebo ($p = 0.09$).

To further assess the effect of nesiritide on renal function, a meta-analysis of completed trials was performed [110]. During the FDA review of nesiritide in 1999, the agency defined clinically relevant worsening renal function as an increase

**Table 11.2** Effects of nesiritide and nitroglycerin on the incidence of worsening renal function in the VMAC trial. ($S_{Cr}$ = serum creatinine) [69].

| | Nitroglycerin | Nesiritide fixed dose | Nesiritide adjustable dose |
|---|---|---|---|
| *n* | 216 | 211 | 63 |
| # (%) with ↑ $S_{Cr}$ of >0.5 mg/dL | 45 (21%) | 59 (28%) | 15 (24%) |
| # (%) with abnormal $S_{Cr}$ within first week | 13 (6%) | 18 (9%) | 6 (10%) |
| # (%) with abnormal $S_{Cr}$ at last value | 21 (10%) | 30 (14%) | 10 (14%) |

# number

in serum creatinine of at least 0.5 mg/dL. When nesiritide was reviewed again in 2001, the same definition was applied by the agency. The FDA data indicated that doses of nesiritide ≤0.03 µg/kg/min significantly increased the risk of worsening renal function (RR = 1.52, 95% CI 1.16–2.00, $p$ = 0.003) relative to any control therapy (which included positive inotropes, vasodilator, or placebo therapy) (Figure 11.2). Similar risks were apparent when analyses were restricted to lower doses of nesiritide (≤0.015) or after comparison to a control group that included patients randomized to inotropic therapy or nesiritide at doses higher than the approved dose range (0.06 µg/kg/min).

Following the publication of this analysis, the manufacturer of nesiritide reviewed its effects at the standard dose (2 µg/kg bolus, 0.01 µg/kg/min infusion) and reported an estimated 35% higher risk of worsening renal function associated with nesiritide (95% CI = 0.88–2.06, $p = 0.17$) (Darlene Horton, Scios Inc. personal communication). Only VMAC utilized this dose and measured serum creatinine on follow-up. With the small number of patients available for this analysis ($n = 265$), these data have been cited as showing no adverse effect on renal function [135–137], when in reality, they demonstrate a lack of proven safety even at this, the standard starting dose. To date, no dose of nesiritide has been shown to be neutral or beneficial on renal function in a multi-center, randomized, double blind clinical trial. Despite the expectation that nesiritide would be beneficial for renal function, the trend toward worsened renal function – even at this low dose – certainly does not provide any evidence to suggest renal protection with nesiritide. Whether the worsening renal function reflects a secondary hemodynamic effect or primary renal injury is unknown but the prognostic importance of worsening renal function mandates further investigation in appropriately powered clinical trials [64], ideally designed to assess the effects both during the hospitalized period and for several weeks thereafter, when the risk appears to continue.

## Mortality risk

To date, no prospective mortality trial for the use of nesiritide in hospitalized acutely decompensated heart failure patients has been performed. A preliminary analysis evaluated the safety of standard dose nesiritide by pooling data from the only two randomized, double-blind studies that were designed prospectively to collect mortality data within 30 days after nesiritide administration, (VMAC [63] and PROACTION [111]). Within 30 days, patients treated with nesiritide appeared to be at higher risk of death. (Figure 11.3a) [112]. This analysis focused on the safety of standard dose nesiritide in trials where the control group did not mandate inotrope use. Within VMAC, the nesiritide treatment groups did have more frequent use of the inotrope dobutamine, yet adjusting for this imbalance did not change the estimate of risk appreciably. The apparent increased risk of death associated with nesiritide in this analysis of double-blind trials with prespecified 30-day mortality endpoints stood in contrast to the apparent decrease relative to dobutamine that had been previously reported in the post hoc subgroup analysis from an open-label trial [113].

Nesiritide was evaluated in one additional randomized, double-blind study that included patients with acutely decompensated heart failure. The Nesiritide Study Group Efficacy Trial

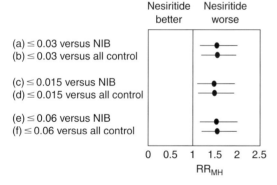

Figure 11.2 Relative risk of worsening renal function with nesiritide, evaluating effects relative to non-inotrope-based (NIB) or any control therapies. (a) Nesiritide ≤0.03 µg/kg/min versus non-inotrope-based controls; (b) nesiritide ≤0.03 µg/kg/min versus all control therapies, including inotropes; (c) nesiritide ≤0.015 µg/kg/min versus non-inotrope-based controls; (d) nesiritide ≤ 0.015 µg/kg/min versus all control therapies, including inotropes; (e) nesiritide ≤ 0.06 µg/kg/min versus non-inotrope-based controls; (f) nesiritide ≤0.06 µg/kg/min versus all control therapies, including inotropes [110].

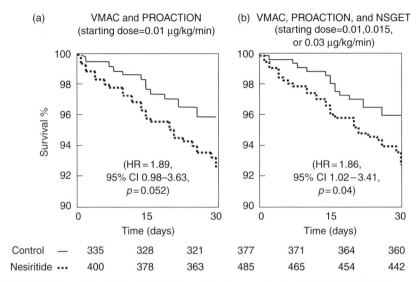

**Figure 11.3** Risk of death associated with nesiritide therapy based on randomized double-blind trials (assessed by Log Rank test). (a) Comparison of standard dose nesiritide to control therapy, based on VMAC [63] and PROACTION [111] studies [112] and (b) Comparison of any dose nesiritide to control therapy (addition of NSGET study [62]) [114]. [Adapted with permission from J Sackner-Bernstein]

(NSGET), compared a 6-h infusion of placebo with nesiritide – with dosing including a smaller bolus but a higher infusion rate than is currently recommended [62]. (providing for similar amount of total drug exposure over 12–24 h). While the NSGET trial was designed to measure outcomes at 21 days, FDA files also report on outcomes through 30 days of follow-up. None of these three trials mandated that control therapy include a positive inotropic agent and these three trials are the only ones that studied acutely decompensated heart failure patients using a double-blind study design. Confirming results of the initial meta-analysis based on only the first two studies [112] and in accordance with the QUORUM guidelines for meta-analyses, the final report included all three of these studies. Nesiritide was associated with an estimated 80% higher risk of death within 30 days of its use (RR = 1.81, 95% CI, 1.01–3.27, $p = 0.04$ by Log Rank, RR = 1.80, 95% CI, 0.98–3.31, $p = 0.057$ by Cox Proportional Hazards) [114] (Figure 11.3b).

A post-hoc, retrospective analysis was recently reported from the ADHERE registry, an uncontrolled, unblinded registry of patients hospitalized with acute decompensated heart failure [115]. While the unadjusted risk of in hospital death

was significantly increased for patients receiving nesiritide, statistical adjustment based on several factors of proven prognostic importance resulted in a lower mortality for nesiritide treated patients compared to those receiving dobutamine or milrinone; mortality was similar for patients treated with nesiritide versus nitroglycerin. However, observational analyses can only adjust for measured differences between groups. There are no statistical methods to account for unmeasured differences that may lead a physician to choose to use one medication rather than another. The experience of hormone replacement therapy – better outcome in observational studies [116] but increased risk in prospective, randomized, double-blind clinical trials [117,118] – strongly argues for caution in drawing conclusions from this study. The hormone replacement therapy example is particularly relevant owing to early work demonstrating favorable effects of the therapy on biomarkers of recognized prognostic importance [119]. Therefore, despite the registry data from ADHERE, its inherent limitations do not mitigate the need for an adequately powered clinical trial to establish both efficacy and risk at clinically relevant doses in prospective patient populations [64,114,120].

Based upon a review of data provided by the manufacturer of nesiritide, a committee was convened by Dr Eugene Braunwald at the request of Scios as a result of recent publications questioning the risks of nesiritide therapy [110,114]. The committee recommended marked curtailment of the outpatient intermittent use and continuous inpatient use of nesiritide and recommended that a large scale trial be undertaken to establish the risks of worsening renal function and death [64]. Although other agents used for acutely decompensated heart failure have not undergone such formal safety assessments, this is no reason to exclude nesiritide from such tests, particularly when there are several lines of evidence suggesting that nesiritide is associated with an increased risk of death and no proof that it is clinically superior to other available therapies.

## Outpatient therapy

Intermittent outpatient infusions of nesiritide for patients with advanced symptomatic chronic heart failure became a common practice despite limited clinical trial data [120]. FUSION-I is the single trial completed with FUSION-II targeted for completion in late 2007. FUSION-I evaluated the feasibility of intermittent infusions in 210 patients using an open-label study design where patients were randomized to no infusions, standard dose nesiritide for 4–6 h, or low dose infusions for similar duration (1 μg/kg/min bolus followed by infusion at 0.005 μg/kg/min). Patients were eligible for study participation even if they had received nesiritide infusions within the prior 6 months [121]. Patients were treated at a frequency determined by investigator discretion based on hydration status and symptoms, from twice weekly to once every other week. Inotrope use was permitted and was administered to 58% of control patients and 1.4% of the nesiritide groups.

The study showed that infusions were generally well-tolerated, with 79% continuing to receive infusions at the end of the 12-week protocol. Although aldosterone and endothelin levels were reduced acutely after a nesiritide infusion, there were no significant changes reported over the duration of the study in basal levels. Although the investigators' assessment of well-being showed significant benefit for patients receiving standard-dose nesiritide, patients' perception indicated no difference between nesiritide and standard care, with no distinction between therapies based on global well-being or Minnesota living with heart failure questionnaire [121].

Although analysis of the prospectively defined high-risk subgroup suggested a reduction in the combined risk of all-cause mortality and all-cause hospitalization, the data reinforce another disturbing trend, that of a narrow window of therapeutic safety. As was the case in the comparison to the inotrope dobutamine, where modest doses of nesiritide seemed safer but a slight increase in dose had a similar mortality risk as dobutamine, so did the data appear from this high-risk subgroup. The subset of patients ($n = 24$) receiving 0.005 μg/kg/min infusion appeared to be at lower risk than standard care ($p = 0.019$), while those receiving standard dose nesiritide (2 μg/kg bolus followed by 0.01 μg/kg/min infusion) had a risk more similar to those patients in the standard care group [122].

FUSION-II is designed as a larger trial ($n = 900$) in which patients will be randomized in double-blind fashion to placebo, low dose or standard dose nesiritide. Unfortunately, this trial is unlikely to have the statistical power to address safety issues with sufficient confidence for physicians to be able to interpret the relative value of utilizing this therapy in clinical practice. The suggestion of the narrow window for safety in the high-risk strata of FUSION-I makes this limitation of the FUSION-II study design very important to recognize.

In addition, this report of a narrow dose range for safety in the FUSION-I database parallels prior reports in the inpatient setting [63,113]. Such a trend is a strong signal warning of the likelihood of risk with nesiritide use.

## Alternative agents and administrative routes

Small studies have examined the feasibility of twice daily subcutaneous injection of nesiritide and several ANP analogs [71,77,123], have been studied. Recently, a novel natriuretic peptide, d-type (DNP) has been identified in snake venom. When administered to dogs DNP markedly reduced filling pressures and systemic blood pressure, maintained renal blood flow, and enhanced urinary sodium excretion without affecting cardiac output [124]. Its pharmacologic activity in human tissue has also been demonstrated [125]. Of note, DNP does not appear to be degraded by neutral endopeptidase [126], yet contains both diuretic and vasodilatory effects [124,126].

A phase 2 study demonstrated hemodynamic benefits of urodilatin in patients with heart failure [138]. The preliminary report suggested no signal of renal risk, but did not disclose the protocol for surveillance, i.e., the frequency of measurement of serum creatinine, definitions of relevant worsening of renal function, etc.

Further studies will be required to delineate the clinical applicability of alternate modes of administration and alternative therapeutic agents to affect the natriuretic pathway.

## Conclusion

The multiple roles of natriuretic peptides in the pathophysiology of heart failure and the effects of pharmacologic administration of recombinant forms makes this pathway one of great interest. However, because of their novel mechanisms of action and protean cardiovascular effects, adequately powered randomized clinical trials that focus on safety and efficacy are needed to better understand their role in the clinical armamentarium for the treatment of heart failure [64,83,120]. In the absence of a specific clinical trial that accurately defines the safety of nesiritide, the meta-analyses [110,112,114] suggest that caution is warranted in using nesiritide in patients with acutely decompensated heart failure. While registry data such as that from ADHERE may seem reassuring [115], clinicians must recognize the inherent flaws in open-label, non-randomized registries. Therefore, adequately powered, randomized, double-blind clinical trials must be performed to assess the safety of nesiritide before the drug can be used widely for the treatment of heart failure, as would be the mandate for any drug developed for acutely decompensated heart failure. Pending the results of appropriately powered clinical trials, the Braunwald committee advocated [64] that nesiritide's use should be limited to the immediate and short-term therapy of patients admitted for worsening heart failure. Hopefully, additional trials will help clinicians to better understand the clinical roles natriuretic peptides in the future by defining their safety and effectiveness.

## References

1 Muntwyler J, Abetel G, Gruner C, Follath F. One-year mortality among unselected outpatients with heart failure. *Eur Heart J* 2002;**23**:1861–1866.

2 Mann DL. Mechanisms and models in heart failure: A combinatorial approach. *Circulation* 1999;**100**:999–1008.

3 Lucas C, Johnson W, Hamilton M *et al.* Freedom from congestion predicts good survival despite previous class IV symptoms of heart failure. *Am Heart J* 2000;**140**:840–847.

4 Bayliss J, Norell M, Canepa-Anson R, Sutton G, Poole-Wilson P. Untreated heart failure: clinical and neuroendocrine effects of introducing diuretics. *Br Heart J* 1987;**57**:17–22.

5 Packer M, Gottlieb SS, Kessler PD. Hormone-electrolyte interactions in the pathogenesis of lethal cardiac arrhythmias in patients with congestive heart failure. Basis of a new physiologic approach to control of arrhythmia. *Am J Med* 1986;**80**:23–29.

6 Plavinik FL, Rodrigues CI, Zanella MT, Ribeiro AB. Hypokalemia, glucose intolerance, and hyperinsulinemia during diuretic therapy. *Hypertension* 1992;**19**:II26–29.

7 Monrad E, Baim D, Smith H, Lanoue A. Milrinone, dobutamine, and nitroprusside: comparative effects on hemodynamics and myocardial energetics in patients with severe congestive heart failure. *Circulation* 1986;**73**:III168–174.

8 Elkayam U, Kulick D, McIntosh N, Roth A, Hsueh W, Rahimtoola SH. Incidence of early tolerance to hemodynamic effects of continuous infusion of nitroglycerin in patients with coronary artery disease and heart failure. *Circulation* 1987;**76**:577–584.

9 Dies F, Krell MJ, Whitlow P *et al.* Intermittent dobutamine in ambulatory outpatients with chronic cardiac failure. *Circulation* 1986;**74**:II–38 (Abstract).

10 Packer M, Carver JR, Rodeheffer RJ *et al.* Effect of oral milrinone on mortality in severe chronic heart failure. The PROMISE Study Research Group. *N Engl J Med* 1991;**325**:1468–1475.

11 Silver MA, Maisel A, Yancy CW *et al.* BNP Consensus Panel 2004: A clinical approach for the diagnostic, prognostic, screening, treatment monitoring, and therapeutic roles of natriuretic peptides in cardiovascular diseases. *Congest Heart Fail* 2004;**10**:1–30.

12 de Bold AJ, Borenstein HB, Veress AT, Sonnenberg H. A rapid and potent natriuretic response to intravenous injection of atrial myocardial extract in rats. *Life Sci* 1981;**28**:89–94.

13 de Bold AJ, Flynn TG. Cardionatrin I – a novel heart peptide with potent diuretic and natriuretic properties. *Life Sci* 1983;**33**:297–302.

14 Flynn TG, de Bold ML, de Bold AJ. The amino acid sequence of an atrial peptide with potent diuretic and natriuretic properties. *Biochem Biophys Res Commun* 1983;**117**:859–865.

15 Sudoh T, Kangawa K, Minamino N, Matsuo H. A new natriuretic peptide in porcine brain. *Nature* 1988;**332**:78–81.

16 Hosoda K, Nakao K, Mukoyama M et al. Expression of brain natriuretic peptide gene in human heart. Production in the ventricle. *Hypertension* 1991;**17**:1152–1155.

17 Yasue H, Yoshimura M, Sumida H et al. Localization and mechanism of secretion of B-type natriuretic peptide in comparison with those of A-type natriuretic peptide in normal subjects and patients with heart failure. *Circulation* 1994;**90**:195–203.

18 Sudoh T, Minamino N, Kangawa K, Matsuo H. C-type natriuretic peptide (CNP): a new member of natriuretic peptide family identified in porcine brain. *Biochem Biophys Res Commun* 1990;**168**:863–870.

19 Suga S, Nakao K, Itoh H et al. Endothelial production of C-type natriuretic peptide and its marked augmentation by transforming growth factor-beta. Possible existence of 'vascular natriuretic peptide system'. *J Clin Invest* 1992;**90**:1145–1149.

20 Stingo AJ, Clavell AL, Heublein DM, Wei CM, Pittelkow MR, Burnett JC, Jr. Presence of C-type natriuretic peptide in cultured human endothelial cells and plasma. *Am J Physiol* 1992;**263**:H1318–H1321.

21 Suga S, Nakao K, Hosoda K et al. Receptor selectivity of natriuretic peptide family, atrial natriuretic peptide, brain natriuretic peptide, and C-type natriuretic peptide. *Endocrinology* 1992;**130**:229–239.

22 Koller KJ, Goeddel DV. Molecular biology of the natriuretic peptides and their receptors. *Circulation* 1992;**86**:1081–1088.

23 Maack T, Suzuki M, Almeida FA et al. Physiological role of silent receptors of atrial natriuretic factor. *Science* 1987;**238**:675–678.

24 Lang RE, Tholken H, Ganten D, Luft FC, Ruskoaho H, Unger T. Atrial natriuretic factor – a circulating hormone stimulated by volume loading. *Nature* 1985;**314**:264–266.

25 Ruskoaho H. Atrial natriuretic peptide: synthesis, release, and metabolism. *Pharmacol Rev* 1992;**44**:479–602.

26 Rosenzweig A, Seidman CE. Atrial natriuretic factor and related peptide hormones. *Annu Rev Biochem* 1991;**60**:229–255.

27 Maeda K, Tsutamoto T, Wada A, Hisanaga T, Kinoshita M. Plasma brain natriuretic peptide as a biochemical marker of high left ventricular end-diastolic pressure in patients with symptomatic left ventricular dysfunction. *Am Heart J* 1998;**135**:825–832.

28 Tsuruda T, Boerrigter G, Huntley BK et al. Brain natriuretic peptide is produced in cardiac fibroblasts and induces matrix metalloproteinases. *Circ Res* 2002;**91**:1127–1134.

29 Wei CM, Heublein DM, Perrella MA et al. Natriuretic peptide system in human heart failure. *Circulation* 1993;**88**:1004–1009.

30 Akioka K, Takeuchi K, Yanagi S et al. Prognostic value of Doppler transmittal flow patterns and cardiac natriuretic peptides in patients with chronic congestive heart failure admitted for episodes of acute decompensation. *Heart Vessels* 2000;**15**:53–60.

31 Koglin J, Pehlivanli S, Schwaiblmair M, Vogeser M, Cremer P, vonScheidt W. Role of brain natriuretic peptide in risk stratification of patients with congestive heart failure. *J Am Coll Cardiol* 2001;**38**:1934–1941.

32 McDonagh TA, Cunningham AD, Morrison CE et al. Left ventricular dysfunction, natriuretic peptides, and mortality in an urban population. *Heart* 2001;**86**:21–26.

33 Cheng V, Kazanagra R, Garcia A et al. A rapid bedside test for B-type peptide predicts treatment outcomes in patients admitted for decompensated heart failure: a pilot study. *J Am Coll Cardiol* 2001;**37**:386–391.

34 Harrison A, Morrison LK, Krishnaswamy P et al. B-type natriuretic peptide predicts future cardiac events in patients presenting to the emergency department with dyspnea. *Ann Emerg Med* 2002;**39**:131–138.

35 Anand IS, Fisher LD, Chiang YT et al. Changes in brain natriuretic peptide and norepinephrine over time and mortality and morbidity in the Valsartan Heart Failure Trial (Val-HeFT). *Circulation* 2003;**107**:1278–1283.

36 Logeart D, Thabut G, Jourdain P et al. Predischarge B-type natriuretic peptide assay for identifying patients at high risk of re-admission after decompensated heart failure. *J Am Coll Cardiol* 2004;**43**:635–641.

37 de Lemos JA, McGuire DK, Drazner MH. B-type natriuretic peptide in cardiovascular disease. *Lancet* 2003;**362**:316–322.

38 Sonnenberg JL, Sakane Y, Jeng AY et al. Identification of protease 3.4.24.11 as the major atrial natriuretic factor degrading enzyme in the rat kidney. *Peptides* 1988;**9**:173–180.

39 Wilkins MR, Unwin RJ, Kenny AJ. Endopeptidase-24.11 and its inhibitors: potential therapeutic agents

for edematous disorders and hypertension. *Kidney Int* 1993;**43**:273–285.

40 Good JM, Peters M, Wilkins M, Jackson N, Oakley CM, Cleland JG. Renal response to candoxatrilat in patients with heart failure. *J Am Coll Cardiol* 1995;**25**:1273–1281.

41 Kimmelstiel CD, Perrone R, Kilcoyne L *et al.* Effects of renal neutral endopeptidase inhibition on sodium excretion, renal hemodynamics and neurohormonal activation in patients with congestive heart failure. *Cardiology* 1996;**87**:46–53.

42 Cleland JG, Swedberg K. Lack of efficacy of neutral endopeptidase inhibitor ecadotril in heart failure. The International Ecadotril Multi-centre Dose-ranging Study Investigators. *Lancet* 1998;**351**:1657–1658.

43 Rouleau JL, Pfeffer MA, Stewart DJ *et al.* Comparison of vasopeptidase inhibitor, omapatrilat, and lisinopril on exercise tolerance and morbidity in patients with heart failure: IMPRESS randomised trial. *Lancet* 2000;**356**:615–620.

44 Packer M, Califf RM, Konstam MA *et al.* Comparison of omapatrilat and enalapril in patients with chronic heart failure: the Omapatrilat Versus Enalapril Randomized Trial of Utility in Reducing Events (OVERTURE). *Circulation* 2002;**106**:920–926.

45 Kostis JB, Packer M, Black HR, Schmieder R, Henry D, Levy E. Omapatrilat and enalapril in patients with hypertension: the Omapatrilat Cardiovascular Treatment vs. Enalapril (OCTAVE) trial. *Am J Hypertens* 2004;**17**:103–111.

46 Coats AJ. Omapatrilat–the story of Overture and Octave. *Int J Cardiol* 2002;**86**:1–4.

47 Richards AM, Nicholls MG, Ikram H, Webster MW, Yandle TG, Espiner EA. Renal, haemodynamic, and hormonal effects of human alpha atrial natriuretic peptide in healthy volunteers. *Lancet* 1985;**1**:545–549.

48 Tikkanen I, Fyhrquist F, Metsarinne K, Leidenius R. Plasma atrial natriuretic peptide in cardiac disease and during infusion in healthy volunteers. *Lancet* 1985;**2**:66–69.

49 Cody RJ, Atlas SA, Laragh JH *et al.* Atrial natriuretic factor in normal subjects and heart failure patients. Plasma levels and renal, hormonal, and hemodynamic responses to peptide infusion. *J Clin Invest* 1986;**78**:1362–1374.

50 Holmes SJ, Espiner EA, Richards AM, Yandle TG, Frampton C. Renal, endocrine, and hemodynamic effects of human brain natriuretic peptide in normal man. *J Clin Endocrinol Metab* 1993;**76**:91–96.

51 van der Zander K, Houben AJ, Hofstra L, Kroon AA, de Leeuw PW. Hemodynamic and renal effects of low-dose brain natriuretic peptide infusion in humans: a randomized, placebo-controlled crossover study. *Am J Physiol Heart Circ Physiol* 2003;**285**:H1206–H1212.

52 Mattingly MT, Clavell AL, Brandt RR, Wei CM, Barclay PL, Burnett JC, Jr. Potentiation of the renal actions of canine brain natriuretic peptide by neutral endopeptidase inhibition. *Am J Hypertens* 1994;**7**:14A (Abstract).

53 Kenny AJ, Bourne A, Ingram J. Hydrolysis of human and pig brain natriuretic peptides, urodilatin, C-type natriuretic peptide and some C-receptor ligands by endopeptidase-24.11. *Biochem J* 1993;**291**:83–88.

54 NDA 20-920 Cardio-renal advisory committee briefing document (3749B2_01_Scios-1999.pdf). US FDA, 1999. http://www.fda.gov/cder/audiences/acspage/ cardiovascularmeetings1.htm. (Accessed 28 September 2001)

55 Natrecor product insert. 2001. http://www.natrecor.com/ 919_Revised_Promotional_PI.pdf. (Accessed 25 August 2002)

56 Schreiner GF, Protter AA. B-type natriuretic peptide for the treatment of congestive heart failure. *Curr Opin Pharmacol* 2002;**2**:142–147.

57 Kudo T, Baird A. Inhibition of aldosterone production in the adrenal glomerulosa by atrial natriuretic factor. *Nature* 1984;**312**:756–757.

58 Akabane S, Matsushima Y, Matsuo H, Kawamura M, Imanishi M, Omae T. Effects of brain natriuretic peptide on renin secretion in normal and hypertonic saline-infused kidney. *Eur J Pharmacol* 1991;**198**:143–148.

59 Yoshimura M, Yasue H, Morita E *et al.* Hemodynamic, renal, and hormonal responses to brain natriuretic peptide infusion in patients with congestive heart failure. *Circulation* 1991;**84**:1581–1588.

60 Abraham WT, Lowes BD, Ferguson DA *et al.* Systemic hemodynamic, neurohormonal, and renal effects of a steady- state infusion of human brain natriuretic peptide in patients with hemodynamically decompensated heart failure. *J Card Fail* 1998;**4**:37–44.

61 Hayashi M, Tsutamoto T, Wada A *et al.* Intravenous atrial natriuretic peptide prevents left ventricular remodeling in patients with first anterior acute myocardial infarction. *J Am Coll Cardiol* 2001;**37**:1820–1826.

62 Colucci WS, Elkayam U, Horton D *et al.* Intravenous nesiritide, a natriuretic peptide, in the treatment of decompensated congestive heart failure. Nesiritide Study Group. *N Engl J Med* 2000;**343**:246–253.

63 Publication Committee for the VMAC Investigators (Vasodilation in the Management of Acute CHF). Intravenous nesiritide vs. nitroglycerin for treatment of decompensated congestive heart failure: a randomized controlled trial. *JAMA* 2002;**287**:1531–1540.

64 Panel of Cardiology Experts Provides Recommendations to Scios Regarding NATRECOR, press release from Scios Inc., 13 June 2005. Scios Inc., 2005. http://www.sciosinc.com/scios/pr_1118721302. (Accessed 22 June 2005)

65 Marcus LS, Hart D, Packer M *et al.* Hemodynamic and renal excretory effects of human brain natriuretic peptide infusion in patients with congestive heart failure. A double-blind, placebo-controlled, randomized crossover trial. *Circulation* 1996;**94**:3184–3189.

66 Mills R, TH L, Horton D. Sustained hemodynamic effects of an infusion of nesiritide (human b-type natriuretic peptide) in heart failure: a randomized, double-blind, placebo-controlled clinical trial. Natrecor Study Group. *J Am Coll Cardiol* 1999;**34**: 155–162.

67 3749b2_02_01-FDA-Combined Medical & Statistical Review.pdf. US FDA, 1999. http://www.fda.gov/cder/audiences/acspage/cardiovascularmeetings1.htm. (Accessed 28 September 2001)

68 Nieminen MS. Pharmacological options for acute heart failure syndromes: current treatments and unmet needs. *Eur Heart J* 2005;**7**:B20–B4.

69 3749b2_02_02-FDA-Medical Review.pdf, NDA 20-920. US FDA, 2001. http://www.fda.gov/cder/audiences/acspage/cardiovascularmeetings1.htm. (Accessed 28 September 2001)

70 Michaels AD, Klein A, Madden JA, Chatterjee K. Effects of intravenous nesiritide on human coronary vasomotor regulation and myocardial oxygen uptake. *Circulation* 2003;**107**:2697–2701.

71 Kuga H, Ogawa K, Oida A *et al.* Administration of atrial natriuretic peptide attenuates reperfusion phenomena and preserves left ventricular regional wall motion after direct coronary angioplasty for acute myocardial infarction. *Circ J* 2003;**67**:443–448.

72 Asakura M, Jiyoong K, Minamino T, Shintani Y, Asanuma H, Kitakaze M. Rationale and design of a large-scale trial using atrial natriuretic peptide (ANP) as an adjunct to percutaneous coronary intervention for ST-segment elevation acute myocardial infarction: Japan-Working groups of acute myocardial infarction for the reduction of Necrotic Damage by ANP (J-WIND-ANP). *Circ J* 2004;**68**:95–100.

73 Udelson JE, Konstam MA. Relation between left ventricular remodeling and clinical outcomes in heart failure patients with left ventricular systolic dysfunction. J Card Fail 2002;8(6 Suppl):S465-71.

74 Tamura N, Ogawa Y, Chusho H *et al.* Cardiac fibrosis in mice lacking brain natriuretic peptide. *Proc Natl Acad Sci USA* 2000;**97**:4239–4244.

75 Hama N, Itoh H, Shirakami G *et al.* Rapid ventricular induction of brain natriuretic peptide gene expression in experimental acute myocardial infarction. *Circulation* 1995;**92**:1558–1564.

76 Kawakami R, Saito Y, Kishimoto I *et al.* Overexpression of brain natriuretic peptide facilitates neutrophil infiltration and cardiac matrix metalloproteinase-9 expression after acute myocardial infarction. *Circulation* 2004;**110**:3306–3312.

77 Kikuchi M, Nakamura M, Suzuki T, Sato M, Takino T, Hiramori K. Usefulness of carperitide for the treatment of refractory heart failure due to severe acute myocardial infarction. *Jpn Heart J* 2001;**42**:271–280.

78 Aronson D, Burger AJ. Intravenous nesiritide (human B-type natriuretic peptide) reduces plasma endothelin-1 levels in patients with decompensated congestive heart failure. *Am J Cardiol* 2002;**90**:435–438.

79 Abramson BL, Ando S, Notarius CF, Rongen GA, Floras JS. Effect of atrial natriuretic peptide on muscle sympathetic activity and its reflex control in human heart failure. *Circulation* 1999;**99**:1810–1815.

80 Brunner-La Rocca HP, Kaye DM, Woods RL, Hastings J, Esler MD. Effects of intravenous brain natriuretic peptide on regional sympathetic activity in patients with chronic heart failure as compared with healthy control subjects. *J Am Coll Cardiol* 2001;**37**:1221–1227.

81 Meyer DJ, Jr., Huxley VH. Differential sensitivity of exchange vessel hydraulic conductivity to atrial natriuretic peptide. *Am J Physiol* 1990;**258**:H521–H528.

82 Rutlen DL, Christensen G, Helgesen KG, Ilebekk A. Influence of atrial natriuretic factor on intravascular volume displacement in pigs. *Am J Physiol* 1990;**259**:H1595–H1600.

83 Drazner M, McGuire DK, de Lemos JA. Nesiritide in acute heart failure. *Lancet* 2003;**362**:998–999.

84 Cowley AJ, Skene AM. Treatment of severe heart failure: quantity or quality of life? A trial of enoximone. Enoximone Investigators. *Br Heart J* 1994;**72**: 226–230.

85 Lubsen J, Just H, Hjalmarsson AC *et al.* Effect of pimobendan on exercise capacity in patients with heart failure: main results from the Pimobendan in Congestive Heart Failure (PICO) trial. *Heart* 1996;**76**:223–231.

86 Hampton JR, van Veldhuisen DJ, Kleber FX *et al.* Randomised study of effect of ibopamine on survival in patients with advanced severe heart failure. Second Prospective Randomised Study of Ibopamine on Mortality and Efficacy (PRIME II) Investigators. *Lancet* 1997;**349**:971–977.

87 Cohn JN, Goldstein SO, Greenberg BH *et al.* A dose-dependent increase in mortality with vesnarinone among patients with severe heart failure. Vesnarinone Trial Investigators. *N Engl J Med* 1998;**339**: 1810–1816.

88 NDA 20-920: cardiovascular and renal drugs advisory committee briefing document (3749b2_01_Scios.pdf). Scios, 2001. http://www.fda.gov/cder/audiences/acspage/cardiovascularmeetings1.htm. (Accessed 25 August 2001)

89 Burger AJ, Horton DP, LeJemtel T *et al.* Effect of nesiritide (B-type natriuretic peptide) and dobutamine on ventricular arrhythmias in the treatment of

patients with acutely decompensated congestive heart failure: the PRECEDENT study. *Am Heart J* 2002;**144**: 1102–1108.

90 Azevedo ER, Newton GE, Parker AB, Floras JS, Parker JD. Sympathetic responses to atrial natriuretic peptide in patients with congestive heart failure. *J Cardiovasc Pharmacol* 2000;**35**:129–135.

91 McCullough PA, Soman SS, Shah SS *et al.* Risks associated with renal dysfunction in patients in the coronary care unit. *J Am Coll Cardiol* 2000;**36**:679–684.

92 Gibson CM, Pinto DS, Murphy SA *et al.* Association of creatinine and creatinine clearance on presentation in acute myocardial infarction with subsequent mortality. *J Am Coll Cardiol* 2003;**42**:1535–1543.

93 Hillege HL, van Gilst WH, van Veldhuisen DJ *et al.* Accelerated decline and prognostic impact of renal function after myocardial infarction and the benefits of ACE inhibition: the CATS randomized trial. *Eur Heart J* 2003;**24**:412–420.

94 Chertow GM, Levy EM, Hammermeister KE, Grover F, Daley J. Independent association between acute renal failure and mortality following cardiac surgery. *Am J Med* 1998;**104**:343–348.

95 Mangano CM, Diamondstone LS, Ramsay JG, Aggarwal A, Herskowitz A, Mangano DT. Renal dysfunction after myocardial revascularization: risk factors, adverse outcomes, and hospital resource utilization. The Multicenter Study of Perioperative Ischemia Research Group. *Ann Intern Med* 1998;**128**:194–203.

96 Keeley EC, Kadakia R, Soman S, Borzak S, McCullough PA. Analysis of long-term survival after revascularization in patients with chronic kidney disease presenting with acute coronary syndromes. *Am J Cardiol* 2003;**92**:509–514.

97 Nakayama Y, Sakata R, Ura M, Itoh T. Long-term results of coronary artery bypass grafting in patients with renal insufficiency. *Ann Thorac Surg* 2003;**75**:496–500.

98 Hillege HL, Girbes AR, de Kam PJ *et al.* Renal function, neurohormonal activation, and survival in patients with chronic heart failure. *Circulation* 2000;**102**:203–210.

99 Al-Ahmad A, Rand WM, Manjunath G *et al.* Reduced kidney function and anemia as risk factors for mortality in patients with left ventricular dysfunction. *J Am Coll Cardiol* 2001;**38**:955–962.

100 McAlister FA, Ezekowitz J, Tonelli M, Armstrong PW. Renal insufficiency and heart failure: prognostic and therapeutic implications from a prospective cohort study. *Circulation* 2004;**109**:1004–1009.

101 Mahon NG, Blackstone EH, Francis GS, Starling RC, 3rd, Young JB, Lauer MS. The prognostic value of estimated creatinine clearance alongside functional capacity in ambulatory patients with chronic congestive heart failure. *J Am Coll Cardiol* 2002;**40**:1106–1113.

102 Dries DL, Exner DV, Domanski MJ, Greenberg B, Stevenson LW. The prognostic implications of renal insufficiency in asymptomatic and symptomatic patients with left ventricular systolic dysfunction. *J Am Coll Cardiol* 2000;**35**:681–689.

103 Krumholz HM, Chen YT, Vaccarino V *et al.* Correlates and impact on outcomes of worsening renal function in patients ≥65 years of age with heart failure. *Am J Cardiol* 2000;**85**:1110–1113.

104 Butler J, Forman DE, Abraham WT *et al.* Relationship between heart failure treatment and development of worsening renal function among hospitalized patients. *Am Heart J* 2004;**147**:331–338.

105 Smith GL, Vaccarino V, Kosiborod M *et al.* Worsening renal function: what is a clinically meaningful change in creatinine during hospitalization with heart failure? *J Card Fail* 2003;**9**:13–25.

106 Gottlieb SS, Abraham W, Butler J *et al.* The prognostic importance of different definitions of worsening renal function in congestive heart failure. *J Card Fail* 2002;**8**:136–141.

107 Aronson D, Horton D, Burger JJ. Prognostic significance of deteriorating renal function in patients with decompensated heart failure. *JACC* 2004;**43**:180A.

108 Butler J, Emerman C, Peacock WF, Mathur VS, Young JB. The efficacy and safety of B-type natriuretic peptide (nesiritide) in patients with renal insufficiency and acutely decompensated congestive heart failure. *Nephrol Dial Transplant* 2004;**19**:391–399.

109 Wang DJ, Dowling TC, Meadows D *et al.* Nesiritide does not improve renal function in patients with chronic heart failure and worsening serum creatinine. *Circulation* 2004;**110**:1620–1625.

110 Sackner-Bernstein JD, Skopicki HA, Aaronson KD. Risk of worsening renal function with nesiritide in patients with acutely decompensated heart failure. *Circulation* 2005;**111**:1487–1491.

111 Peacock W, Emerman C, Group PS. Safety and efficacy of nesiritide in the treatment of decompensated heart failure in observation patients. *J Am Coll Cardiol* 2003;**41**:336A.

112 Sackner-Bernstein J, Kowalski M, Fox M. Is there risk associated with the use of nesiritide for acute heart failure? *J Am Coll Cardiol* 2003;**41**:161A.

113 Silver M, Horton D, Ghali J, Elkayam U. Effect of nesiritide versus dobutamine on short-term outcomes in the treatment of patients with acutely decompensated heart failure. *J Am Coll Cardiol* 2002;**39**:798–803.

114 Sackner-Bernstein JD, Kowalski M, Fox M, Aaronson K. Short-term risk of death after treatment with nesiritide for decompensated heart failure: a pooled analysis of randomized controlled trials. *JAMA* 2005;**293**:1900–1905.

115 Abraham WT, Adams KF, Fonarow GC *et al.* In-hospital mortality in patients with acute decompensated heart failure requiring intravenous vasoactive medications: an analysis from the Acute Decompensated Heart Failure National Registry (ADHERE). *J Am Coll Cardiol* 2005;**46**:57–64.

116 Stampfer MJ, Colditz GA, Willett WC *et al.* Postmenopausal estrogen therapy and cardiovascular disease. Ten-year follow-up from the nurses' health study. *N Engl J Med* 1991;**325**:756–762.

117 Rossouw JE, Anderson GL, Prentice RL *et al.* Risks and benefits of estrogen plus progestin in healthy postmenopausal women: principal results From the Women's Health Initiative randomized controlled trial. *JAMA* 2002;**288**:321–333.

118 Hulley S, Grady D, Bush T *et al.* Randomized trial of estrogen plus progestin for secondary prevention of coronary heart disease in postmenopausal women. Heart and Estrogen/progestin Replacement Study (HERS) Research Group. *JAMA* 1998;**280**:605–613.

119 Effects of estrogen or estrogen/progestin regimens on heart disease risk factors in postmenopausal women. The Postmenopausal Estrogen/Progestin Interventions (PEPI) Trial. The Writing Group for the PEPI Trial. *JAMA* 1995;**273**:199–208.

120 Topol EJ. Nesiritide – not verified. *N Engl J Med* 2005;**353**:113–116.

121 Yancy CW, Saltzberg MT, Berkowitz RL *et al.* Safety and feasibility of using serial infusions of nesiritide for heart failure in an outpatient setting (from the FUSION I trial). *Am J Cardiol* 2004;**94**:595–601.

122 Future Directions in the Management of Heart Failure: The FUSION Trials. WebMD, 2004. http://www.medscape.com/viewprogram/3530_pnt. (Accessed 27 July 2005)

123 Tsuneyoshi H, Nishina T, Nomoto T *et al.* Atrial natriuretic peptide helps prevent late remodeling after left ventricular aneurysm repair. *Circulation* 2004;**110**:II174–II179.

124 Lisy O, Lainchbury JG, Leskinen H, Burnett JC, Jr. Therapeutic actions of a new synthetic vasoactive and natriuretic peptide, dendroaspis natriuretic peptide, in experimental severe congestive heart failure. *Hypertension* 2001;**37**:1089–1094.

125 Khurana VG, Wijdicks EF, Heublein DM *et al.* A pilot study of dendroaspis natriuretic peptide in aneurysmal subarachnoid hemorrhage. *Neurosurgery* 2004;**55**:69–75.

126 Chen HH, Lainchbury JG, Burnett JC, Jr. Natriuretic peptide receptors and neutral endopeptidase in mediating the renal actions of a new therapeutic synthetic natriuretic peptide dendroaspis natriuretic peptide. *J Am Coll Cardiol* 2002;**40**:1186–1191.

127 Bestle MH, Olsen NV, Christensen P, Jensen BV, Bie P. Cardiovascular, endocrine, and renal effects of urodilatin in normal humans. *Am J Physiol* 1999;276(3 Pt 2):R684–95.

128 Hirsch JR, Meyer M, Magert HJ *et al.* cGMP-dependent and -independent inhibition of a K+ conductance by natriuretic peptides: molecular and functional studies in human proximal tubule cells. *J Am Soc Nephrol* 1999;10(3):472–80.

129 Kentsch M, Ludwig D, Drummer C, Gerzer R, Muller-Esch G. Haemodynamic and renal effects of urodilatin bolus injections in patients with congestive heart failure. *Eur J Clin Invest* 1992;22(10):662–9.

130 Forssmann WG, Richter R, Meyer M. The endocrine heart and natriuretic peptides: histochemistry, cell biology, and functional aspects of the renal urodilatin system. *Histochem Cell Biol* 1998;110(4):335–57.

131 Allgren RL, Marbury TC, Rahman SN *et al.* Anaritide in acute tubular necrosis. Auriculin Anaritide Acute Renal Failure Study Group. *N Engl J Med* 1997;336(12):828–34.

132 Schmitt M, Gunaruwan P, Payne N *et al.* Effects of exogenous and endogenous natriuretic peptides on forearm vascular function in chronic heart failure. *Arterioscler Thromb Vasc Biol* 2004;24(5):911–7.

133 Cohn JN, Goldstein SO, Greenberg BH *et al.* A dose-dependent increase in mortality with vesnarinone among patients with severe heart failure. Vesnarinone Trial Investigators. *N Engl J Med* 1998;339(25):1810–6.

134 Torre-Amione G, Young JB, Colucci WS *et al.* Hemodynamic and clinical effects of tezosentan, an intravenous dual endothelin receptor antagonist, in patients hospitalized for acute decompensated heart failure. *J Am Coll Cardiol* 2003;42(1):140–7.

135 Mehra MR. Acute decompensated heart failure treatment: optimizing patient outcomes. Medscape.com; 2005. http://www.medscape.com/viewprogram/4459_pnt (Accessed November 27, 2005).

136 Adams KF. Acute decompensated heart failure treatment: optimizing patient outcomes. Medscape.com; 2005. http://www.medscape.com/viewprogram/ 4459_pnt (Accessed November 27, 2005).

137 Yancy CW. Is nesiritide safe and effective for acute heart failure? Protagonist. HFSA Annual Scientific Sessions. Boca Raton, FL; September 20, 2005.

138 Cleland JG, Coletta AP, Lammiman M *et al.* Clinical trials update from the European Society of Cardiology meeting 2005: CARE-HF extension study, ESSENTIAL, CIBIS-III, S-ICD, ISSUE-2, STRIDE-2, SOFA, IMAGINE, PREAMI, SIRIUS-II and ACTIVE. *Eur J Heart Fail* 2005;7(6):1070–5.

# CHAPTER 12

# Immune modulatory therapies in heart failure: using myocarditis to gain mechanistic insights

*Grace Chan, Koichi Fuse,* MD, PHD, *Mei Sun,* MD, PHD, *Bill Ayach,* MSC *& Peter P. Liu,* MD

## Inflammatory mechanisms underlying heart failure

### Evidence of inflammatory activation in heart failure

Heart failure has previously been thought of as a hemodynamic or neurohormonal disease. However recent data suggest that there is an active inflammatory component that participates in the progression of the disease [1–4]. This finding is interesting as recent discoveries in the areas of atherosclerosis and coronary artery disease have also suggested an important role for the inflammatory pathways in their pathophysiology [5,6].

The evidence of inflammatory activation in heart failure comes both from measurements in the peripheral circulation as well as the finding of markers of inflammation in the heart [1,7,8]. For example, in patients with moderate to severe heart failure symptoms, investigators have documented the presence of elevated levels of proinflammatory cytokines including tumor necrosis factor-alpha (TNFα) and selected interleukins in the peripheral circulation. Furthermore, there is evidence from numerous sources that inflammatory signals are activated in the heart both in patients with heart failure [9,10] as well as in animal models of heart failure [11–13]. In addition, transgenic over expression of the proinflammatory cytokine TNFα effects the development of cardiac dilatation, extracellular matrix remodeling, reexpression of the fetal gene program, inflammatory exudates, abnormal

calcium homeostasis, and early death due to heart failure [14,15]. The cardiotoxic effects of TNFα overexpression can be attenuated early, but not late, in the development of cardiac dilatation and failure by treatment with TNF soluble receptor, an anti-TNF monoclonal antibody, or selective mutation of the TNF receptor 1 [16]. Recently, we have developed a heterotopic heart transplant model and documented that the generation of TNF secondary to cardiac injury can directly lead to cardiac dilatation [12]. This is partially ameliorated by selective removal of TNF with a soluble receptor.

### Stretch and mechanical stress activate inflammatory cytokines

Cytokines such as TNFα and IL-6 are rapidly released following direct myocardial mechanical stretch (Figure 12.1). Kapadia *et al.* have shown that direct hemodynamic stretch can trigger myocardial production of TNFα *de novo* within 30 min [17]. Mechanical stimulus acts through potential mechanosensors (integrins, cytoskeleton, and sarcolemmal proteins) and converts into three major intracellular cross-talking signal transduction pathways, MAPK, JAK-STAT, and calcineurin-dependent pathways. These pathways activate cognate downstream nuclear transcription factors, such as NF-κB and AP-1, which are required for the induction of most cytokine genes, including TNFα and IL-6 [18].

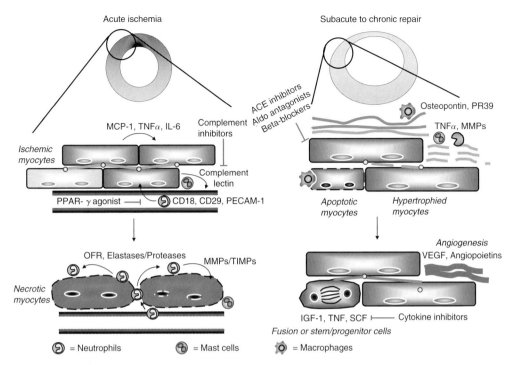

**Figure 12.1** (a) The contributions of immune and inflammatory signals towards cardiac remodeling post-ischemia and infarction, leading to heart failure. Acutely following ischemia, mechanical stress and free radicals induce local production of cytokines such as macrophage chemoattractant protein (MCP-1), TNF and IL-6. These in turn activate complement and lectin, and leads to adhesion and migration of inflammatory cells through CD18 and CD29 activation with the blood vessel wall. These processes can be potentially inhibited by anti-inflammatory strategies, such as peroxisome proliferators activated receptor (PPAR-γ) agonist or complement inhibitors. These subsequently lead to activation of proteases, including elastase and matrix metalloproteinases (MMPs) or tissue inhibitor of metalloproteinases (TIMP). (b) More chronically, the myocytes may die through necrosis and apoptosis, and the matrix dissolution and rebuilding also take place. During this time the ventricle may significantly dilate, and can be inhibited by pharmacological agents such as angiotensin modulators, aldosterone antagonists, and beta-blockers. However, it is through the elaboration of growth factors such as insulin growth factor (IGF-1), stem cell factor (SCF), and TNF that may also promote the migration of stem cells or endothelial progenitor cells into the injured area.

## Ischemia and oxidative stress activate inflammation

Ischemia and oxidative stress are also potential stimuli that can upregulate cytokine production as part of an intrinsic or an innate stress response against myocardial injury in the setting of heart failure [19]. In rodent models of myocardial infarction, within the first hours to 1 day, there is robust upregulation of intramyocardial cytokines including TNFα, IL-1β, and IL-6 mRNA expression in the infarct area (up to 50-fold) as well as in the noninfarcted myocardium (up to 15-fold) [1,20]. Reactive oxygen species can also directly induce myocardial TNFα production via the p38 MAPK pathway and in turn mediate myocardial dysfunction and apoptosis [21].

## Activation of cytokines leads to further activation of cytokines

Cytokines also have the unique ability to self-amplify, through positive feedback loop targeting the transcription factor NF-κB. For example, the upregulation of cytokines such as TNFα in a localized area of the myocardium, can easily induce further TNFα upregulation in neighboring normal myocardium leading to amplified cytokine effects. Irwin *et al.* demonstrated that TNFα mRNA was maximally detectable acutely in the infarct and peri-infarct zones during the first days of post-MI. In contrast, by day 35 late post-MI, the "contralateral normal zone" in the infarcted hearts showed the highest level of TNFα expression [11].

To definitively demonstrate that cytokines such as TNFα can upregulate remote regions in the heart through a "virtual" network, we have recently used a novel heterotopic cardiac transplant model, where myocardial infarction was imposed on the heart in the abdomen while the native recipient heart, totally undisturbed by surgery, is observed during subsequent days of follow-up [12]. Most surprisingly, the otherwise uninfarcted and undisturbed recipient heart demonstrated a significant decrease in LV fractional shortening and increase in LV end-diastolic dimension following infarction in the abdominal heart. This set of unusual observations were significantly abolished by the intravenous administration of the TNFα soluble receptor, etanercept, and the resulting inhibition of TNFα bioactivity. This suggests that cytokines such as TNFα can activate a remote amplification network that mediates myocardial remodeling not only in areas of acute injury but also in remote regions and areas of the heart thereby effecting global cardiac structure and function.

## Impact of inflammation on cardiac structure and function

### Inflammatory effects on myocyte function

Cytokines are capable of depressing LV performance and myocyte contractility both directly and indirectly. TNFα and IL-6 can attenuate myocyte contractility directly through the immediate reduction of systolic cytosolic $[Ca^{2+}]$ via alterations in sarcoplasmic reticulum function, effects that are reversible upon the removal of the cytokine exposure [22]. On the other hand, TNFα is also capable of depressing myocyte contractility indirectly through nitric oxide dependent attenuation of myofilament $Ca^{2+}$ sensitivity [23].

Alternatively, TNF provokes negative inotropic effects in myocytes partially through the neutral sphingomyelinase pathway. Within minutes following cardiac injury, TNF depresses systolic function by altering calcium-induced calcium release by the sarcoplasmic reticulum and by disrupting the L-type calcium channel [24]. In this phase, the binding of TNF to TNFR1 leads to the release of sphingolipid metabolite (stress-induced second messenger) via sphingomyelin degeneration. Oral

and coworkers also reported that sphingosine production correlated directly with calcium imbalance [25]. Furthermore, blockade of sphingosine production negatively regulated TNFα-induced contractile dysfunction.

## Inflammatory effect on myocyte survival

Cytokines such as TNFα appear to have a significant pleotropic effect on the host cells with the potential for *apoptosis* on one hand versus cellular preservation and hypertrophy on the other. The net balance between these two opposing processes defines the net cellular remodeling.

The activation of cytokines, particularly in high concentrations, or other death promoting signals can activate death domain-related signaling pathways. In response to TNFα, TNF-R1 trimerized and death domain containing molecule TRADD is recruited to the cytoplasmic regions of the receptors [26]. TRADD recruits the downstream signaling adaptor molecules Fas-associated death domain (FADD), which in turn activates procaspase 8 and initiates cell death by destroying the cell's own repair mechanisms.

Conversely, the cytoprotective effect of TNFα may converge through the activation of the transcription factors NF-κB and stress-activated protein kinase (SAPK)/c-Jun N-terminal kinase (JNK), leading to the activation of cytoprotective gene expression. TRAFs, such as TRAF2, interact with and activate downstream signaling molecules such as NF-κB-inducing kinase (NIK), a member of the serine/threonine mitogen-activated protein kinase (MAPK) kinase (MEK) kinase (MEKK) family [27,28]. NIK phosphorylates inhibitor of κB (IκB) kinase IKK leading to NF-κB translocation to the nucleus and activation of genes involved in cellular inflammation, growth, and survival [29,30].

The hypertrophic effect of TNFα was demonstrated in several independent studies. Physiologically relevant concentrations of TNFα provoke a hypertrophic response by increasing the synthesis of both structural and contractile proteins in adult feline cardiac myocytes [31]. Moreover, transgenic mice with cardiac specific overexpressing TNFα developed cardiac hypertrophy [13]. The cardioprotective action of TNFα is best illustrated in mice with combined genetic ablation of the TNF-R1 and TNF-R2 receptors. TNF-R1 and TNF-R2 double-receptor-knockout mice undergoing left coronary ligation had significantly larger infarct size and increased myocyte apoptosis when compared to normal control mice. However, mice overexpressing TNFα on a background of selective ablation of TNF-R2 had a worse outcome than mice in which both TNFR1 and TNFR2 were intact[15].

## Effect of inflammation of matrix turnover

Cytokines, such as TNF or interleukins, can directly increase the transcription of matrix metalloproteinases (Figure 12.1). Matrix metalloproteinases are present in the myocardial interstitium normally in the inactive form and can be activated by free radicals, cytokines, and hypoxia and can be counter regulated to a certain extent by tissue inhibitors of MMPs or TIMPs [32]. The activation of MMP is initially responsible for collagen degradation and subsequently matrix deposition. In transgenic mice overexpressing TNFα, which develops dilated cardiomyopathy with time, their myocardium demonstrates increased MMP activity by gelatin zymography [33].

Finally, some members of the membrane-bound, such as TACE, can process the extracellular production of cytokines, such as TNF. We have tested inhibitors of the proinflammatory MMP-12 or elastase and found that elastase inhibition can significantly improve the ventricular function and remodeling in an ischemic model of heart failure [34]. This confirms our earlier testing of this strategy in blocking inflammation and ventricular function in a model of myocarditis [35]. These results are also supported by the finding that inhibition of MMP improves cardiac function in models of dilated cardiomyopathy.

## Myocarditis as a model to understand inflammation and heart failure

Myocarditis is defined as inflammation of the heart muscle and may be a more common cause of heart failure and dilated cardiomyopathy in the adult than is generally recognized. The incidence of myocarditis is estimated at 1 to 5% of *all deaths* [36–38] and about $\frac{1}{3}$ of cases of dilated

cardiomyopathy. Enteroviral infection remains one of the common causes of myocarditis representing about 25% prevalence by polymerase chain reaction (PCR) [39–41]. Enteroviruses commonly linked with myocarditis are coxsackievirus group B (CVB), especially the B3 serotype, adenovirus, and more recently parvovirus and hepatitis C virus.

Myocarditis is a classic model in which to examine the triggers and consequences of cardiac inflammation and heart failure. Myocarditis can result from a diverse repertoire of etiologies, but regardless of the infecting organism the infection triggers subsequent immune activation which is believed to be the essential factor leading to the development of heart failure. We have divided the myocarditis process into an initial brief viral phase, followed by an immune phase, and finally a cardiomyopathy phase incorporating cardiac remodeling and dilatation [36].

## Role of innate immune system in myocarditis

Innate immunity can be conceptually divided into two broad categories: intrinsic and extrinsic [42]. Extrinsic innate immunity involves cellular systems that respond to the presence of external pathogen or foreign DNA by mobilization *without* the requirement of specific individualized antigenic recognition such as a T-cell receptor. These cells may include macrophages, granulocytes, or natural killer cells that are derived from hematopoietic stem cells and can provide a general defense against external pathogens [43]. Intrinsic innate immunity on the other hand involves the local production of protective mediators such as interferons and defensins by any host cells faced with pathogen, as a result of signaling through cell surface toll-like receptors (TLRs). These TLRs recognize general molecular patterns often associated with invading pathogens or foreign genetic material and trigger a specific network of signaling pathways that leads to production of cytokines and interferons [44]. Recent cloning and identification of entire families of TLRs and their adaptors indicated that each TLR member recognizes a unique general molecular pattern, but share a number of signaling modules. The activation of innate immunity is now thought to also provide the first initial critical step for the subsequent development of acquired immunity through specific antigen recognition via T or B cell receptors and the ultimate production of T-killer cells or production of antigen-specific antibodies.

## Role of acquired immune system in myocarditis

The presence of inflammatory cell infiltration, including macrophages and T-cells, indicates that acquired immunity also plays an important role in the pathogenesis of myocarditis (Figure 12.2). The viral peptide fragments are processed in the golgi apparatus of the host cell and presented to the cell surface in an MHC restricted manner. This promotes T-cell mediated killing through cytokine-mediated signaling [45–47] or perforin-mediated cell death [48,49]. These processes ultimately

produce myocyte damage and the reduction of contractile units in a terminally differentiated organ [50–53].

We have been methodically mapping the major determinants of the host immune system using molecular targeting strategies in knockout mice. Earlier work has demonstrated that components of innate immunity are critical for host survival, yet T-cell signaling and activation are injurious to the host. Through CD4$^-$/CD8$^-$ knockout mice, we have established that both CD4 and CD8 T cells contribute to the host's autoimmune inflammatory disease, accompanied by a shift of cytokine profile from Th1 to Th2 response [53]. Furthermore, we have identified that the T-cell costimulatory tyrosine kinase, p56$^{lck}$, is critical for both virus proliferation in the heart as well activation of the

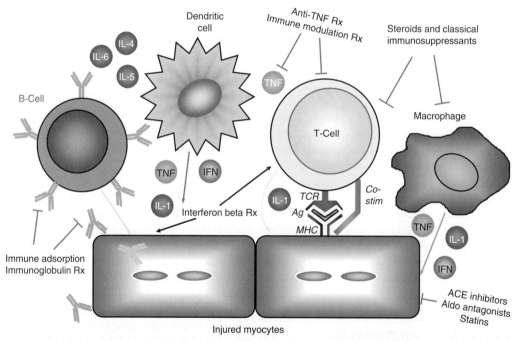

**Figure 12.2** The major pathways for immune activation in the setting of heart failure and potential sites or targets of therapy. The injured myocytes may elaborate cytokines through activation of innate immunity, typically via TLRs. These in turn activate dendritic cells, macrophages, and T-cells leading to activation of acquired immunity. The pathways ultimately also lead to B-cell activation, resulting in autoantibody production that perpetuates the inflammatory state as often found in dilated cardiomyopathy. Multiple sites of action are possible to enhance innate immunity protection and attenuate T- and B-cell activation. These include anti-cytokine or immune modulation therapy, or immune adsorption therapy to remove the auto antibodies. However, interferon $\beta$ may have both host protection and anti-inflammatory role in immune modulation, while the traditional angiotensin and aldosterone inhibitors also have anti-inflammatory properties (IL = interleukin; TCR = Tcellreceptor; Ag = antigen; MHC = major histocompatibility complex; Aldo = aldosterone; IFN = interferon).

T-cells that target the heart [45]. Indeed, p56$^{lck-/-}$ homozygous knockout animals do not develop any myocarditis despite exposure to large doses of the coxsackievirus. More recently, we have identified that p56$^{lck}$ triggers downstream ERK activation in the host target cell and appears to be critical for the determinant of host susceptibility [47]. To validate these observations, we have also investigated the function of the associated tyrosine phosphatase CD45 linked in function to the p56$^{lck}$ kinase and confirmed that CD45$^{-/-}$ animals are also resistant to viral myocarditis [54]. After careful dissection, it was apparent that CD45 is an important src as well as JAK/STAT phosphatase and virally triggered CD45 activation shuts down interferon production. Interferon levels are markedly increased once CD45 is removed and the host is indeed rescued.

## Direct anti-inflammatory strategies

A number of immune modulatory strategies have been used in heart failure in general and inflammatory cardiomyopathies in particular. We have divided the discussion into direct anti-inflammatory strategies that include steroids, anti-TNF, and immune adsorption strategies (Figure 12.2). In addition, there are a number of indirect anti-inflammatory therapies including the classical heart failure treatments such as angiotensin converting enzyme inhibitors, cAMP modulators, and aldosterone antagonists. Interestingly, more recent data on combined antiviral and anti-inflammatory strategies such as immune globulin therapy and more recently interferon therapy have gained increasing attention.

### Steroids and immunosuppressive agents
The first systematic approach to evaluate immune modulatory therapy in heart disease is the original NIH-sponsored myocarditis trial. In this trial, patients with biopsy-proven myocarditis were randomized to receive either conventional therapy, including ACE inhibitors and standard antiheart failure regimen, or the addition of immunosuppressive therapy. The immunosuppressive therapy regimen consisted of steroids, azathioprine, or cyclosporine. The results showed that there was a significant improvement in ejection fraction in both arms of the randomized trial, such that at the end of follow-up period at 4.3 years there was no significant difference between the two arms. The outcome of patients with myocarditis and dilated cardiomyopathy is still poor. In the NIH myocarditis trial, patients with positive diagnosis based on the Dallas biopsy criteria had a mortality of 20% at 1 year and 56% at 4.3 years, with many cases of chronic heart failure, despite optimal medical management [55]. When examining the survival in more detail, there was a trend for improvement in the immunosuppressed arm while the treatment was actively being administered. However, because the immunosuppression was given for only 6 months, and was discontinued thereafter, the effect was not sustained.

In retrospect, this may have represented an overly simplified notion of immune modulation therapy in heart failure. The immunosuppressive regimen used was nonspecific for the innate or acquired arms of immunity. Furthermore, there was no delineation of the viral etiology in the trial itself. The patients who entered the trial were at various stages of development of cardiomyopathy, and the sample size was not adequate in retrospect to detect a transient albeit potentially important benefit over the short term [36].

### Antitumor necrosis factor strategies
In view of the overall contributory role of cytokines such as TNFα in the progression of heart failure in diverse etiologies an attractive hypothesis was that targeted anticytokine therapy would be beneficial in patients with heart failure. In an initial study at two large heart failure centers, etanercept improved heart size and heart function in a group of heart failure patients who were able to accomplish moderate aerobic exercise prior to enrollment (56). However, the results of two subsequent trials assessing the efficacy of the same agent were surprisingly disappointing. The first trial was the Randomized Etanercept North American Strategy to Study Antagonism of Cytokines (RENAISSANCE) trial [57]. In this trial, patients with severe heart failure (class III and IV) and limited functional capacity were randomized to bi- or tri-weekly subcutaneous

injections of a soluble recombinant TNFα receptor (etanercept), or a placebo. The second trial involved the same agent at a slightly different regimen in heart failure patients in Europe, Research into Etanercept Cytokine Antagonism in Ventricular dysfunction (RECOVER). The results of both trials uniformly failed to demonstrate any benefit of the anti-TNF regimen in terms of clinical status, or deaths and hospitalization.

Several possible explanations have been offered to reconcile the surprise finding. The first is that cytokines mediate remodeling and heart failure progression during early stages of heart failure. The patients enrolled in the large phase III anti-TNF trials however were far advanced in their disease, had limited ability to exercise, and presumably had extensive cardiac remodeling. Thus, these patients may not have been able to respond adequately to anti-TNF treatment. Furthermore, these trials were the first to use a biologic agent rather than standard pharmacologic agent for the treatment of heart failure. How the heart failure patient metabolizes biologic agents and how these agents interact with the patient's multitudes of other heart failure drugs are largely unknown. Finally, there is further disquieting suggestion that these anti-cytokine agents may bind to transmembrane TNFα receptors and in turn activate antibody – or complement – dependent immune activation. Mann and colleagues (Mann D, personal communication) have recently demonstrated that the TNF heterodimer is actually stabilized when bound to a dimeric TNF-soluble receptor and can be passively transferred from the soluble receptor to cell surface receptors.

Another possibility is that cytokines such as TNF has both beneficial and harmful effects in the setting of heart failure. The blocking of the cytokine signaling pathways may demonstrate a short-term benefit such as reverse remodeling and improvement in LV function [58], as shown in the earlier pilot trial. However, under continued chronic utilization, the negative effect of TNF removal may ultimately lead to worse cell survival and inability to defend against stress. The challenge in the future is to develop appropriately targeted agents that will be selective in blocking the harmful effects without compromising the beneficial aspects of cytokines.

## Immune adsorption therapy

Another strategy to physically remove potential cardiac depressant factors is immune adsorption therapy through the plasmapheresis of peripheral blood. There have been previous suggestions that in addition to cytokines circulating antibodies may target against specific components of the myocyte under stress, such as the beta-adrenergic receptor, the ATP carrier, or even the myosin molecule, leading to eventual cell dysfunction and cell death. Various strategies have been developed to capture these cardiodepressant factors or antibodies, and colleagues from Germany have been most active in this arena.

In one earlier randomized trial using immune adsorption therapy 34 patients were randomized to standard therapy or immune adsorption therapy aimed to remove antibodies against the beta-adrenergic receptor [59]. After 1 year of treatment, the treated group demonstrated a change of LV ejection fraction from a mean of 22.3% to 37.9% whereas the placebo or standard treatment arm did not show any significant improvement. There was also accompanying improvement in patients' symptomatic status.

More recently, other groups have demonstrated further specificity by identifying the IgG-3 subclass of antibodies to be particularly responsible for cardiac depression [60,61]. Patient's who had effective removal of the IgG-3 class of antibodies are particularly those who demonstrated improvement in ejection fraction.

However, these innovative approaches have not been subjected to a large randomized trial examining the hard endpoints such as deaths or hospitalization. Nevertheless, this does represent another novel approach towards the removal of proinflammatory factors in heart failure, and at least offers a potential proof of concept that continued strategic focus on this approach may ultimately be beneficial for patients with severe heart failure.

## Indirect anti-inflammatory strategies

### Immune modulation therapy

In view of the fact that direct anti-cytokine therapy has not been successful alternative strategies have been sought to abrogate cytokine effects through indirect strategies. A novel technique involving taking a patient's own whole blood, irradiating it with ultraviolet radiation, and reinjecting it back into the same patient intramuscularly has been shown to decrease markers of inflammation in a single small study. The mechanisms are not clear but it is thought that the irradiation triggers apoptosis in the white blood cells in the blood, and in turn induces tolerance or anergy in activated immune cell clones.

A preliminary study involved 75 heart failure patients in functional class III or IV who were randomized to receive either immune modulation therapy or placebo on top of standard therapy for 6 months [62]. At the end of follow-up period, there was no difference in the primary endpoint of 6-min walk test but surprisingly there was a significant reduction in the risk of death ($p = 0.022$) and hospitalization ($p = 0.008$) in the immune modulation group. There was also a suggestion of improved quality of life in the treated patients. This is an intriguing result from a very small preliminary study and has resulted in the initiation of a large follow-up mortality/morbidity study involving over 3000 patients. This study may provide important information about the role of this innovative approach to modulate immune activation in patients with heart failure.

## ACE inhibitors/Beta blockers

What is less well-realized is the fact that the traditional heart failure therapies may already have significant anti-inflammatory effect. Take, for example, ACE inhibitors which together with beta-blockers, represent the cornerstones of modern heart failure therapy. It has been well-documented that angiotensin is a potent proinflammatory and prooxidative agent. ACE inhibitors have been shown to decrease the expression of adhesion molecules on the surface of the endothelium. ACE inhibitors also have general anti-inflammatory properties in terms of inflammatory cell mobilization and cytokine release. The effect of ACE inhibitors in heart failure and atherosclerosis are consistent with its effect on inflammation.

Although beta-blockers have traditionally been associated with blockade of the adverse effects of continuous activation of the adrenergic system there is a recent appreciation that they may also have impact on inflammatory cytokine signaling. In a canine model of heart failure, it has been demonstrated that the effective use of beta-blockade in this setting can significantly reduce cytokine gene expression in the myocardium [63]. This reduction in cytokine expression is accompanied by improvements in ventricular function and reverse remodeling of the ventricle.

## Cyclic AMP modulators

There have been suggestions that cyclic AMP levels could modulate the production of cytokines such as TNF$\alpha$ and IL1$\beta$. Indeed, the phosphodiesterase inhibitor, pentoxyphyllin, demonstrates salutary effects on heart failure signs and symptoms while substantially lowering circulating TNF$\alpha$ levels [64–66]. Other inhibitors of cytokine production that may also utilize this system may include amiodarone, ouabain, and thalidomide. In addition, a recent report suggests that estrogen may constitutively downregulate TNF$\alpha$ expression.

Studies to date have also demonstrated that adenosine is a potent inhibitor of TNF$\alpha$ expression by neonatal myocytes, adult myocytes, rodent papillary muscle preparations, and adult human heart via activation of the adenosine $A_2$ receptor [67]. This effect appears to be partially selective for the heart as adenosine's anti-cytokine effects in white cells is mediated via the $A_3$ adenosine receptor [68]. This concept was further supported by Loh *et al.* [69] who demonstrated improved survival in heart failure patients having a common mutation in at least one allele of the AMP deaminase gene. In the peripheral muscle, and presumably in the heart, patients with this mutation have diminished AMP deaminase activity resulting in decreased metabolism of AMP to inosine and enhanced production of adenosine. Thus, investigators have hypothesized that adenosine agonists might have therapeutic utility in the management of patients with heart failure because of their anti-cytokine effects.

## Aldosterone antagonists

In addition to ACE inhibitors and beta-blockers showing a benefit in heart failure through anti-inflammatory processes the aldosterone antagonists also may have major anti-inflammatory action in heart failure. The importance of aldosterone antagonists have been underscored by the RALES trial in which patients with severe heart failure were randomized to low-dose spironolactone or placebo. The results showed a dramatic 30% reduction in all-cause mortality. More recently, this result was further supported by the EPHESUS trial, in which patients with heart failure post-myocardial infarction were randomized to a daughter compound of spironolactone, eplerenone [70]. Despite the concomitant use of state-of-art therapy for myocardial infarction these patients had an additional 16% reduction in all-cause mortality. These trials underscored the importance of aldosterone antagonism in the setting of heart failure, but the precise mechanisms are not well-appreciated.

Our laboratory has new evidence to suggest that aldosterone is a major proinflammatory factor in the injured myocardium. The use of an aldosterone antagonist, such as eplerenone, may significantly decrease the effect of inflammatory factors on cardiac remodeling as well as on the activation of MMPs. Therefore the combined use of these agents may very well significantly impact on myocardial inflammatory signal activation post-cardiac injury. The dramatic benefit that we have seen with agents such as aldosterone antagonists may be due, at least in part, to the ability of these agents to block inflammatory pathways.

### HMG-CoA reductase inhibitors (Statins)

The HMG-CoA reductase inhibitors are universally prescribed for patients with coronary artery disease because of an abundant amount of data demonstrating their long-term benefits. However, the role of statins in patients with heart failure but without coronary disease is less certain. Retrospective analyses of large randomized trials of heart failure patients have demonstrated that the utilization of statins appears to benefit all classes of heart failure patients. This has also been observed in large administrative databases derived from cohorts of heart failure patients.

The mechanism of this benefit has not been obvious until one realizes from recent cholesterol lowering trials that in addition to the lowering of serum cholesterol the statins appeared to have marked anti-inflammatory properties. The most consistent evidence to support this notion is through the lowering of a surrogate marker of inflammation, C-reactive protein. In fact, more recent trials of statin therapy have identified that

those who are able to lower their C-reactive protein tended to be those patients who benefit the most from statin therapy. There is also a suggestion that satin therapy may dissociate the lipid rafts on the cell membrane, where the inflammatory signals aggregate [71]. Therefore, statins may have previously unrecognized important anti-inflammatory benefits. This hypothesis is now being tested in other inflammatory and autoimmune diseases.

As a result of these intriguing observations and the new insights into the mechanism of statin's benefits there are large-scale randomized trials evaluating statins in heart failure. The GISSI-5 and other large trials testing statins versus placebo will hopefully provide to the answer to guide clinical therapy in 2 to 3 years.

## Combined anti-viral and anti-inflammatory strategies

### Immunoglobulin therapy

Many causes of acute onset dilated cardiomyopathy, including peri-partum cardiomyopathy, are likely the result of a combination of autoimmune and inflammatory processes in the myocardium, possibly triggered by a transient viral infection. Instead of anti-cytokine therapy or active immune suppression a possible strategy is to induce passive immunization, through the infusion of immune globulins. In cases of pediatric heart failure, particularly myocarditis, uncontrolled studies suggested a potential benefit with intravenous immune globulins [72].

Retrospective analysis suggested that patients with peri-partum cardiomyopathy who received intravenous immune globulin had better ventricular function during follow-up [58]. To test this hypothesis more thoroughly and prospectively in adults, McNamara and Feldman conducted a randomized double blinded trial involving 62 patients with acute heart failure and randomized the patients to receive 2 g/kg intravenous immune globulin or placebo. Patients were followed to assess changes in LVEF from the baseline to 6 months and 12 months. Overall, there was impressive improvement of LVEF from 0.25 to 0.41 at 6 months and to 0.42 at 12 months. However, this improvement was identical in both the immune globulin and placebo arms of the trial. The transplant-free survival was 92% at 1 year.

Therefore, in this study, the patients demonstrated significant improvement independent of therapy. This rapid improvement obscured any possibility of demonstrating a treatment effect. In retrospect, the evaluation of this agent in a more advanced chronic cardiomyopathy population with evidence of inflammation in the heart may have produced a more promising result.

### Interferon therapy

Type I interferons (interferon a and b) are antiviral through their ability to phosphorylate interferon stimulated genes (ISGs). These ISGs include $2'-5'$ PAS and PKR, which together can lead to degradation of viral RNA, and the small GTPase Mx that can limit coxsackieviral infection through interference of accumulation of viral RNA and coat protein. Interferon $\beta$ has been shown to be most effective in animal models of viral myocarditis and we have demonstrated recently that interferon $\beta$ knockout animals ($IFN^{-b-/-}$) have a higher viral titer, increased inflammatory cell infiltrate, increased mortality, and worse cardiac function [73].

To determine if this strategy can be applied to patients, Kuhl et al. have evaluated 22 patients with dilated cardiomyopathy and biopsy evidence of viral persistence [74]. The patients were treated with subcutaneous interferon $\beta$ for a period of 24 weeks. The interferon treatment was able to eliminate the viral genome from all of the patients, and improved ventricular function in 15 of 22 patients. The mean LVEF improved from 44.6% to 53.1% ($p < 0.001$). Overall, the patients also improved in clinical status. These encouraging phase II results have paved the way for an ongoing worldwide phase III trial of interferon $\beta$ in patients with dilated cardiomyopathy, and should offer a very interesting opportunity for evaluating the role of interferon in heart failure.

### Future directions

The concept of immune activation and inflammatory cytokines contributing to heart failure has now been well-established. Indeed, both in experimental models and in humans there is considerable evidence that inflammation is an important component of the pathophysiology of heart failure and progressive left ventricular remodeling. Unfortunately, pharmacologic approaches to treat the inflammatory processes in the heart has not proven to be beneficial in patients with heart failure. This lack of success may be due to a failure to recognize the appropriate target or targets, the side-effect profile of anti-inflammatory agents, or the inability to develop appropriately targeted therapies. For example, broad suppression of the immune/inflammatory system may be detrimental in healing and thus might have untoward long-term consequences. Thus, the challenge might now be to develop targeted approaches. In addition, it will be important to gain an increased understanding of the complex pathways that are involved in cardiac inflammation and immunity in order to identify the appropriate targets.

## References

1 Torre-Amione G, Kapadia S, Lee J et al. Tumor necrosis factor-alpha and tumor necrosis factor receptors in the failing human heart. Circulation 1996;**93**:704–711.

2 Sun M, Dawood F, Wen WH et al. Excessive tumor necrosis factor activation post-infarction contributes to susceptibility to myocardial rupture and left ventricular dysfunction. Circulation 2004;**110**:3221–3228.

3 Nian M, Lee P, Khaper N, Liu P. Inflammation and cytokines in post-myocardial infarction remodeling. Circ Res 2004;**94**:1543–1553.

4 Vasan RS, Sullivan LM, Roubenoff R et al. Framingham Heart Study. Inflammatory markers and risk of heart failure in elderly subjects without prior myocardial infarction: the Framingham Heart Study. Circulation 2003;**107**:1486–1491.

5 Ridker PM, Cushman M, Stampfer MJ, Tracy RP, Hennekens CH. Inflammation, aspirin, and the risk of cardiovascular disease in apparently healthy men. N Engl J Med. 1997;**336**:973–979.

6 Albert MA, Danielson E, Rifai N, Ridker PM, Investigators P. Effect of statin therapy on C-reactive protein levels: the pravastain inflammation/CRP evaluation (PRINCE): a randomized trial. JAMA 2001;**286**:91–93.

7 Puhakka M, Magga J, Hietakorpi S et al. Interleukin-6 and tumor necrosis factor alpha in relation to myocardial infarct size and collagen formation. J Card Fail 2003;**9**:325–332.

8 Feldman AM, Combes A, Wagner D et al. The role of tumor necrosis factor in the pathophysiology of heart failure. J Am Coll Cardiol 2000;**35**:537–544.

9 Ferrari R, Bachetti T, Confortini R et al. Tumor necrosis factor soluble receptors in patients with various

degrees of advanced congestive heart failure. *Circulation* 1995;**92**:1479–1486.

10 Kapadia S, Lee J, Torre-Amione G, Birdsall HH, Ma TS, Mann DL. Tumor necrosis factor-alpha gene and protein expression in adult feline myocardium after endotoxin administration. *J Clin Invest* 1995;**96**:1042–1052.

11 Irwin M, Mak S, Mann D *et al.* Tissue expression and immunolocalization of tumour necrosis factor-alpha in post infarction-dysfunctional myocardium. *Circulation* 1999;**99**:1492–1498.

12 Nakamura H, Umemoto S, Naik G *et al.* Induction of left ventricular remodeling and dysfunction in the recipient heart after donor heart myocardial infarction: new insights into the pathologic role of tumor necrosis factor-alpha from a novel heterotopic transplant-coronary ligation rat model. *J Am Coll Cardiol* 2003;**42**:173–181.

13 Frangogiannis NG, Smith CW, Entman ML. The inflammatory response in myocardial infarction. *Cardiovasc Res* 2002;**53**:31–47.

14 Kubota T, McTiernan CF, Frye CS, Demetris AJ, Feldman AM. Cardiac-specific overexpression of tumor necrosis factor-alpha causes lethal myocarditis in transgenic mice. *J Card Fail* 1997;**3**:117–124.

15 Sivasubramanian N, Coker ML, Kurrelmeyer KM *et al.* Left ventricular remodeling in transgenic mice with cardiac restricted overexpression of tumor necrosis factor. *Circulation* 2001;**104**:826–831.

16 Higuchi Y, McTiernan CF, Frye CV, McGowan BS, Chan TO, Feldman AM. Tumor necrosis factor receptors 1 and 2 differentially regulate survival, cardiac dysfunction, and remodeling in transgenic mice with tumor necrosis factor-alpha-induced cardiomyopathy, *Circulation* 2004;**109**:1892–1897.

17 Kapadia SR, Oral H, Lee J, Nakano M, Taffet GE, Mann DL. Hemodynamic regulation of tumor necrosis factor-alpha gene and protein expression in adult feline myocardium. *Circ Res.* 1997;**81**:187–195.

18 Beg AA, Baltimore D. An essential role for NF-kappaB in preventing TNF-alpha-induced cell death. *Science* 1996;**274**:782–784.

19 Mann DL. Stress-activated cytokines and the heart: from adaptation to maladaptation. *Annu Rev Physiol* 2003;**65**:81–101.

20 Deten A, Volz HC, Briest W, Zimmer HG. Cardiac cytokine expression is upregulated in the acute phase after myocardial infarction. Experimental studies in rats. *Cardiovasc Res* 2002;**55**:329–340.

21 Meldrum DR, Dinarello CA, Cleveland JCJ *et al.* Hydrogen peroxide induces tumor necrosis factor alpha-mediated cardiac injury by a p38 mitogen activated protein kinase-dependent mechanisms. *Surgery* 1998;**124**:291–296.

22 Yokoyama T, Vaca L, Rossen RD, Durante W, Hazarika P, Mann DL. Cellular basis for the negative inotropic effects

of tumor necrosis factor-alpha in the adult mammalian heart. *J Clin Invest* 1993;**92**:2303–2312.

23 Goldhaber JI. Free radicals enhance $Na^+/Ca^{2+}$ exchange in ventricular myocytes. *Am J Physiol* 1996;**271**:H823–H833.

24 Krown KA, Yasui K, Brooker MJ *et al.* TNF alpha receptor expression in rat cardiac myocytes: TNF alpha inhibition of L-type $Ca^{2+}$ current and $Ca^{2+}$ transients. *FEBS Lett* 1995;**376**:24–30.

25 Oral H, Dorn GWn, Mann DL. Sphingosine mediates the immediate negative inotropic effects of tumor necrosis factor-alpha in the adult mammalian cardiac myocyte. *J Biol Chem* 1997;**272**:4836–4842.

26 MacEwan DJ. TNF ligands and receptors – a matter of life and death. *Br J Pharmacol* 2002;**135**:855–875.

27 Pimentel-Muinos FX, Seed B. Regulated commitment of TNF receptor signaling: a molecular switch for death or activation. *Immunity* 1999;**11**:783–793.

28 Malinin NL, Boldin MP, Kovalenko AV, Wallach D. MAP3K-related kinase inolved in NF-kappaB induction by TNF, CD95. *Nature* 1997;**385**:540–544.

29 Liu ZG, Hsu H, Goeddel DV, Karin M. Dissection of TNF receptor 1 effector function: JNK activation is not linked to apoptosis while NF-kB activation prevents cell death. *Cell* 1996;**87**:565–576.

30 Natoli G, Costanzo A, Ianni A. *et al.* Activation of SAPK/JNK by TNF receptor 1 through a noncytotoxic TRAF2-dependent pathway. *Science* 1997;**275**:200–203.

31 Yokoyama T, Nakano M, Bednarczyk JL, McIntyre BW, Entman M, Mann DL. Tumor necrosis factor-alpha provokes a hypertrophic growth response in adult cardiac myocytes. *Circulation* 1997;**95**:1247–1252.

32 Creemers EE, Cleutjens JP, Smits JF, Daemen MJ. Matrix metalloproteinase inhibition after myocardial infarction: a new approach to prevent heart failure? *Circ Res* 2001;**89**:201–210.

33 Li YY, Kadokami T, Wang P, McTiernan CF, Feldman AM. MMP inhibition modulates TNF-alpha transgenic mouse phenotype early in the development of heart failure. *Am J Physiol Heart Circ Physiol* 2002;**282**:H983–H989.

34 Ohta K, Nakajima T, Cheah AY *et al.* Elafin overexpressing mice have improved cardiac function after myocardial infarction. *Am J Physiol Heart Circ Physiol* 2004;**287**:4286–4292.

35 Lee JK, Zaidi SHE, Liu P *et al.* A serine elastase inhibitor reduces inflammation and fibrosis and preserves cardiac function following experimental murine myocarditis. *Nat Med* 1998;**4**:1383–1391.

36 Liu P, Mason J. Advances in the understanding of myocarditis. *Circulation* 2001;**104**:1076–1082.

37 Morens DM, Pallansch MA. Epidemiology of Enteroviral Infections. In: Rotbart HA, ed. *Human Enterovirus Infections*. ASM Press, Washington, DC, 1995:3–23.

38 Martino TA, Liu P, Petric M, Sole MJ. Enteroviral myocarditis and dilated cardiomyopathy: A review of clinical and experimental studies. In: Rotbart HA, ed. *Human Enterovirus Infections*. ASM Press, Washington, DC, 1995:291–351.

39 Pauschinger M, Bowles NE, Fuentes-Garcia FJ *et al.* Detection of adenoviral genome in the myocardium of adult patients with idiopathic left ventricular dysfunction. *Circulation* 1999;**99**:1348–1354.

40 Li YY, Feng Y, McTiernan CF *et al.* Downregulation of matrix metalloproteinases and reduction in collagen damage in the failing human heart after support with left ventricular assist devices. *Circulation* 2001; **104**:1147–1152.

41 Jin O, Sole MJ, Butany JW *et al.* The detection of enterovirus RNA in myocardial biopsies from patients with myocarditis and cardiomyopathy using gene amplification by the polymerase chain reaction. *Circulation* 1990;**82**:8–16.

42 Ayach B, Fuse K, Martino T, Liu P. Dissecting mechanisms of innate and acquired immunity in myocarditis. *Curr Opin Cardiol* 2003;**18**:175–181.

43 Dai WJ, Bartens W, Kohler G, Hufnagel M, Kopf M, Brombacher F. Impaired macrophage listericidal and cytokine activities are responsible for the rapid death of Listeria monocytogenes-infected IFN-gamma receptor-deficient mice. *J Immunol* 1997;**158**:5297–5304.

44 Hemmi H, Takeuchi O, Kawai T *et al.* A Toll-like receptor recognizes bacterial DNA. *Nature* 2000;**408**:740–745.

45 Liu P, Aitken K, Kong YY *et al.* Essential role for the tyrosine kinase p56lck in coxsackievirus B3 mediated heart disease. *Nat Med* 2000;**6**:429–434.

46 Wada H, Saito K, Kanda T *et al.* Tumor necrosis factor-alpha (TNF-alpha) plays a protective role in acute viralmyocarditis in mice: A study using mice lacking TNF-alpha. *Circulation* 2001;**103**:743–749.

47 Opavsky MA, Martino T, Rabinovitch M *et al.* Enhanced ERK-1/2 activation in mice susceptible to coxsackievirus-induced myocarditis. *J Clin Invest* 2002;**109**:1561–1569.

48 Seko Y, Matsuda H, Kato K *et al.* Expression of intercellular adhesion molecule-1 in murine hearts with acute myocarditis caused by coxsackievirus B3. *J Clin Invest* 1993;**91**:1327–1336.

49 Seko Y, Shinkai Y, Kawasaki A *et al.* Expression of perforin in infiltrating cells in murine hearts with acute myocarditis caused by coxsackievirus B3. *Circulation* 1991;**84**:788–795.

50 Kishimoto C, Abelmann WH. In vivo significance of T cells in the development of Coxsackievirus B3 myocarditis in mice. Immature but antigen-specific T cells aggravate cardiac injury. *Circ Res* 1990;**67**:589–598.

51 Zoller J, Partridge T, Olsen I. Interactions between cardiomyocytes and lymphocytes in tissue culture: an in vitro model of inflammatory heart disease. *J Mol Cell Cardiol* 1994;**26**:627–638.

52 Henke A, Huber S, Stelzner A, Whitton JL. The role of CD8$^+$ T lymphocytes in coxsackievirus B3-induced myocarditis. *J Virol* 1995;**69**:6720–6728.

53 Opavsky MA, Penninger J, Aitken K *et al.* Susceptibility to myocarditis is dependent on the response of $\alpha\beta$ T lymphocytes to coxsackieviral infection. *Circ Res* 1999;**85**:551–558.

54 Irie-Sasaki J, Sasaki T, Matsumoto W *et al.* CD45 is a JAK phosphatase and negatively regulates cytokine receptor signaling. *Nature* 2001;**409**:349–354.

55 Mason JW, O'Connell JB, Herskowitz A *et al.* Investigators MTT. A clinical trial of immunosuppressive therapy for myocarditis. *N Engl J Med* 1995;**333**: 269–275.

56 Bozkurt B, Torre-Amione G, Warren MS *et al.* Results of targeted anti-tumor necrosis factor therapy with etanercept (ENBREL) in patients with advanced heart failure. *Circulation* 2001;**103**:1044–1047.

57 Mann DL, McMurray JJ, Packer M *et al.* Targeted anticytokine therapy in patients with chronic heart failure: results of the Randomized Etanercept Worldwide Evaluation (RENEWAL). *Circulation* 2004;**109**:1594–1602.

58 Deswal A, Bozkurt B, Seta Y *et al.* Safety and efficacy of a soluble P75 tumor necrosis factor receptor (Enbrel, etanercept) in patients with advanced heart failure. *Circulation* 1999;**99**:3224–3226.

59 Muller J, Wallukat G, Dandel M *et al.* Immunoglobulin adsorption in patients with idiopathic dilated cardiomyopathy. *Circulation* 2000;**101**:385–391.

60 Staudt A, Bohm M, Knebel F *et al.* Potential role of autoantibodies belonging to the immunoglobulin G-3 subclass in cardiac dysfunction among patients with dilated cardiomyopathy. *Circulation* 2002;**106**: 2448–2453.

61 Staudt A, Schaper F, Stangl V *et al.* Immunohistological changes in dilated cardiomyopathy induced by immunoadsorption therapy and subsequent immunoglobulin substitution. *Circulation* 2001;**103**:2681–2686.

62 Torre-Amione G, Sestier F, Radovancevic B, Young J. Effects of a novel immune modulation therapy in patients with advanced chronic heart failure: results of a randomized, controlled, phase II trial. *J Am Coll Cardiol* 2004;**44**:1181–1186.

63 Prabhu SD, Chandrasekar B, Murray DR, Freeman GL. Beta-adrenergic blockade in developing heart failure: effects on myocardial inflammatory cytokines, nitric oxide, and remodeling. *Circulation* 2000;**101**:2103–2109.

64 Sliwa K, Woodiwiss A, Kone VN *et al.* Therapy of ischemic cardiomyopathy with the immunomodulating agent pentoxifylline: results of a randomized study. *Circulation* 2004;**109**:750–755.

65 Skudicky D, Bergemann A, Sliwa K, Candy G, Sareli P. Beneficial effects of pentoxifylline in patients with idiopathic dilated cardiomyopathy treated with angiotensin-converting enzyme inhibitors and carvedilol: results of a randomized study. *Circulation* 2001;**103**: 1083–1088.

66 Sliwa K, Skudicky D, Candy G, Wisenbaugh T, Sareli P. Randomised investigation of effects of pentoxifylline on left-ventricular performance in idiopathic dilated cardiomyopathy. *Lancet* 1998;**351**:1091–1093.

67 Wagner DR, McTiernan C, Sanders VJ, Feldman AM. Adenosine inhibits lipopolysaccharide-induced secretion of tumor necrosis factor-alpha in the failing human heart. *Circulation* 1998;**97**:521–524.

68 Sajjadi FG, Takabayashi K, Foster AC, Domingo RC, Firestein GS. Inhibition of TNF-alpha expression by adenosine: role of A3 adenosine receptors. *J Immunol* 1996;**156**:3435–3442.

69 Loh E, Rebbeck TR, Mahoney PD, DeNofrio D, Swain JL, Holmes EW. Common variant in AMPD1 gene predicts improved clinical outcome in patients with heart failure. *Circulation* 1999;**99**:1422–1425.

70 Pitt B, Remme W, Zannad F *et al*. EP-AMIHFEaSS Investigators. Eplerenone, a selective aldosterone blocker, in patients with left ventricular dysfunction after myocardial infarction. *N Engl J Med* 2003;**348**:1309–1321.

71 Ehrenstein MR, Jury EC, Mauri C. Statins for atherosclerosis – as good as it gets? *N Engl J Med* 2005;**352**: 73–75.

72 Drucker N, Colan S, Lewis A *et al*. Gamma globulin treatment of acute myocarditis in the pediatric population. *Circulation* 1994;**89**:252.

73 Deonarain R, Cerullo D, Fuse K, Liu PP, Fish EN. Protective role for interferon- beta in coxsackievirus B3 infection. *Circulation* 2004;**110**:3540–3543.

74 Kuhl U, Pauschinger M, Schwimmbeck PL *et al*. Interferon-beta treatment eliminates cardiotropic viruses and improves left ventricular function in patients with myocardial persistence of viral genomes and left ventricular dysfunction. *Circulation* 2003;**107**:2793–2798.

## CHAPTER 13

# The role of vasopressin and vasopressin antagonists in heart failure

*Olaf Hedrich,* MD*, Marvin A. Konstam,* MD, FACC *&*
*James Eric Udelson,* MD, FACC

## Introduction

In addition to the components of other well-defined neuroendocrine systems that play an important role in the pathophysiology of heart failure (HF), such as the sympathetic nervous system (SNS) and the renin–angiotensin–aldosterone system (RAAS), arginine vasopressin (AVP) has recently attracted attention as a potentially important neurohormonal mediator of the HF syndrome in humans [1]. A neurohypophysial hormone, vasopressin (also called antidiuretic hormone or ADH), helps regulate free water reabsorption, body fluid osmolality, blood volume, blood vessel vasoconstriction, and myocardial contractile function [2,3]. These biological functions are subtended by two distinct receptors ($V_{1a}$ and $V_2$), which in turn activate intracellular second messenger pathways with diverse effects [4]. Accordingly, this system represents a novel target for the treatment of HF and several vasopressin antagonists are currently under development [5].

This chapter focuses on the pathophysiology of vasopressin in HF, the pharmacology of vasopressin receptor antagonists, and a review of current clinical trial data.

## Pathophysiology

### Synthesis and release of vasopressin

Human vasopressin, a 9-amino acid peptide with arginine in position 8, is synthesized as a pre-pro-hormone by vasopressinergic neurons of the supraoptic and paraventricular nuclei in the hypothalamus [6]. Post-translational modification of this large primary precursor occurs in these neurons. The modified precursor is transported along axons to the neuronal terminals in the posterior pituitary (neurohypophysis), undergoing cleavage by endopeptidases into the mature hormone [7]. Once it reaches the nerve terminal membrane it is stored in secretory granules and is then released into the circulation by means of exocytosis in response to either osmotic or nonosmotic stimuli [8,9].

Under ordinary physiological conditions plasma osmolality is the major factor governing release of vasopressin. Exquisitely sensitive osmoreceptor cells located in the hypothalamus reflect even minute changes in osmolality by alterations in their volume causing the stimulation of secretory neurons in the hypothalamus [9]. The degree of vasopressin secretion from the neurohypophyseal axon terminals is directly determined by the degree of change of osmolality.

A variety of nonosmotic stimuli can also lead to the release of vasopressin, though in nondisease states these factors play a less significant role than does osmolality. Circulatory homeostasis is monitored in part by high-pressure mechanoreceptors located in the carotid sinus, left ventricle, aortic arch, and renal juxtaglomerular apparatus [9,10]. In response to events such as decreased arterial blood pressure, profound hypovolemia, shock, or renal hypoperfusion, vasopressin production and

185

release are stimulated by afferent stimuli via cranial nerves IX and X. In contrast, if pressure increases production and release of vasopressin is reduced.

Once released into the venous circulation draining the neurohypophysis (via the dural, cavernous, and inferior petrosal sinuses) vasopressin circulates unbound to plasma proteins (although it does bind to specific receptors on platelets), and is degraded by endo- and amino-peptidases. The circulating half-life of vasopressin is 5–15 min.

## Vasopressin receptors

There are three distinct vasopressin receptors (V-R) through which vasopressin exerts its biological effects (Table 13.1)[4]. All have seven trans-membrane spanning domains and are G-protein-coupled, but they have distinct pharmacological profiles and intracellular second messenger systems [11]. $V_1$ receptors have two subtypes, $V_{1a}$ and $V_{1b}$. In addition to the $V_1$ receptors, $V_2$ receptors have also been identified and characterized. $V_{1a}$ and $V_2$ receptors are the primary receptors involved in various physiological processes including regulation of vascular tone, body fluid regulation, and cardiovascular contractility.

The $V_{1a}$ ("vascular") receptors are located on several diverse cell types including vascular smooth muscle and cardiomyocytes, and it is through this receptor that vasopressin assists in maintaining and regulating vascular tone and myocardial function [3]. Binding of vasopressin to the $V_{1a}$ receptor subtypes leads to activation of the phosphoinositide pathway, activation of a host of protein kinases (including protein kinase C, p42/p44 MAP kinase, PI 3-kinase, and calcium/calmodulin-dependent kinase II), mobilization of cytosolic calcium, and activation of the $Na^+$–$H^+$exchanger [4,12]. Shortly after agonist binding receptor internalization occurs.

The $V_2$ ("renal") receptors are expressed on the basolateral membrane of the renal collecting ducts, and mediate the antidiuretic effects of vasopressin. Intracellular events triggered by binding of vasopressin to the $V_2$ receptor include activation of adenylyl cyclase and subsequent generation of intracellular cyclic adenosine monophosphate, activation of protein kinase A, and "shuttling" of aquaporin 2 water channels (AQP-2) from cytoplasmic vesicles to the luminal surface of the renal collecting duct cells where they are inserted into the cell membrane and facilitate water transport across the collecting duct cells (Figure 13.1) [13,14]. $V_2$ receptor agonism also appears to promote increased *de novo* synthesis of AQP-2 channels.

The $V_{1b}$ ("pituitary") receptors are expressed on the surfaces of corticotropic cells in the anterior pituitary, where they potentiate the release of adrenocorticotropic hormone (ACTH). It is beyond the scope of this chapter to consider the effects mediated by this receptor at length, but ACTH-mediated aldosterone secretion and subsequent sodium reabsorption may indirectly lead to fluid accumulation which may worsen heart failure.

Table 13.1 Vasopressin receptor subtypes.

| Receptor subtypes (alternative nomenclature) | Site of action | AVP activation effects |
|---|---|---|
| $V_{1a}$ ($V_1$-vascular receptor, $V_1R$) | Vascular smooth muscle cells<br>Platelets<br>Lymphocytes and monocytes<br>Adrenal cortex | Vasoconstriction<br>Platelet aggregation<br>Coagulation factor release<br>Glycogenolysis |
| $V_2$ ($V_2$-renal receptor, $V_2R$) | Basolateral membrane of distal nephron and renal collecting duct | Free water reabsorption |
| $V_{1b}$ ($V_3$-pituitary receptor, $V_3R$) | Anterior pituitary | ACTH and $\beta$-endorphin release |

AVP: arginine vasopressin; ACTH: adrenocorticotropic hormone.
*Source:* Modified from [5].

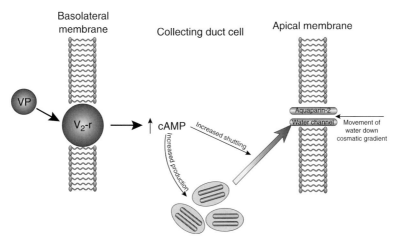

**Figure 13.1** Intracellular events in renal collecting duct cells in response to $V_2$ receptor stimulation. Upon binding with vasopressin, the $V_2$ receptor (on the basolateral membrane of the renal collecting duct cells) causes activation of adenylyl cyclase and subsequent synthesis of intracellular cAMP. AQP-2 water channels are "shuttled" from their cytoplasmic vesicles to the apical membrane, where they facilitate movement of free water across the apical membrane down an osmotic gradient. AQP-2 synthesis is also increased. Reproduced from [14].

### Physiologic effects of vasopressin

From a cardiovascular standpoint the major effects of vasopressin to be considered are (1) its indirect effects on circulating blood volume (and interstitial fluid volume) through mediation of water retention ($V_2$-related characteristics) and (2) its direct and indirect effects on the blood vessels and myocardium bringing about a change in hemodynamics ($V_{1a}$-related characteristics).

### Body fluid regulation

Under normal physiological conditions, continuous changes in plasma osmolality modulate the release of vasopressin from the neurohypophysis by means described earlier. Through its effects on the $V_2$ receptor and the subsequent chain of intracellular events, increased "shuttling" and synthesis of AQP-2 channels then occurs. Thus, the permeability of the collecting duct is effectively increased allowing water to be reabsorbed and ultimately returned to the intravascular circulation. This is the primary function of vasopressin in physiological conditions.

An increases in plasma osmolality increases the plasma concentration of vasopressin in a linear manner [9]. The mean plasma osmolality that acts as a set point above which vasopressin concentration increases in response to further increases in osmolality is termed the "osmotic threshold". In humans, the osmotic threshold has been shown to be approximately 280 to 290 mOsm/kg $H_2O$ [9]. There appears to be no level of osmolality below which its release is truly completely suppressed. While the osmotic threshold is subject to considerable inter-individual variability it forms part of a very reproducible system within any given individual, and governs plasma osmolality with exquisite sensitivity and gain. For example, if plasma becomes hypertonic (serum [$Na^+$] >142 mEq/L) the plasma vasopressin concentration rises from approximately 2.5 pg/mL in isotonic conditions to above 5 pg/mL and urine becomes maximally concentrated (1200 mOsm/kg $H_2O$). If, on the other hand, the same individual becomes hypotonic (serum [$Na^+$] <135 mEq/L), vasopressin becomes undetectable in the plasma and urine becomes maximally dilute (50 mOsm/kg $H_2O$) in the collecting duct [6]. Even changes in plasma osmolality, as minimal as a few percent, result in significant changes in vasopressin concentration and urine osmolality. Thus, vasopressin is a major influence in the control of plasma osmolality.

### Vascular tone regulation

Vasopressin, along with the sympathetic nervous system and RAAS, helps regulate vascular tone via the $V_{1a}$ receptors located ubiquitously on the surfaces of vascular smooth muscle cells. It is a potent direct arteriolar vasoconstrictor [15] causing significant increases in systemic vascular resistance (SVR) [16]. As suggested by animal studies vasopressin may also indirectly potentiate the vasoconstrictive effects of angiotensin-II and norephinephrine [17], although this effect is less well-defined in humans. In the face of hypotensive or hypovolemic stress vasopressin is essential in maintaining vascular tone, and its release is triggered by baroreceptor-mediated reflexes as described earlier. Elevations in plasma vasopressin concentration in response to blood pressure reduction appear to be exponential, in contrast to the linear increases of osmoregulated vasopressin release.

Despite vasopressin's potent vasoconstrictive properties a *physiological* increase *in vivo* usually does not cause an increase in arterial blood pressure [16]. This interesting observation may be explained by the fact that vasopressin also augments the sinoartic baroreceptor reflex. This effect is mediated through $V_2$ receptor stimulation with consequent lowering of both heart rate and cardiac output to maintain a constant blood pressure [18]. Therefore, under "normal" circumstances, stimulation of both $V_{1a}$ and $V_2$ receptors causes elevation of SVR without increasing the arterial blood pressure. An extreme *supraphysiological* increase in plasma vasopressin level is required before an elevation in arterial pressure can result [19]. Under such circumstances, $V_{1a}$-mediated increases in vascular tone overshadow the $V_2$-mediated baroreceptor reflex augmentation.

### Cardiovascular contractility

Vasopressin's effects on the myocardium are less well-appreciated than its other hemodynamic effects, and must again be interpreted against the background of possible reflex-mediated responses. The effects of vasopressin on cardiac contractility appear to be mediated solely by $V_{1a}$ receptor agonism [20].While a dose-dependent increase in intracellular calcium is seen when individual myocytes are exposed to elevated concentrations of vasopressin [21] whether net positive or negative cardiac inotropy is achieved depends on the systemic concentration of vasopressin attained.

The effects of vasopressin on cardiac contractility appear to be related to plasma concentration of vasopressin, much like the observed effects on

the vasculature. In a variety of animal models subjecting the myocardium to supraphysiological doses of vasopressin resulted in a reduction in cardiac contractility [20,22,23]. This reduction in contractile function is felt to be secondary to relative coronary ischemia due to $V_{1a}$-mediated coronary vasoconstriction occurring at high concentrations of vasopressin [22]. When coronary perfusion is maintained in the presence of modest elevations of vasopressin within physiological range a positive (yet transient) inotropic response has been demonstrated [20]. Therefore, in the physiological state, small increases in cardiac contractility can occur with elevations of vasopressin concentration within physiological range, while supraphysiological concentrations may result in a reduction in myocardial contractility.

## Vasopressin in heart failure

### General concepts

Several studies have shown a significant elevation in plasma vasopressin concentration in the setting of heart failure [5,24–26]. In the neuroendocrine substudy of the Studies of Left Ventricular Dysfunction (SOLVD) patients with left ventricular dysfunction were shown to have higher levels of vasopressin [as well as norepinephrine, plasma renin activity (PRA), and atrial natriuretic peptide] than did control patients [26]. Patients with asymptomatic left ventricular (LV) dysfunction (LV ejection fraction ≤35%) had higher mean plasma vasopressin levels (AVP = 2.2 pg/mL) than their controls (AVP = 1.8 pg/mL). Interestingly, individuals with mild to moderate symptoms of HF had even higher mean levels (AVP = 3.0 pg/mL) than their asymptomatic counterparts. The important observation to be made from these data is that neuroendocrine activation of vasopressin in the setting of LV dysfunction occurs even in the absence of clinical symptoms and increases in proportion to the severity of the syndrome, similar to observations made about the SNS and RAAS. A summary of vasopressin levels in several major HF populations is presented in Table 13.2. As may be appreciated, not all studies nor all patients in these studies demonstrate consistently elevated vasopressin levels compared to normals. However, these levels may be "inappropriately" elevated in HF relative to

**Table 13.2** Vasopressin levels measured by radio-immunosorbent assay (RIA) in heart failure and other populations.

| Reference | Patients | Mean AVP levels (pg/mL) | Comments |
|---|---|---|---|
| [44] | CHF, $n = 10$ | $2.4 \pm 0.6$ | Vasodilators held $\times$48 h |
|  | Normals | $1.1 \pm 0.2$ |  |
| [27] | CHF, $n = 10$ | $2.3 \pm 0.8$ |  |
| [28] | CHF, $n = 14$ | $4.6 \pm 0.3$ | On diuretics |
|  | HTN, $n = 8$ | $2.9 \pm 0.1$ | On diuretics |
|  | CAD, $n = 11$ | $3.4 \pm 0.2$ | Not on diuretics |
| [24] | CHF, $n = 31$ | $9.5 \pm 0.9$ | Vasodilators/diuretics held |
|  | Normals, $n = 51$ | $4.7 \pm 0.7$ | $\times$48 h, low Na diet |
| [29] | CHF, $n = 15$ | $11.6 \pm 5.5$ | Elevated baseline levels in |
|  | Normals, $n = 9$ | $5.3 \pm 2.3$ | HF patients did not increase in response to orthostatic stress |
| [25] | CHF, $n = 9$ | $4.6 \pm 2.1$ | At serum [Na] 137 mEq/L |
| [31] | CHF, $n = 20$ |  |  |
|  | "High AVP" for Posm | $14.5 \pm 8.8$ |  |
|  | "Low AVP" for Posm | $3.9 \pm 1.0$ |  |
| [36] | Asx LVD, $n = 534$ | $1.8 \pm 6.7$ | SAVE Trial population, 27% "activated", i.e. $>1.96$ SD above age-matched controls |
| [30] | Normals, $n = 12$ | $1.1 \pm 0.2$ |  |
| [26] | CHF, $n = 80$ | 3.5 | Range 2.3–4.4 |
|  | Asx LVD, $n = 147$ | 2.6 | Range 1.7–3.0 |
|  | Normals, $n = 54$ | 2.9 | Range 1.4–2.3 (SOLVD population) |
| [30] | CHF, $n = 42$ | $3.0 \pm 2.5$ |  |
|  | Normals, $n = 10$ | $1.0 \pm 0.4$ |  |
| [66] | CHF, $n = 142$ | Median levels 2.1–2.9 |  |

AVP = arginine vasopressin; CHF = congestive heart failure; HTN = hypertension; CAD = coronary artery disease; Asx LVD = asymptomatic left ventricular dysfunction; Posm = plasma osmolality; SOLVD = Studies of Left Ventricular Dysfunction.

the state of plasma volume or osmolality, although studies are not often analyzed as such [31].

The mechanisms underlying the elevation of plasma vasopressin in heart failure are unclear. Whereas in the physiological state, as described above, there is a close relationship between plasma vasopressin levels and osmolality this relationship appears to be disrupted in heart failure. Several studies have found that vasopressin levels do indeed decrease with decreasing plasma osmolality but that overall they remained at higher levels than expected even when hypo-osmolality occurred [32,33]. This net increase in vasopressin level occurs even though plasma osmolality is often reduced compared to normal subjects. In a population of patients with HF who received an osmotic load by means of mannitol infusion vasopressin levels were demonstrated to increase to a greater degree than in non-HF subjects, and baseline levels of vasopressin relative to plasma osmolality were found to be higher in the HF patients (who also demonstrated lower baseline osmolality) than in their normal counterparts [34]. Although dysregulated, the overall sensitivity of the system appears to remain intact but with an "upward shift" in plasma vasopressin levels.

If it is assumed that osmotic sensitivity remains intact in heart failure patients then the elevated levels of vasopressin encountered may be explained on the basis of an ongoing increase in the nonosmotic stimulation of vasopressin release. Changes in tone of cardiopulmonary baroreceptors (as has been described in chronic heart failure) have been shown to modulate osmotic stimulation of vasopressin release [35], and it may be on this basis that inappropriately high levels of vasopressin for prevailing osmolality are encountered in heart failure. Alternatively (or perhaps additionally) reduction in arterial blood pressure may stimulate mechanoreceptor-mediated pathways of vasopressin release. In the setting of hemodynamic derangements encountered in heart failure the mechanoreceptor-mediated release of vasopressin therefore may outweigh the osmoreceptor response to decreased osmolality to result in a net increase in vasopressin levels seen in these patients.

It has been postulated that an "interfering substance" present in HF somehow disrupts the effects of vasopressin at the renal level. Neurohumoral responses of the sympathetic nervous, renin–angiotensin–aldosterone, natriuretic peptide, and nitric oxide systems alter the synthesis of prostaglandins, which have been shown to modulate the effects of vasopressin [36]. Atrial natriuretic peptide (ANP) is known to be one of the most potent antagonists of the renal effects of vasopressin *in vitro* [37]. Whether these effects are present to any significant degree *in vivo* remains unclear. There exist other, more direct, associations between vasopressin and neurohormones activated in heart failure, described in more detail in later sections.

## Pathophysiologic effects of vasopressin in heart failure

As demonstrated earlier, vasopressin levels in heart failure tend to be elevated and the degree of elevation appears to mirror the severity of the clinical syndrome. To assess whether vasopressin is truly a neuroendocrine pathogen in the development and progression of heart failure consideration must be given to its potential pathophysiologic role, and its association with long-term outcomes [38,39]. While it is presently unclear whether chronically elevated vasopressin levels unfavorably affect outcome measures in heart failure both experimental and clinical data suggest that this hormone mediates important pathophysiologic functions in heart failure, and may play a role in progression of

the disease [1,5,38]. Furthermore, in multivariate analysis, vasopressin levels obtained 1-month after myocardial infarction in patients enrolled in the Survival and Ventricular Enlargement (SAVE) Study correlated independently with severe heart failure (RR = 1.6), recurrent myocardial infarction (RR = 2.3), and a combined endpoint measure of cardiovascular mortality or heart failure or myocardial infarction (RR = 1.6) [40]. This tends to suggest that vasopressin levels in this setting do have some prognostic significance.

### Effects on water balance

Through the complex and currently incompletely defined system of interactions between osmotic and nonosmotic pathways characterized earlier, elevated plasma vasopressin concentrations appear to be associated with impaired free water excretion in patients with heart failure [25,32]. These processes are thought to be subtended by $V_2$ receptor-mediated increases in AQP-2 water channels in the renal collecting ducts [41].

In an experimental chronic heart failure model, AQP-2 expression in the renal collecting duct was upregulated [42,43]. When comparing rats with mild, compensated heart failure without elevated left ventricular end-diastolic pressure (LVEDP) or reduced plasma sodium concentration rats with an elevated LVEDP and reduced plasma sodium were found to have a significantly increased expression of AQP-2 mRNA [42]. While these observations are helpful in explaining the clinical observations of volume expansion and hyponatremia in heart failure the role for implicating vasopressin in these processes is strengthened by further experimental observations regarding selective inhibition of $V_2$ receptors in animals with heart failure.

The previously mentioned rat study found that administration of an oral selective nonpeptide $V_2$ receptor antagonist OPC-31260 (5 - dimethylamino-1-[4-(2-methylbenzoylamino) benzoyl]-2, 3, 4, 5-tetrahydro-1H-benzazepine hydrochloride) resulted in a reduction of AQP-2 protein expressed in the collecting duct [42]. In another experimental model using rats with ischemia-induced CHF manifesting impaired systolic function, left ventricular remodeling, and increased lung and heart weights, animals were treated with OPC-31260 for 6 months [44].

Chronic $V_2$ receptor blockade in these rats increased urine volume and decreased urine osmolality without modifying myocardial remodeling, cardiac function, or survival.

The VPA-985 (5-fluoro-2-methyl-N-[4-(5H-pyrrolo[2,1-c][1,4] benzodiazepin-10(11H)-ylcarbonyl)-3-chlorophenyl]benzamide), a specific and selective nonpeptide $V_2$ receptor antagonist has been shown to be a potent aquaretic compound in dogs and rats [45]. Furthermore, in humans, a randomized, placebo-controlled study administering VPA-985 resulted in a significant, dose-related increase in water excretion and resulting elevation of serum sodium concentration and serum osmolality in patients with advanced HF [46].In this study, an observed reduction in urinary AQP-2 protein levels suggested that the observed aquaresis may have been secondary to a reduction in AQP-2 expression at the level of the renal collecting duct.

Cumulatively, these observations suggest that antagonism of $V_2$ receptor subtypes may represent an alternative target in managing water retention in CHF.

### Effects on hemodynamics

As noted earlier, under normal physiologic conditions, the vasoconstrictive effects of vasopressin are usually not associated with appreciable changes in arterial blood pressure at plasma levels within physiological range [16]. When vasopressin is infused intravenously in patients with HF, however, a variety of hemodynamic effects have been observed [47]. In the setting of stepwise increments in vasopressin infusion statistically significant and dose-dependent increases in SVR and pulmonary capillary wedge pressure (PCWP) occur, along with decreases in stroke volume (SV) and cardiac output (CO) (Figure 13.2).

These hemodynamic effects are primarily thought to be mediated through activation of $V_{1a}$ receptors on vascular smooth muscle cells, which promotes an increase in afterload by means of arteriolar vasoconstriction [15,48]. However, indirect effects mediated by $V_2$ receptor agonism may result in increased water retention, which increases circulating blood volume and hence preload, with concomitant increases in PCWP and left ventricular filling pressure. The increase in SVR appears

to be one major force driving a reduction in CO in heart failure patients given their heightened sensitivity to changes in afterload. At the myocyte level vasopressin may be positively inotropic; yet, when factoring in the effects of vasoconstriction on the coronary arteries resulting in decreased coronary flow elevated levels of vasopressin may on balance have a negatively inotropic effect on the failing heart, with an attending decline in SV and CO [38].

Supportive evidence for these hypotheses once again comes from observational data employing selective $V_{1a}$ receptor antagonists *in vivo* [48], where significant improvements in SVR and CO were recorded when vasopressin levels were elevated (Figure 13.2). In animal series, similar results were reported. In a model of CHF induced by rapid ventricular pacing in dogs administration of the nonpeptide vasopressin antagonist OPC-21268 (1-(1-[4-(3-acetylaminopropoxy) benzoyl]-4- piperidyl)-3,4-dihydro-2(1H)- quinolone) resulted in significantly increased cardiac output and reduced total peripheral resistance [49]. A porcine model of CHF revealed improved ventricular loading conditions when the nonpeptide $V_1$ receptor antagonist SR49059 ((2S) 1-[ (2R3S ) -5-chloro - 3-(2-chloro-phenyl)-1-(3,4- dimethoxy benzene- sulfonyl ) - 3-hydroxy-2,3- dihydro 1H-indole-2-carbonyl]-pyrrolidine-2- carboxamide) was administered, with reduced left ventricular end-diastolic dimension and peak wall stress [50].

### Effects on the myocardium

Vasopressin has been implicated in cardiac remodeling, and structural changes in myocardium exposed to high levels have been demonstrated in both neonatal and adult myocytes [51–53]. In cultured neonatal rat myocardial cells cellular hypertrophy by means of enhanced protein synthesis (including the proto-oncogene c-fos mRNA) has been observed [51,52]. By means of exposure to $V_{1a}$ receptor antagonists the observed hypertrophy was significantly inhibited [51,52]. In adult animals, similar changes have been demonstrated in isolated, perfused rat hearts [53]. In addition to cellular hypertrophy, deposition of collagen appears to be enhanced by exposure to vasopressin. Again, these effects in the intact animal models were

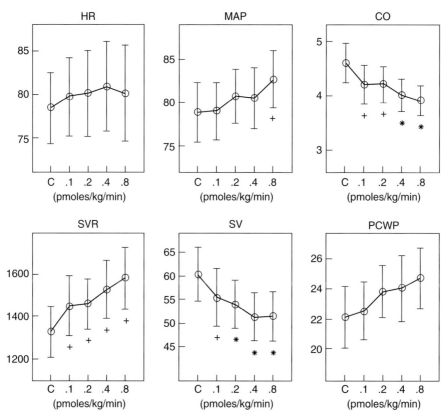

**Figure 13.2** Hemodynamic effects of vasopressin in HF. Overall hemodynamic responses to infused arginine vasopressin. Data are shown as mean ± SD for each infusion rate. The mean basal plasma arginine vasopressin level was 6.4 ± 2.7 pg/mL, and increased to 63 ± 39 pg/mL at peak infusion rate. During the infusion, heart rate (HR, bpm) and mean arterial pressure (MAP, mmHg) did not change, except for a small increase in blood pressure at the highest infusion rate. A statistically significant decline in cardiac output (CO, L/min) and stroke volume (SV, mL) was recorded, as was a statistically significant increase in systemic vascular resistance (SVR, dynes s/cm$^5$). There was significant overall variation ($p < 0.01$) in the pulmonary capillary wedge pressure (PCWP, mmHg), but no individual pairs attained statistical significance. Right atrial pressure and pulmonary artery pressure (not shown) did not change. $^+p < 0.05$; $^*p < 0.01$; C denotes control group (no vasopressin). Reproduced from [47].

ameliorated by the presence of a $V_{1a}$ receptor antagonist [54], suggesting that this receptor is central in the pathophysiology of vasopressin-mediated myocardial remodeling.

As described previously, by means of a series of intracellular events, myocardial $V_{1a}$ receptor agonism results in an increase in intracellular calcium concentration as well as protein kinase C activity [51,52], which is thought to be central in mediating the observed hypertrophic myocardial cell growth not unlike effects ascribed to angiotensin II. Whether these structural changes translate into clinically significant outcomes in heart failure, or contribute to progression of the disease, is currently unknown.

**Effects on other regulatory systems**

Interactions between vasopressin and other neuroendocrine systems active in the pathophysiology of HF continue to be defined. Although the precise mechanisms are not fully understood it has been postulated that the cardiac effects of vasopressin may be enhanced during RAAS inhibition. This is of potential importance given that early (peptide) vasopressin antagonist studies were performed in patients who were not necessarily on ACE-inhibitors, suggesting that vasopressin inhibition may become progressively more important as other neurohormonal systems are blocked. Stated alternatively, the hemodynamic effects of vasopressin in experimental studies are more obvious in the milieu of decreased sympathetic nervous system or RAAS activity. This may have potentially significant implications for drug safety evaluation given the current era of focused neuroendocrine antagonism in heart failure [16].

The RAAS and SNS both are potentiated by vasopressin, particularly at high plasma concentrations, and both systems in turn activate synthesis of vasopressin [38,41]. After intracerebral injection of angiotensin II in rats increases in vasopressin concentration that were statistically significant have been observed [55]. Endothelin-1 has been identified as a further stimulus to vasopressin release, and may additively increase afterload by means of its vasoconstricting properties [56].

## Vasopressin antagonists

More comprehensive neurohormonal antagonism beyond ACE-inhibition, $\beta$-adrenergic receptor-blockade, and aldosterone antagonism holds promise in modulating the long-term effects (and possibly outcome) of HF. As demonstrated in animal studies and human HF trials to date blockade of vasopressin receptors may be beneficial in this regard. In an effort to harness the potentially beneficial effects of decreasing the activity of vasopressin in this syndrome selective and potent vasopressin receptor antagonists have been developed in recent years, several of which have reached the stage of human clinical trials designed to determine both short-term and long-term efficacy (Table 13.3). Although vasopressin receptor antagonists have been available for several years early animal studies utilized peptide analogs that were limited in their potential for long-term use by their relative species specificity in terms of receptor affinity, inadequate oral bioavailability, and short half-lives [5,57]. These characteristics hindered their further advancement to human trials.

Newer, nonpeptide antagonists of $V_{1a}$ and $V_2$ receptors, as well as dual $V_{1a}/V_2$ receptor antagonists, have been developed by employing a complementary approach of random drug screening and structure-based drug design [57]. These agents possess properties that have allowed further study for long-term use, including excellent oral bioavailability, good receptor specificity, and

Table 13.3 Vasopressin receptor blockers currently being investigated.

| $V_{1a}$ | $V_2$ | $V_{1a}/V_2$ |
|---|---|---|
| Relcovaptan (SR-49059) | Tolvaptan (OPC-41061) | Conivaptan (YM-087) |
| OPC-21268 | Lixivaptan (VPA-985) | JTV-605 |
| | OPC-31260 | CL-385-004 |
| | SR-121463 | |
| | VP-343 | |
| | FR-161282 | |

sustained intermediate term effects in experimental and human models. Currently, several agents are undergoing clinical investigation for conditions as diverse as heart failure, systemic hypertension, peripheral vascular disease, as well as for hyponatremia due to hepatic cirrhosis, nephrotic syndrome, and the syndrome of inappropriate secretion of ADH (SIADH) [2,34,57].

## Clinical trials of vasopressin receptor antagonists

### $V_2$ receptor antagonists

From a pathophysiological point of view antagonism of $V_2$ receptors may be expected to result in a reduction in overall body fluid volume by means of enhanced aquaresis, and possibly thereby correction of hyponatremia (although the pathophysiology resulting in hyponatremia is complex and involves factors such as renal perfusion and impairment of renal function by diuretics). Several studies employing selective nonpeptide $V_2$ receptor antagonists have demonstrated beneficial effects in the acute and long-term treatment of HF, and are described here in further detail.

$V_2$ receptor antagonism has been demonstrated to result in stimulation of aquaresis in humans, with net loss of free water. Unlike with the administration of loop diuretics antagonism of $V_2$ receptors appears not to increase activation of the RAAS [58].

The first orally active nonpeptide $V_2$ receptor antagonist studied in humans (OPC 31260), which displaces vasopressin more potently from its $V_2$ receptors than from its $V_1$ receptors, was demonstrated to significantly induce aquaresis with an associated increase in plasma sodium and osmolality in a rat model previously described [42]. In humans, however, selectivity of this agent for $V_2$ receptors is dramatically diminished, inducing diuresis with similar potency as furosemide [59]. This limited effect has hindered the development of this drug for use in heart failure.

### Tolvaptan

(OPC-41061;(±)-7-chloro-5-hydroxy-1-[2-methyl-4- (2methylbenzoylamino) benzoyl]-2, 3, 4, 5-tetra-hydro-1H-1-benzazepine) is a specific and selective nonpeptide $V_2$ receptor antagonist without intrinsic agonist properties, shown to have potent aquaretic properties in an animal model [60]. In cloned human receptors the $V_2 : V_{1a}$ receptor selectivity was 29 : 1 [60]. Tolvaptan's half-life is between 6 and 8 h. Dose-dependent responses demonstrated in rats include markedly increased free water clearance, significantly less urinary loss of sodium than furosemide, and no significant effect on serum creatinine or BUN [58]. In comparison with furosemide serum sodium increased in a dose-dependent fashion in those animals given tolvaptan [58] highlighting the drug's potential benefit in hyponatremia.

A randomized, placebo-controlled preliminary investigation of 83 New York Heart Association (NYHA) functional class II and III patients with CHF and congestion who were taken off background diuretic therapy, salt restricted, and given either tolvaptan (30 mg/day), furosemide (80 mg/day), or a combination for 7 days aimed at comparing tolvaptan with furosemide for volume reduction [61]. Tolvaptan-treated patients demonstrated a significant decline in body weight and increase in urine output when compared with furosemide, while serum sodium increased within normal range without a change in serum potassium.

In hospitalized, hyponatremic heart failure patients tolvaptan administration across a broad dosage range (10–60 mg/day) was significantly better than water restriction in normalizing serum sodium, both from a viewpoint of rapidity and degree of correction [62]. Maintenance of normal serum sodium levels in these patients was demonstrated for the 25-day duration of the trial (Figure 13.3).

In a small open-label, randomized, placebo-controlled, crossover study in patients with mild to moderate CHF designed to assess the effects of tolvaptan and furosemide on renal function and renal hemodynamics [63] tolvaptan was found to increase urine output, glomerular filtration rate (GFR), and renal blood flow (RBF) to statistical significance. By comparison, furosemide increased urine output to a comparable degree, but at the expense of a decreasing GFR and RBF. This result supports current opinion that $V_2$ receptor antagonism may help preserve renal function in HF patients while promoting diuresis.

Prospective randomized trials published to date assessing the clinical utility of tolvaptan have focused on its use in chronic HF [64], and more recently in patients admitted with acutely decompensated heart failure to evaluate its short- and intermediate-term effects [64].

In a double-blinded study conducted in a group of 254 HF patients the efficacy of tolvaptan to remove excessive fluid when added to a diuretic was assessed [62]. Three oral doses of tolvaptan (30 mg, 45 mg, or 60 mg) given daily for 25 days were evaluated. The study enrolled patients irrespective of left ventricular ejection fraction (LVEF). All patients had clinical evidence of volume overload, and included those with systolic dysfunction (LVEF <40%), preserved systolic function (LVEF >40%), and those who did not have an assessment of ejection fraction (44% of the cohort). The majority of patients were in NYHA functional class II or III, and there was a high background prevalence of ACE-inhibitor or angiotensin receptor blocker use with a lower proportion of patients on $\beta_2$-receptor antagonists (71% versus 26%). Patients were not fluid restricted, and their loop diuretics were continued at stable dose (furosemide dose averaged 85 mg/day). Interestingly, abnormally elevated plasma concentrations of vasopressin (>8.0 pg/mL) were observed at baseline in only 6.3% of the patient population. Hyponatremia at baseline (defined as serum sodium ≤136 mEg/L) was encountered in approximately 30% of the population [65].

This study demonstrated a significant decrease in body weight and edema in modestly volume-overloaded CHF patients, increased urinary volume, and normalization of hyponatremia [62].

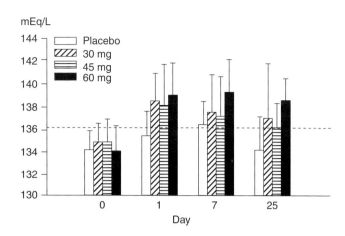

**Figure 13.3** Effects of tolvaptan on serum sodium concentration in hyponatremic HF patients. This figure demonstrates the mean absolute changes in serum sodium concentration over time in a series of HF patients with hyponatremia (defined as serum $Na^+$ <136 mEq/L) treated with tolvaptan. These patients experienced greater increases in serum sodium than their normonatremic counterparts, and serum sodium concentration remained within normal range during the study. Reproduced from [62].

These effects were all sustained over the full course of therapy. A statistically significant decrease in body weight was observed on the first day when compared with placebo ($p < 0.001$), which was not dose dependent, and was similar in extent in all patients regardless of LVEF. This reduction was maintained until the end of the study period. Although fluid intake was increased in tolvaptan-treated patients compared with placebo net fluid losses were also greater in these patients ($p < 0.05$ at each dose). Urinary findings appeared to be dose dependent: urine osmolality decreased significantly in a dose-dependent fashion at day 1 and mean decreases in urine sodium from baseline were significantly greater in tolvaptan-treated patients ($p < 0.05$). Interestingly, although tolvaptan is thought to exert purely aquaretic effects, total urinary sodium excretion in the first 24 h rose significantly when compared with placebo, raising the possibility of a volume-mediated effect. The urinary effects were observed in both normo- and hyponatremic patients [65]. Serum sodium increased modestly at day 1 (<4 mEq/L and within the normal range) in tolvaptan-treated patients ($p < 0.0001$). In the hyponatremic subgroup this was greater than in the normonatremic patients, and was sustained in 82% by the end of the treatment period (versus 40% of placebo-treated patients, $p < 0.05$) (Figure 13.3). In the normonatremic tolvaptan-treated cohort serum sodium returned to baseline values by the end of the treatment period after an initial small rise, while in the hyponatremic patients levels persisted in the normal range. No significant changes in serum potassium levels or renal function were reported. Only dry mouth, thirst, and polyuria were encountered with significantly higher frequency in the tolvaptan treated group than in the placebo group.

The above study did not attempt to assess neurohormonal effects of tolvaptan nor did the length of study and number of adverse events observed allow for any evaluation of effects on outcome. Results from the Acute and Chronic Therapeutic Impact of a Vasopressin Antagonist in Congestive Heart Failure (ACTIV in CHF) trial, in which the acute and intermediate-term clinical effects of tolvaptan in patients hospitalized for HF were evaluated, have recently been published [64]. These are summarized below, and may assist in broadening our understanding of the role of tolvaptan in managing hospitalized, volume overloaded HF patients.

In the multicenter, randomized, double blind, placebo-controlled ACTIV in CHF trial three oral, once-daily doses of tolvaptan (30 mg, 60 mg, or 90 mg) were compared with placebo in patients hospitalized with acute decompensated heart failure. From 45 centers in the United States and Argentina 319 patients were enrolled. The main inclusion criteria were admission for worsening HF with signs of systemic congestion after initial standard in hospital therapy including diuretics, and an LVEF <40%. Patients received the study drug in both an inpatient and outpatient setting up to 10 days in hospital (after which if the patient was still in hospital the treatment was deemed to have failed) followed by a 7-week (49–51 days) outpatient period. The inhospital (acute) endpoint was a change in body weight at 24 h after the administration of the first dose of study drug. The outpatient (intermediate-term) endpoint was worsening HF at 60 days after randomization, defined as hospitalization for heart failure, unscheduled visits for HF to an emergency department or outpatient facility resulting in an intensification of therapy, or death. Apart from a slightly higher prevalence of prior percutaneous intervention or coronary artery bypass grafting ($p = 0.02$) and male gender ($p = 0.04$) in the placebo group there were no significant differences between the groups. Background use of ACE-inhibitors (83%) and $\beta$-receptor antagonists (42%) was similar among the groups.

Body weight decreased significantly from baseline in all tolvaptan-treated groups on day one when compared with placebo, decreased further during the course of hospitalization, and remained stable after discharge (Figure 13.4). This effect appeared not to be dose dependent. Similarly, urine volume on day one was significantly higher in all groups treated with tolvaptan than placebo, and this effect also was maintained throughout the period of hospitalization. Signs and symptoms of HF improved in all patients during the period of hospitalization, although when compared with placebo only dyspnea was significantly less often encountered by discharge ($p = 0.04$). Diuretic use (defined by furosemide equivalents) decreased in all groups after discharge, but the mean dosage reduction was not significant. Serum sodium increased slightly (mean increase between 2.77 and 3.50 mEq/L) in the tolvaptan-treated groups, whereas a small decrease (mean $-0.20 \pm 3.12$ mEq/L) was encountered in placebo-treated patients. Hyponatremia (defined as serum sodium concentration <136 mEq/L) was observed in 16% of patients randomized to tolvaptan. Serum sodium concentrations were observed to rise rapidly, and often normalize, in this cohort. Adverse events were relatively frequent in all groups with thirst encountered more frequently in tolvaptan-treated patients ($p = 0.07$). Interestingly, serious adverse events requiring drug discontinuation were also encountered slightly more frequently in the tolvaptan-treated cohort, although this did not reach statistical significance ($p = 0.06$).

In the ACTIV in CHF trial, tolvaptan did not cause a decline in renal function and no changes in serum potassium were noted. The absence of adverse effects on renal function seen in this trial and other preliminary investigations [63] is potentially important, as worsening renal function during hospitalization for decompensated HF is common [66] and associated with an unfavorable hospital course and outcome.

While no significant differences were observed in rates of rehospitalization or outpatient visits for heart failure there was a trend toward longer event-free survival in the tolvaptan groups compared to placebo. In post hoc subgroup analysis patients with elevated BUN levels and severe systemic congestion who were treated with tolvaptan experienced lower total mortality rates, although it should be noted that the study was not sufficiently powered or prospectively designed to assess mortality and these results should be viewed in this light.

An important point to be noted from this trial is that acutely decompensated HF patients with elevated BUN or severe congestion were at very high risk for short-term mortality (22.5% and 17.8% respectively). Whether the possible mortality benefit observed with tolvaptan in these groups is significant requires confirmation in appropriately powered studies.

In summary, the above outlined trial data suggest that tolvaptan possesses several properties of significant potential benefit in the treatment of chronic heart failure; these include decreasing body weight and therefore congestion by increasing urine output, maintaining serum sodium concentration within normal range in normonatremic patients normalizing serum sodium concentration in hyponatremic patients, and preventing a concomitant decline in renal function or significant electrolyte derangement commonly encountered with traditional diuretic regimens. Several of these beneficial effects seem to be maintained beyond the initial administration of the drug, as demonstrated by a decrease in diuretic dosage achieved in the ACTIV in CHF patient group during a prolonged follow-up period. Currently, phase 3 studies are underway to further assess the potential for benefit of tolvaptan in acute decompensated HF (particularly from a standpoint of mortality and outcome), as well as for the specific treatment of hyponatremia associated with a variety of conditions including HF.

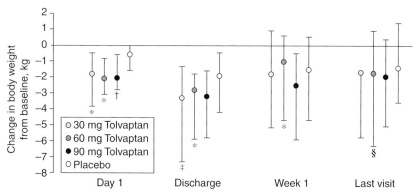

**Figure 13.4** Weight response to tolvaptan in heart failure. Median changes in body weight over time in response to tolvaptan orally for up to 60 days as observed in the ACTIV in CHF Trial. A significantly greater reduction in median body weight was observed in patients treated with tolvaptan than in those treated with placebo on day 1; this effect was dose-independent and was observed at tolvaptan doses of 30 mg ($p = 0.002$;*), 60 mg ($p = 0.002$;*), and 90 mg ($p = 0.009$;†). By discharge, body weight reductions in the 30 mg ($p = 0.006$;‡) and 60 mg ($p = 0.002$;*) groups remained significantly greater than in the placebo group. At last visit, the 60 mg tolvaptan group sustained the significant reduction in body weight when compared with those treated with placebo ($p = 0.008$;§). Reproduced from [64].

*Lixivaptan*
(VPA-985; 5-fluoro-2-methyl-N-[4-(5H-pyrrolo [2,1-c][1,4]benzodiazepin-10(11H)-yl carbonyl)- 3-chlorophenyl]benzamide) is another specific, nonpeptide, orally active antagonist of the $V_2$ receptor currently undergoing evaluation for efficacy in HF and hepatic cirrhosis [67]. Its binding affinity for $V_2$ receptors is approximately 100 times greater than for $V_1$ receptors. Dose-dependent increases in urine output, free water clearance, and serum sodium concentration have been demonstrated in human studies of single doses of lixivaptan administered to patients with NYHA class II and III HF [46]. Lixivaptan has been evaluated in a multiple dose study of 44 patients with hyponatremia (etiologies of which included cirrhosis, CHF, and SIADH) receiving doses of 25 mg, 125 mg, or 250 mg orally twice daily for 7 days [68]. The observed effects included a significant overall aquaretic response compared with placebo, with significant dose-related increases in free water clearance ($p < 0.05$) and serum sodium ($p < 0.05$), without significant changes in orthostatic blood pressure or serum creatinine levels. This agent may therefore hold promise in correcting abnormal renal water handling and hyponatremia in conditions associated with water retention. Of note is that, although safe and effective at lower doses, the higher dose (250 mg) resulted in significant dehydration requiring withholding of doses in

50% of the patients receiving this dose. Further studies are required to determine the optimal dose and indication for this new vasopressin antagonist.

## $V_{1a} V_2$ receptor antagonists
Due to the hemodynamic effects attributed to activation of the $V_{1a}$ receptor in heart failure there lies a theoretical advantage in antagonizing both the $V_{1a}$ and $V_2$ receptor simultaneously. The result is conceivably a synergistic effect on systemic hemodynamic and renal parameters. The most extensively studied dual receptor vasopressin antagonist is conivaptan (YM087).

*Conivaptan*
(YM087; 4′-[(2-methyl-1,4,5,6-tetrahydroimidazo [4,5-d][1][benzazepin-6-yl)-carbonyl]-2-phenyl- benzanilide monochloride) is a nonpeptide vasopressin antagonist with high affinity for both $V_{1a}$ and $V_2$ receptors. Its binding affinities ($K_i$ values) in radioligand competition binding assays are 3.36 ng/mL and 0.59 ng/mL respectively [57], suggesting more potent $V_2$ inhibition than $V_{1a}$ inhibition. Conivaptan may be administered by oral and intravenous routes, and its oral bioavailability is approximately 44% [68]. In animal models, potent aquaretic and effective inhibitory pressor responses have been demonstrated to occur in a

dose-dependent manner. The effects of conivaptan on urinary parameters in the rat model, either with or without captopril, has been shown to bring about a statistically significant increase in both volume and urine sodium concentration when compared with placebo [69]. These results were sustained after a 25-day period of administration of conivaptan. Additionally, interesting experimental data has emerged from studies of conivaptan's effects on neonatal rat cardiomyocytes [52]. Decreased intracellular free calcium and mitogen-activated protein kinase activity were observed to occur in a dose-dependent manner suggesting a reduction of intracellular protein synthesis and, by extrapolation, perhaps of cardiomyocyte hypertrophy. These observations are bolstered by the results of a rat infarct study of ventricular mass after 4 weeks of treatment with conivaptan, captopril, or combination [69]. Conivaptan-treated rats demonstrated a statistically significant decrease in right ventricular mass when compared to placebo, and the combination of captopril and conivaptan yielded a greater decrease in both left and right ventricular mass, suggesting that vasopressin inhibition may play a role in remodeling after myocyte injury.

Human studies with conivaptan demonstrate that single dose dual $V_{1a}/V_2$ antagonism results in significant, positive aquaretic and hemodynamic effects in patients with HF. In a multicenter study of 142 patients with severe heart failure (NYHA Class III or IV, LVEF 21–26%) conivaptan was administered as a single intravenous dose (10, 20, or 40 mg) and compared with placebo in an effort to evaluate its hemodynamic effects [70]. Patients were mostly male (75%), caucasian (60%), and were of an average age of 60 years. Background diuretic use was high (95–100% across the randomized groups), as was ACE-inhibitor (84–86%) and $\beta$-adrenergic blocker (44–50%) use.

Pulmonary artery catheterization was used to assess hemodynamic changes, which required the eligible patients to have a PCWP of $\geq 16$ mmHg and a cardiac index of $\leq 2.8$ L/min/m$^2$ at baseline. Both PCWP and right atrial pressure (RAP) were significantly reduced after drug administration in the 20 mg ($p < 0.01$) and 40 mg ($p < 0.05$) conivaptan groups when compared with placebo, without significant change in cardiac index, pulmonary artery pressures, systemic or pulmonary vascular resistance, systemic arterial pressure, or heart rate. The peak effect on PCWP was sustained for approximately 8 h after administration.

Urine output in the conivaptan-treated group was significantly greater than in the placebo group ($p < 0.001$), and demonstrated a dose-dependent response that peaked at 2 to 3 h after the dose was administered (Figure 13.5). Similarly, urine osmolality was significantly reduced by all doses of conivaptan ($p < 0.05$), without a significant change in serum osmolality, serum sodium, or serum potassium levels (although there was a small, dose-dependent trend toward higher serum sodium in the conivaptan groups). The hemodynamic and urine output effects were evaluated in relation to baseline serum sodium and AVP concentration. Both AVP and serum sodium concentrations were normal on average, and there was no significant correlation between conivaptan effects and baseline

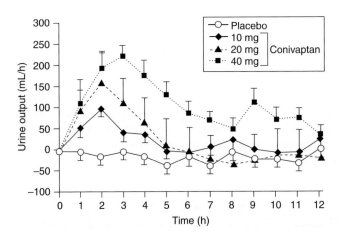

**Figure 13.5** Urinary output in response to conivaptan administration. Urine output rates for the groups randomized to conivaptan or placebo. There was a dose-dependent increase in urine flow rates with increasing conivaptan dose ($p < 0.001$). Reproduced from [70].

levels of either. This suggests that the effects of conivaptan are apparent in a patient population beyond merely those with hyponatremia or elevated vasopressin levels. Side effects of conivaptan were few, and there were overall fewer side effects than that in the placebo group; the most frequently encountered side effect was headache (7.9% with placebo versus 5.8% with conivaptan).

A preliminary study of oral conivaptan in relation to potential effects on functional capacity yielded less-promising results [71]. A total of 343 patients were randomized to conivaptan versus placebo in this study, which sought to determine the safety and effect of dual $V_{1a}/V_2$ receptor antagonism on functional capacity (determined by time to reach 70% of peak $VO_2$ during treadmill exercise testing) during 3 months of oral administration of conivaptan. Side effects again were encountered slightly more frequently in the conivaptan group when compared with placebo (12.8% versus 4.3% respectively), but conivaptan did not demonstrate efficacy in terms of improving exercise tolerance or quality of life.

In summary, conivaptan has been demonstrated to have promising properties for the treatment of HF particularly with regard to increasing urine output and consequently improving hemodynamic parameters of congestion, as well as normalization of serum sodium concentrations in hyponatremic subjects. The intravenous form of conivaptan is undergoing continued development for potential use in hyponatremic states [specifically the syndrome of inappropriate ADH secretion (SIADH) and CHF] and acute decompensated HF [72]. Recent data suggest that intravenous administration of conivaptan is not only well-tolerated but also causes a significant improvement in serum sodium in hyponatremic subjects [73].

## Summary and future directions

As the role of vasopressin in promoting the pathologic effects of HF has become clearer new pharmacologic modalities are undergoing development in order to allow antagonism of this neurohormonal mediator. Selective nonpeptide vasopressin antagonists have been developed that have shown to have several beneficial effects on the clinical syndrome of HF. These include a reduction in body fluid volume by promotion of aquaresis with maintenance of electrolyte homeostasis (with consequent symptomatic and hemodynamic improvements) and correction of hyponatremia (in HF as well as other hyponatremic states). The major properties of several vasopressin antagonists currently under development are summarized in (Table 13.4). Of potentially major importance is that vasopressin antagonism has been shown to largely maintain renal function in acute decompensated HF while procuring the above effects. Since volume reduction with diuretics is often accompanied by hyponatremia and renal function impairment (both of which have been associated with poor outcomes) this property may prove to be invaluable in managing HF in the future. Current investigations are focusing on establishing the safety and efficacy

**Table 13.4** Properties of vasopressin receptor blockers.

|  | Tolvaptan (OPC-41061) | Lixivaptan (VPA-985) | SR-121463 | Conivaptan (YM-087) |
|---|---|---|---|---|
| Receptor | $V_2$ | $V_2$ | $V_2$ | $V_{1a}/V_2$ |
| Selectivity ($K_i V_{1a} : K_i V_2$) | 29:1 | 100:1 | 100:1 | 10:1 |
| Administration route | Oral | Oral | Oral | Intravenous |
| Urine volume | ↑ | ↑ | ↑ | ↑ |
| Urine osmolality | ↓ | ↓ | ↓ | ↓ |
| Sodium excretion/24 h | ↔ | ↔Low dose ↑High dose | ↔ | ↔ |
| Manufacturer | Otsuka | Wyeth-Ayerst | Sanofi | Yamanouchi |

↑increases; ↓ decreases; ↔ remains overall unchanged.
*Source:* Adapted from [5].

of several of these agents in acute decompensated HF and chronic HF confirming their beneficial effects in maintenance of renal function in decompensated HF, and determining their potential for improving outcomes in HF. In addition to traditional methods of neurohormonal blockade vasopressin antagonism may become an important tool in the pharmacologic armamentarium against the syndrome of HF.

# References

1 Schrier RW, Abraham W. Hormones and hemodynamics in heart failure. *N Engl J Med* 1999;**341**:577–585.

2 Thibonnier M. Vasopressin receptor antagonists in heart failure. *Curr Opin Pharmacol* 2003;**3**:683–687.

3 Penit J, Faure M, Jard S. Vasopressin and angiotensin II receptors in rat aortic arch smooth muscle cells in culture. *Am J Physiol* 1983;**244**:E72–E82.

4 Carmichael MC, Kumar R. Molecular biology of vasopressin receptors. *Semin Nephrol* 1994;**14**:341–348.

5 Lee CR, Watkins MI, Patterson JH *et al.* Vasopressin: A new target for the treatment of heart failure. *Am Heart J* 2003;**146**:9–18.

6 Guyton AC. The kidneys and body fluids. In: Guyton AC, Hall JE, eds. *Textbook of Medical Physiology.* WB Saunders Company, Philadelphia, PA, 1996; 308–372.

7 Reeves WB, Bichet DG, Andreoli TE. Posterior pituitary and water metabolism. In: Wilson TD, Foster DW, Kronenberg HM, eds. *Williams Textbook of Endocrinology.* WB Saunders Company, Philadelphia, PA, 1998:341–348.

8 Katz AM. Neurohumoral responses and the hemodynamic defense reaction. In: Katz AM. *Physiology of the Heart,* 3rd edn. Lippincott Williams & Wilkins, Philadelphia, PA, 2001: 287–311.

9 Schrier RW, Berl T, Anderson RJ. Osmotic and non-osmotic control of vasopressin release. *Am J Physiol* 1979;**236**:F321–F332.

10 Gilmore JP. Contribution of baroreceptors to the control of renal function. *Circ Res* 1964;**14**:301–317.

11 Thibonnier M, Conarty DM, Preston JA, Wilkins PL, Berti-Mattera LN, Mattera R. Molecular pharmacology of human vasopressin receptors. *Adv Exp Med Biol* 1998;**449**:251–276.

12 Thibonnier M. Signal transduction of V1-vascular vasopressin receptors. *Regul Pept* 1992;**38**:1–11.

13 Nielsen S, Chou CL, Marples D, Christensen EI, Kishore BK, Knepper MA. Vasopressin increases water permeability of kidney collecting duct by inducing translocation of aquaporin-CD water channels to plasma membrane. *Proc Natl Acad Sci USA* 1995;**92**:1013–1017.

14 Kalra PR, Anker SD, Coats AJS. Water and sodium regulation in chronic heart failure: the role of natriuretic peptides and vasopressin. *Cardiovasc Res* 2001;**51**:495–509.

15 Monos E, Cox RH, Peterson CH. Direct effects of physiologic doses of arginine vasopressin on the arterial wall in vivo. *Am J Physiol* 1978;**243**:H167–H173.

16 Goldsmith SR. Vasopressin as vasopressor. *Am J Med* 1987;**82**:1213–1219.

17 Ishikawa S, Goldberg J, Schrier D, Aisenberg G, Schrier R. Interrelationship between subpressor effects of vasopressin and other vasoactive hormones in the rat. *Miner Electrolyte Metab* 1984;**10**:184–189.

18 Ebert TJ, Cowley AW, Skelton M. Vasopressin reduces cardiac function and augments cardiopulmonary baroreflex resistance increases in man. *J Clin Invest* 1986;**77**:1136–1142.

19 Montani JP, Liard JF, Schoun J, Mohring J. Hemodynamic effects of vasopressin infused into the vertebral circulation of conscious dogs. *Circ Res* 1980;**47**:346–350.

20 Walker BR, Childs ME, Adams EM. Direct cardiac effects of vasopressin: role of $V_1$- and $V_2$-vasopressinergic receptors. *Am J Physiol* 1988;**255**:H261–H265.

21 Xu YJ, Gopalakrishnan V. Vasopressin increases cytosolic free $[Ca^{2+}]$ in the neonatal rat cardiomyocyte. Evidence for $V_1$ subtype receptors. *Circ Res* 1991;**69**:239–245.

22 Khayyal MA, Eng C, Franzen D *et al.* Effects of vasopressin on the coronary circulation: reserve and regulation during ischemia. *Am J Physiol* 1985;**248**:H516–H522.

23 Fujisawa S, Iijima T. On the inotropic actions of arginine vasopressin in ventricular muscle of the guinea pig heart. *Jpn J Pharmacol* 1999;**81**:309–312.

24 Goldsmith SR, Francis GS, Cowley AW, Levine TB, Cohn JN. Increased plasma arginine vasopressin levels in patients with congestive heart failure. *J Am Coll Cardiol* 1983;**1**:1385–1390.

25 Szatalowicz VL, Arnold PE, Chaimovitz C, Bichet D, Schrier RW. Radioimmunoassay of plasma arginine vasopressin in hyponatremic patients with congestive heart failure. *N Engl J Med* 1981;**305**:263–266.

26 Francis GS, Benedict C, Johnstone DE *et al.* Comparison of neuroendocrine activation in patients with left ventricular dysfunction with and without congestive heart failure. A substudy of the Studies of Left Ventricular Dysfunction (SOLVD). *Circulation* 1990;**82**:1724–1729.

27 Nicod P, Waeber B, Bussien JP *et al.* Acute hemodynamic effect of a vascular antagonist of vasopressin in patients with congestive heart failure. *Am J Cardiol* 1985;**55**:1043–1047.

28 Pruszczynski W, Vahanian A, Ardaillou R, Acar J. Role of antidiuretic hormone in impaired water excretion of patients with congestive heart failure. *J Clin Endocrinol Metab* 1984;**58**:599–605.

29  Goldsmith SR, Francis GS, Levine TB, Cowley AW Jr, Cohn JN. Impaired response of plasma vasopressin to orthostatic stress in patients with congestive heart failure. *J Am Coll Cardiol* 1983;**2**:1080–1083.

30  Gavras H, Ribeiro AB, Kohlmann O *et al*. Effects of a specific inhibitor of the vascular action of vasopressin in humans. *Hypertension* 1984;**6**:I156-I160.

31  Kramer BK, Schweda F, Riegger GAJ. Diuretic treatment and diuretic resistance in heart failure. *Am J Med* 1999;**106**:90–96.

32  Goldsmith SR, Cowley AW, Francis GS, Cohn JN. Arginine vasopressin and the renal response to water loading in congestive heart failure. *Am J Cardiol* 1986;**58**:295–299.

33  Bichet DG, Kortas C, Mettauer B *et al*. Modulation of plasma and platelet vasopressin by cardiac function in patients with heart failure. *Kidney Int* 1986;**29**:1188–1196.

34  Uretsky BF, Verbalis JG, Generalovich T, Valdes A, Reddy PS. Plasma vasopressin response to osmotic and hemodynamic stimuli in heart failure. *Am J Physiol* 1985;**248**:H396–H402.

35  Goldsmith SR, Dodge-Brown D, Cowley AW. Nonosmotic influences on the osmotic stimulation of vasopressin in humans. *Am J Physiol* 1987;**252**:H85–H88.

36  Smith WL, Watanabe T, Garcia-Perez A, Sonnenburg WK. The renal collecting tubule as a model for examining the mechanism of action of prostaglandins: interactions between prostaglandin E2 and vasopressin. In: Hayash O, Yamamoto S, eds. *Advances in Prostaglandin, Thromboxane and Leukotriene Research*. Raven, New York, NY, 1985:673–675.

37  Dillingham MA, Anderson RJ. Inhibition of vasopressin action by atrial natriuretic factor. *Science* 1986;**231**:1572–1573.

38  Goldsmith SR. Vasopressin: a therapeutic target in congestive heart failure? *J Card Fail* 1999;**5**:347–356.

39  Francis GS, Tang WHW. Vasopressin receptor antagonists. Will the "vaptans" fulfill their promise? *JAMA* 2004;**291**:2017–2018.

40  Rouleau JL, de Champlain J, Klein M *et al*. Activation of neurohumoral systems in postinfarction left ventricular dysfunction. *J Am Coll Cardiol* 1993;**22**:390–398.

41  Schrier RW, Martin PY. Recent advances in the understanding of water metabolism in heart failure. *Adv Exp Med Biol* 1998;**449**:415–426.

42  Xu DL, Martin PY, Ohara M *et al*. Upregulation of aquaporin-2 water channel expression in chronic heart failure rat. *J Clin Invest* 1997;**97**:1500–1505.

43  Berl T. Water channels in health and disease. *Kidney Int* 1998;**53**:1417–1418.

44  Burrell LM, Phillips PA, Risvanis J, Chan RK, Aldred KL, Johnston CI. Long-term effects of nonpeptide vasopressin $V_2$ antagonist OPC-31260 in heart failure in the rat. *Am J Physiol* 1998;**275**:H176–H182.

45  Chan PS, Coupet J, Park HC *et al*. VPA-985, a nonpeptide orally active and seleactive vasopressin $V_2$ receptor antagonist. In: Zingg HH, Bourque CW, Bichet D, eds. *Vasopressin and Oxytocin. Molecular, Cellular, and Clinical Advances*, Vol 449. Plenum Press, New York, NY, 1998:439–443.

46  Abraham WT, Oren RM, Crisman TS *et al*. Effects of an oral, nonpeptide, selective V2 receptor vasopressin antagonist in patients with chronic heart failure (Abstract). *J Am Coll Cardiol* 1997;**29**:169A.

47  Goldsmith SR, Francis SG, Cowley AW, Goldenberg I, Cohn JN. Hemodynamic effects of infused arginine vasopressin in congestive heart failure. *J Am Coll Cardiol* 1986;**8**:779–783.

48  Creager MA, Faxon DP, Cutler SS, Kohlman O, Ryan TJ, Gavras H. Contribution of vasopressin to vasoconstriction in patients with congestive heart failure: comparison with the renin-angiotensin system and the sympathetic nervous system. *J Am Coll Cardiol* 1986;**7**:758–765.

49  Naitoh M, Suzuki H, Murakami M *et al*. Effects of oral AVP receptor antagonists OPC-21268 and OPC-31260 on congestive heart failure in conscious dogs. *Am J Physiol* 1994;**267**:H2245–H2254.

50  Clair MJ, King MK, Goldberg AT *et al*. Selective vasopressin, angiotensin II, or dual receptor blockade with developing congestive heart failure. *J Pharmacol Exp Ther* 2000;**293**:852–860.

51  Nakamura Y, Haneda T, Osaki J *et al*. Hypertrophic growth of cultured neonatal rat heart cells mediated by vasopressin $V_{1a}$ receptor. *Eur J Pharmacol* 2000;**391**:39–48.

52  Tahara A, Tomura Y, Wada K *et al*. Effect of YM087, a potent nonpeptide vasopressin antagonist, on vasopressin-induced protein synthesis in neonatal rat cardiomyocyte. *Cardiovasc Res* 1998;**38**:198–205.

53  Fuzukawa J, Haneda T, Kikuchi K. Arginine vasopressin increases the rate of protein synthesis in isolated perfused adult rat heart via the $V_1$ receptor. *Mol Cell Biochem* 1999;**195**:93–98.

54  Bird E, Sasseville V, Dorso C *et al*. Significant reduction in cardiac fibrosis and hypertrophy in spontaneously hypertensive rats (SHR) treated with a $V_{1a}$ receptor antagonist (Abstract). *Circulation* 2001;**104**:186.

55  Shoji M, Kimura T, Matsui K *et al*. Role of intracerebral angiotensin receptors in the regulation of vasopressin release and the cardiovascular system. *Neuroendocrinology* 1986;**43**:239–244.

56  Yamamoto T, Kimura T, Ota K *et al*. Central effects of endothelin-1 on vasopressin release, blood pressure, and renal solute excretion. *Am J Physiol* 1992;**262**:E856–E862.

57 Thibonnier M, Coles P, Thibonnier A, Shoham M. The basic and clinical pharmacology of nonpeptide vasopressin receptor antagonists. *Annu Rev Pharmacol Toxicol* 2001;**41**:175–202.

58 Hirano T, Yamamura Y, Nakamura S, Onogawa T, Mori T. Effects of the $V_2$-receptor antagonist OPC-41061 and the lop diuretic furosemide alone and in combination in rats. *J Pharmacol Exp Ther* 2000;**292**:288–294.

59 Ohnishi A, Orita Y, Takagi N *et al.* Aquaretic effect of a potent, orally-active, nonpeptide $V_2$ antagonist in men. *J Pharmacol Exp Ther* 1995;**272**:546–551.

60 Yamamura Y, Nakamura S, Ito S *et al.* OPC-41061, a highly potent human vasopressin V2-receptor antagonist: pharmacological profile and aquaretic effect by single and multiple oral dosing in rats. *J Pharmacol Exp Ther* 1998;**287**:860–867.

61 Udelson JE, Orlandi C, O'Brien T, Sequiera R, Ouyang J, Konstam MA. Vasopressin receptor blockade in patients with congestive heart failure: Results from a placebo-controlled, randomized study comparing the effects of tolvaptan, furosemide and their combination. *J Am Coll Cardiol* 2002;**39**:156A

62 Gheorghiade M, Niazi I, Ouyang J *et al.* for the Tolvaptan Investigators. Vasopressinn $V_2$-receptor blockade with tolvaptan in patients with chronic heart failure: Results from a double-blind, randomized trial. *Circulation* 2003;**107**:2690–2696.

63 Burnett JC, Smith WB, Ouyang J, Zimmer CA, Orlandi C. Tolvaptan (OPC-41061), a V2 vasopressin receptor antagonist, protects against the decline in renal function observed with loop diuretic therapy (Abstract). *J Card Fail* 2003;**9**:S12.

64 Gheorghiade M, Gattis WA, O'Connor CM *et al.* Effects of tolvaptan, a vasopressin antagonist, in patients hospitalized with worsening heart failure: a randomized controlled trial. *JAMA* 2004;**291**:1963–1971.

65 Gheorghiade M, Konstam MA, Udelson JE *et al.* Vasopressin receptor blockade with tolvaptan in chronic heart failure: differential effects in normonatremic and hyponatremic patients (Abstract). *J Am Coll Cardiol* 2002;**39**:171A.

66 Forman DE, Butler J, Wang Y *et al.* Incidence, predictors at admission, and impact of worsening renal function among patients hospitalized with heart failure. *J Am Coll Cardiol* 2004;**43**:61–67.

67 Wong F, Blei AT, Blendis LM, Thuluvath PJ. A vasopressin receptor antagonist (VPA-985) improves serum sodium concentration in patients with hyponatremia: a multicenter, randomized, placebo-controlled trial. *Hepatology* 2003;**37**:182–191.

68 Burnier M, Fricker AF, Hayoz D *et al.* Pharmacokinetic and pharmacodynamic effects of YM087, a combined $V_1/V_2$ vasopressin receptor antagonist in normal subjects. *Eur J Clin Pharmacol* 1999;**55**:633–637.

69 Naitoh M, Risvanis J, Balding LC *et al.* Neurohormonal antagonism in heart failure; beneficial effects of vasopressin $V_{1a}$ and $V_2$ receptor blockade and ACE inhibition. *Cardiovasc Res* 2002;**54**:51–57.

70 Udelson JE, Smith WB, Hendrix GH *et al.* Acute hemodynamic effects of conivaptan, a dual $V_{1a}$ and $V_2$ vasopressin receptor antagonist, in patients with advanced heart failure. *Circulation* 2001;**104**:2417–2423.

71 Russell SD, Adams KF, Shaw JP, Gattis WA, O'Connor CM. Results of a twelve week double-blind, placebo controlled, multicenter study of oral conivaptan to assess functional capacity in patients with class III chronic heart failure. *J Card Fail* 2003;**9**:S60.

72 Goldsmith SR, Bisaha JG, Smith N. Evaluating the Efficacy and Safety of the Novel Vasopressin $V_{1a}$ and $V_2$ Receptor Antagonist Conivaptan for the Treatment of Acute Decompensated Chronic Heart Failure: Study Protocol. *J Card Fail* 2004;**10**:S85.

73 Verbalis JG, Bisaha JG, Smith N. Novel Vasopressin $V_{1a}$ and $V_2$ Antagonist (Conivaptan) Increases Serum Sodium Concentration and Effective Water Clearance in Patients with Hyponatremia. *J Card Fail* 2004;**10**:S27.

# CHAPTER 14

# Role of erythropoietin in the correction of anemia in patients with heart failure

*Rebecca P. Streeter,* MD *& Donna M. Mancini,* MD

## Introduction

Anemia is common among patients with chronic heart failure (CHF) and is associated with increased morbidity and mortality. The prevalence of anemia in heart failure varies [1–8] depending on age, patient population, definition of anemia, and CHF severity. Correction of anemia in heart failure patients using erythropoietin, a glycoprotein growth factor produced by the kidney to regulate erythrocyte production, improves exercise capacity and quality of life as well as decreases hospitalizations [7,9,10]. Whether correction of anemia by erythropoietin therapy improves survival remains to be determined. In this chapter the role of erythropoietin in the management of CHF will be explored.

## Epidemiology

Anemia has various definitions but the most frequently used is that of the World Health Organization, which defines anemia as hemoglobin levels <13 g/dL in men or <12 g/dL in women [11]. Given the lack of consensus on a definition of anemia, the prevalence of anemia in heart failure patients as reported in several multicenter trials ranges from 12–61% [1–8]. Table 14.1 summarizes the results from studies that have investigated the links between anemia, morbidity and mortality in heart failure patients.

The relationship between anemia and worsening CHF has been examined in both investigational and observational study populations. Silverberg was the

first to emphasize the high prevalence of anemia in a heart failure population as well as the correlation of anemia with increasing disease severity in a retrospective chart review of 142 patients attending a heart failure clinic [7]. Results obtained from larger studies support Silverberg's initial observations [1,5,6]. Patients with mild CHF are found to be anemic [7] but lower hemoglobin levels are associated with increasing severity of disease as assessed by functional status, and rates of hospitalization.

Not only has anemia been associated with increased morbidity in CHF patients it has repeatedly been associated with increased mortality. Anemia was shown to be a significant independent risk factor for mortality in analyses of 912 NYHA class II–IV patients in the RENAISSANCE trial database, 1130 class IIIB/IV patients in PRAISE [3], 6635 class I–IV patients in SOLVD [4], as well as in a cohort study [5] of 1061 class III/IV patients, and in a population-based cohort [2] of 12 065 patients with new-onset heart failure in Canada.

The time course of the development and/or progression of anemia may prove to be clinically significant. When the change in hemoglobin was examined over time comparison of patients who had an increase in hemoglobin to those with a decrease or no change in hemoglobin revealed a higher mortality rate at 1 year in the latter patients [1]. Other clinical factors may amplify the deleterious effect of anemia. Anemia has been shown to interact significantly with glomerular fitration rate (GFR) implying a synergistic effect of anemia and

**Table 14.1** Prevalence of anemia in clinical trials with outcomes.

| Reference | Patients | Clinical characteristics | Definition of anemia (Hgb, g/dL) (Hct, %) | Prevalence (%) | Outcome anemic versus nonanemic |
|---|---|---|---|---|---|
| [1] | 912 | LVEF <30% NYHA class II–IV | Hb ≤12 | 12 | Mortality rate 28% versus 16% Mortality + hospitalization 56% versus 33% |
| [2] | 12 065 | Population-based new onset CHF | ICD-9 codes 280–289 "all anemia" | 17 | 1 year mortality 38% versus 27% |
| [3] | 1130 | LVEF <30% class IIIB–IV | Lowest quintile of Hct Hct <37.6 | 20 | HR for mortality 1.11 for each 1% ⇓ Hct for Hct <37.6 |
| [4] | 6563 | LVEF ≤35% NYHA class I–IV | Hct ≤39 | 22 | RR for mortality 1.03 for each 1% ⇓ Hct |
| [5] | 1061 | LVEF <40% NYHA class III–IV | Hb = 13 (men) Hb = 12 (women) | 30 | 1-year mortality 44% versus 26% |
| [6] | 2281 | Population-based CHF-discharge diagnosis | Hct ≤37 | 48 | HR for mortality 1.02 for each 1% ⇓ Hct |
| [7] | 142 | LVEF 32% class I–IV | Hb < 12 | 56 | NA |
| [8] | 196 | Class II–IV | Hct < 41 (males) Hct < 38 (females) | 61 | 1 year mortality 59% versus 37% |

CHF = congestive heart failure; Hct = hematocrit; Hgb = hemoglobin; HR = hazard ratio; RR = relative risk; LVEF = left ventricular ejection fraction; ICD = international statistical classification of diseases; ⇓ = decrease.

renal insufficiency on mortality [4]. And finally, anemia itself may contribute to worsening heart failure given that anemia is specifically associated with pump failure death [3,5].

## Pathophysiology

### Causes of anemia in CHF

There are numerous possible mechanisms that can lead to the development of anemia in patients with heart failure. Some potential causes include cytokine release, nutritional factors, renal impairment, medications, and/or sodium and water retention. In CHF, the etiology of anemia is likely to be multifactorial.

Heart failure has been found to be a proinflammatory state with increased cytokine levels in patients with increased disease severity. Circulating cytokines are associated with the development of anemia of chronic disease (ACD) [12], which is characterized by decreased red cell production resulting in a normochromic, normocytic anemia. Cytokines suppress a number of steps in red

blood cell production: production of erythropoietin, mobilization of iron stores for incorporation into hemoglobin, and erythropoiesis, as well as decrease red blood cell survival time in the peripheral circulation [13]. The hypoproliferative bone marrow is thought to result from the effect of cytokines [14]. In CHF patients, blood levels of tumor necrosis factor have been found to be elevated and to correlate with the severity of the anemia [15–17]. The anemia seen in CHF patients, similar to that seen in ACD demonstrates normal red cell morphology and iron stores [14]. Similar to other chronic disease states, erythropoietin levels in patients with CHF tend to be slightly elevated or in the high normal range [18]. It is therefore possible that heart failure may induce the anemia of chronic disease through cytokine-mediation [2,15,19].

Malnutrition may also contribute to the anemia seen in heart failure. Decreased caloric intake may result from anorexia, depression, gastric, intestinal or hepatic congestion, or poor mobility [20–23]. A consistent finding with poor nutritional intake is the association of markers of malnutrition such as lower body mass index and albumin with lower hemoglobin levels in CHF patients [5]. However, when the relationship between hemoglobin and the levels of hematinics, vitamin B12, folate, and iron was examined in 173 unselected patients attending a heart failure clinic only a small number of patients were found to have any hematinic deficiency. Moreover, no correlation was found between hematinic levels and hemoglobin levels in patients with anemia [24]. It seems likely that the role of malnutrition in anemic CHF patients is comparatively minor.

Anemia is associated with chronic renal insufficiency, some degree of which often accompanies CHF due to reduction in renal perfusion. The anemia of chronic kidney disease is thought to reflect decreased functioning renal cell mass resulting in decreased erythropoietin production. Additionally, the use of ACE inhibitors can also reduce the production of erythropoietin in the kidney [25]. While erythropoietin levels are increased above normal values in many anemic CHF patients the increased erythropoietin levels are less than expected for the given degree of anemia and may represent a state of relative hormone deficiency [26]. The prominent role of the kidney, and the complex interplay between heart failure, renal failure, and anemia has been described as the cardio-renal-anemia syndrome. As hypothesized by Silverberg and colleagues, heart failure, renal failure, and anemia produce a vicious cycle whereby each element contributes to worsening organ function [27].

A number of medications commonly used in the management of heart failure patients may contribute to anemia. Antiplatelet agents such as aspirin or clopidogrel as well as anticoagulants such as warfarin may indirectly contribute to anemia by causing iron deficiency secondary to chronic, subacute, blood loss. In contrast, ACE inhibitors may directly contribute to anemia by decreasing erythropoietin production [28]. However, though erythropoietin levels decrease during ACE inhibition, enalapril therapy was not associated with decreased hematocrit when compared to placebo in the SOLVD trial population [4,16]. Furthermore, the presence of anemia seems to be independent of ACE inhibitor use as well as dosing [2,4,5]. It is not known whether angiotensin receptor blockers have the same effect on erythropoietin production as ACE inhibitors.

Lastly and importantly, the high prevalence of anemia in patients with heart failure may be artefactual as the disease itself may cause a pseudoanemia via hemodilution. While a reduced hematocrit may result from reduced red blood cell volume, or true anemia, it also may result from increased plasma volume, or hemodilution, as seen in edematous, hypervolemic states. The prevalence of hemodilution in anemic CHF patients was found to be 46% in a recent study by Androne et al. using the $I^{131}$-tagged albumin technique to assess plasma volume [8]. Of note, congestion, as assessed by volume status on physical examination, was detected in only 50% of patients demonstrated to have plasma volume excess. Therefore, hemodilution may play a role in the anemia associated with CHF despite an absence of overt signs of volume overload. Importantly, those patients with hemodilution tended to have a worse survival compared to those who had true anemia. This is not an unexpected finding given the recent studies demonstrating increased mortality in patients with heart failure and elevated brain natriuretic peptides levels [29–34], which is secreted from the cardiac ventricles in response to volume expansion and pressure overload [35].

## Effects of anemia in CHF

Chronic anemia normally induces increased cardiac output, decreased systemic vascular resistance, widened atriovenous oxygen gradient, and increased plasma volume [36,37]. Such hemodynamic responses are blunted in CHF patients given that cardiac output reserve is limited in response to sympathetic stimulation, vasodilatory reserve is reduced, and oxygen extraction in exercising skeletal muscle is already maximized in nonanemic patients [13]. Yet increased cardiac workload secondary to chronic anemia may lead to ventricular remodeling and progressive heart failure.

Chronic anemia with a hemoglobin <10 g/dL is known to result in increased cardiac output that may lead to left ventricular hypertrophy (LVH) [37,38]. A prospective, multicenter, Canadian cohort study of 446 patients with renal insufficiency demonstrated that in patients with mild to moderately impaired renal function left ventricular growth assessed by baseline and 12-month follow-up echocardiograms occurred in association not only with relative anemia but with decrease in hemoglobin level over time [39]. At baseline, left ventricular mass index was increased in 34% of the cohort comprised of patients with a calculated creatinine clearance between 25 and 75 mL/min. The prevalence of LVH increased with declining renal function. Within each level of progressive renal dysfunction patients with LVH had significantly lower mean hemoglobin levels and significantly greater mean declines in hemoglobin over the course of the study. Each 0.5 g/dL decrease in hemoglobin was associated with an odds ratio of 1.32 for predicting left ventricular growth >20% of baseline or >20 g/m$^2$.

Anand and colleagues recently conducted a retrospective analysis of the RENAISSANCE trial data to examine the relationship between hemoglobin and left ventricular mass in a group of patients with moderate to severe CHF [1]. A subgroup of 69 of the 912 randomized heart failure patients underwent cardiac MRI at baseline and 24 weeks. The mean hemoglobin concentration and left ventricular mass index (LVMI) in the subgroup was 13.6 g/dL and 113 g/m$^2$ respectively. In those subjects whose hemoglobin remained the same or decreased the LVMI increased. In those subjects who showed an increase in hemoglobin concentration over the 24-week period LVMI decreased by 7.5 g/m$^2$ ($p = 0.0008$). The data suggest that a 1 g/dL increase in hemoglobin concentration is associated with a 4.1 g/m$^2$ decrease in LVMI over a 24-week period in patients with moderate to severe CHF and that even small decrease in hemoglobin may contribute to deleterious ventricular remodeling.

Anemia may also exacerbate the development of atherosclerosis by leading to arterial remodeling with arterial enlargement and subsequent intima-media thickening [40,41]. As such, anemia may aggravate existing ischemic heart disease. The ARIC study investigated whether the presence of anemia was a risk factor for cardiovascular disease (CVD) outcomes in the general population [42]. The cohort was comprised of over 14 000 subjects, ages 45–64, from four US communities, who were CVD free at baseline and followed for 6 years. While the anemic men tended to be older with a higher percentage of diabetes, hypertension, LVH, and cardiovascular medication use, and the anemic women had a higher percentage of LVH or hypertension compared with the nonanemic groups the presence of anemia was found to be independently associated with an increased risk of cardiovascular disease, having a hazard ratio of 1.41. Interestingly, the mean hemoglobin levels in the anemic group were not severely diminished, at 12.1 g/dL in men and 11.2 g/dL in women indicating that even mild anemia may have an impact on the development of cardiovascular disease.

Both animal and human studies have demonstrated that the ischemic or hypertrophied heart is more sensitive than the normal heart to decreases in hemoglobin and leads to worsened myocardial ischemia and cardiac function [43,44]. Blood transfusions in elderly patients with acute myocardial infarction were associated with a lower mortality when the initial hematocrit was less than 33% compared to those who were not transfused [45]. Patients with preexisting ischemic heart disease appear to be more susceptible to progressive ventricular remodeling and heart failure resulting from the decreased oxygen carrying capacity of anemic blood.

The cardiovascular demands of anemia generate increased cardiac work from the high output state that may further exacerbate cardiac and peripheral hypoxia leading to the activation of neurohormones and cytokines. Decreased renal perfusion is associated with activation of the renin–angiotensin–aldosterone axis with subsequent salt and water retention, hypervolemia, increased preload, and vasoconstriction, which further stress the cardiac system. Cytokine activation may suppress red cell production in the bone marrow further worsening the anemia. As previously noted, this cycle has been termed the cardio-renal-anemia syndrome [27]. The correction of anemia in patients with CHF may break this cycle [9,13].

## Physiology and pharmacology of erythropoietin

Erythropoietin is a hypoxia-induced glycoprotein hormone that is crucial in the regulation of red blood cell production and tissue oxygen delivery. The majority of the erythropoietin in the body is made in the kidney although there are alternate sources of production. The stimulus for production is impaired oxygen delivery to the kidney, whether by decreased oxygen carrying capacity of the blood or decreased blood flow to the renal parenchyma.

Peri-tubular areas in the renal cortex that appear to be sensitive to changes in oxygen tension drive a feedback loop. Local tissue hypoxia induces the peri-tubular fibroblasts to produce erythropoietin, the structure and signaling mechanisms of which is similar to the family of type I cytokines [26,46–48]. Downregulation of production proceeds from increased oxygen delivery to the kidney. In 1983, the human erythropoietin gene was first cloned. Subsequently, recombinant human erythropoietin was synthesized in 1985 and gained approval for clinical use in 1988 [49].

Erythropoietin is largely used for the treatment of anemia due to chronic kidney failure although it is also indicated for the treatment of anemia secondary to cancer chemotherapy and HIV treatment, and to reduce transfusion requirements in surgical patients. Healthy individuals have used erythropoietin illicitly to improve exercise performance. In end stage kidney disease treatment of anemia has been demonstrated to have a multitude of beneficial effects such as increased cognitive function, quality of life, and exercise tolerance as well as decreased rates of hospitalization and deleterious left ventricular remodeling [35,50–57].

## Administration of erythropoietin for the treatment of anemia

The recommended starting dose of erythropoietin in chronic renal failure is 50–100 U/kg three times a week either intravenously or subcutaneously. Erythropoietin is not recommended in cancer patients unless the baseline serum erythropoietin level is less than 200 mU/mL or in HIV patients unless the baseline serum erythropoietin level is less than 500 mU/mL [58]. It is commonly administered as an IV bolus to hemodialysis patients, although the subcutaneous route may be preferred in other patient populations without preexisting venous access. The onset of activity is approximately 7 to 10 days followed by subsequent increases in red cell parameters within 2–6 weeks [58–60].

According to the European Best Practice Guidelines [61], the goal is to increase hemoglobin at a rate of 1 to 2 g/dL/month to reach a target hemoglobin concentration of 11 g/dL within 4 months of starting treatment. During the correction phase, hemoglobin levels should be monitored every 2–4 weeks. If the change in hemoglobin exceeds 1 g/dL in any 2-week period, or the hemoglobin approaches 12 g/dL, the dose should be reduced by 25%. If the change in hemoglobin is less than 1 g/dL/month doses may be increased by 25%. Following any change in dose hemoglobin should be monitored twice weekly for up to 6 weeks until stable. The target hemoglobin should not exceed 12 g/dL [58].

The elevation of hemoglobin and reticulocyte count is directly proportional to the dose given and the duration of therapy. Initial studies in end stage kidney disease patients indicated that a dose of 150–200 U/kg/week of recombinant human erythropoietin was sufficient to raise hemoglobin levels to between 10 and 12 gm/dL in over 83–90% of patients [26,49,59,60,62]. The maximum dose of erythropoietin that can be given has not been determined, although a greater biologic response is not observed at doses exceeding 300 units/kg three times weekly [60].

Darbepoetin alfa is an analog of epoetin alfa that acts on progenitor stem cells to stimulate red blood cell production [63]. Its structural difference from epoetin alfa slows its clearance and increases its half-life threefold [64]. Studies have shown that dialysis patients treated with epoetin three times weekly could maintain hemoglobin concentrations when given darbepoetin once weekly and dialysis patients who were on epoetin once weekly could maintain hemoglobin concentrations when given darbepoetin every other week [65,66]. The recommended starting dose of darbepoetin is given weekly based on the previous weekly dose of epoetin [63].

Part and parcel of erythropoietin or darbepoetin therapy is hematinic administration with folate and iron supplements. Either absolute or functional iron deficiency can develop during erythropoietin administration. Therefore, adequate iron stores must be maintained as indicated by serum ferritin greater than 100 mcg/L and transferrin saturation greater than 20% [58]. In renal failure patients the National Kidney Foundation recommends that during the correction phase with erythropoietin therapy iron indices should be checked monthly in patients not receiving intravenous iron and at least every 3 months in patients receiving intravenous iron, until the target hemoglobin has been reached [67]. However, the optimal iron supplementation regimen is unclear.

The usual oral dose of iron replacement therapy is 2–3 mg/kg/day of elemental iron in three divided doses. Oral iron absorption is decreased by food, dairy products, and antacids and is frequently complicated by nausea, bloating, constipation, and GI irritation. Oral iron intolerance or insufficiency can be circumvented by the parenteral replenishment of iron stores. Three parenteral iron products, iron dextran, ferric gluconate, and iron sucrose, with varying administration guidelines, are approved for use in the United States. However, the use of iron dextran has been associated with fatal and nonfatal anaphylactic reactions. Data from adverse event reporting and post-marketing studies suggest that ferric gluconate and iron sucrose are safer alternatives compared to iron dextran [68]. Nonetheless, iron injection and IV iron can be safely administered only where resuscitation equipment is available. The reduced risk conferred by the new products must be balanced by their increased cost and greater required number of doses.

## Adverse effects

Concerns have been raised about the safety of the administration of erythropoietin itself. Hypertension occurs in about 25% of renal disease patients treated with erythropoietin [58]. Thrombotic events including myocardial infarction and clotting of arteriovenous fistulas and shunts have also occurred [66]. Indeed, some investigators have suggested that there may be a U-shape response to hemoglobin concentrations with higher morbidity and mortality in patients with both low and high levels. As a result the optimal target hemoglobin level in renal failure patients has yet to be defined given the conflicting data [61].

In 1998, Besarab studied 1233 subjects with congestive heart failure or ischemic heart disease who were undergoing hemodialysis and had hematocrit values of 27–33%. The patients were randomized to either a normal hematocrit group who would receive doses of epoetin to maintain a target hematocrit of 42% or a low hematocrit group who would receive epoetin to maintain a target hematocrit of 30%. After 29 months the study was halted secondary to a higher mortality rate in the normal hematocrit group. Raising the hematocrit to the normal range was associated with a relative risk of 1.3 for death or nonfatal myocardial infarction compared to raising the hematocrit to the lower range. There was no clear explanation to account for the unexpected findings. The authors hypothesized that adequacy of hemodialysis or IV iron therapy may have played a role in the adverse outcomes [50]. Although the data is limited most studies indicate a similar incidence of cardiovascular effects with darbepoetin alfa and epoetin alfa [69].

Whether thrombosis will be a significant adverse outcome of erythropoietin therapy in heart failure patients without renal failure is also unclear. In patients with cancer or HIV infection erythropoietin has generally been well-tolerated [70]. Moreover, many heart failure patients are on antiplatelet or anticoagulant medications as part of their CHF regimen.

## Effects of erythropoietin outside the bone marrow

Aside from its beneficial effect on red blood cell production, erythropoietin is a cytokine that has numerous anti-inflammatory, antiapoptotic, neurotrophic, cardiotrophic, and immuno-modulatory effects. Erythropoietin receptors are found on numerous tissues outside the bone marrow. The localization of the erythropoietin receptor elsewhere in the body may prove to broaden its therapeutic use far beyond the treatment of anemia.

The antiapoptotic and neurotrophic effects of erythropoietin were demonstrated by Brines et al. who administered systemic erythropoietin 24 h before or up to 3 h after the induction of focal brain ischemia [71]. Treatment with erythropoietin reduced brain injury by 50–75%. In the same report, erythropoietin was also noted to be neuroprotective from other insults including trauma, immune-mediated inflammation, and excessive neuronal excitation.

In the cardiovascular system the erythropoietin receptor is widely distributed on smooth muscle cells [72,73], endothelial cells [73–75], and cardiac myocytes [76]. The cardio-protective effects of erythropoietin against ischemic injury have been investigated in several animal models.

In a rabbit infarct model, pretreatment with erythropoietin demonstrated protection against ischemic injury in myoblasts and whole heart preparations [77]. A significant proportion of erythropoietin pretreated myoblasts exhibited increased survival compared with untreated cells. This benefit was reversed upon administration of an inhibitor to the cell survival pathway, Akt. In whole animals, pretreatment with erythropoietin at the time of myocardial infarction induced by coronary artery ligation, enhanced global cardiac function as assessed by LV $dP/dT_{max}$ and significantly reduced infarct size (14 versus 35% for erythropoietin versus saline treated rabbits respectively). Most notably, these effects occurred without a change in hemoglobin suggesting a direct protective effect of erythropoietin in the ischemic heart.

The cardioprotective effect of erythropoietin appears to be due to its ability to mitigate myocardial cell apoptosis. In erythroid cells and neuronal cells stimulation of the erythropoietin receptor has been shown to inhibit apoptosis via specific protein kinase cascades [78]. Erythropoietin-receptor stimulation in both cardiac fibroblasts and intact rabbit hearts activates the JAK2-STAT3 pathway. Ischemia reperfusion also triggers the JAK-STAT pathway but at twice the level associated with erythropoietin-receptor stimulation, suggesting that erythropoietin preconditioning involves known intracellular kinases that may protect the heart against injury and mimic pathways stimulated by ischemia reperfusion itself [78].

Based on the emerging evidence of erythropoietin's role in the response to injury Wright *et al.* characterized the expression of erythropoietin receptors in the heart during ischemia-reperfusion injury [79]. Experiments were done on isolated rat hearts to control for the possibility that cells other than myocytes mediated the cardiac protection apparently conferred by erythropoietin. For the first time, erythropoietin-receptor mRNA transcripts and protein expression were demonstrated in adult cardiac myocytes using reverse transcriptase PCR and immunohistochemical staining techniques. Hearts treated with erythropoietin exhibited significant improvement of contractile function recovery compared

to control hearts after ischemia reperfusion, as assessed by left ventricular developed pressure, an effect which was shown to be concentration dependent. In contrast, in the absence of injury, erythropoietin exerted no significant effect on hemodynamic parameters. ATP levels were significantly better preserved at the end of global ischemia, and recovered to significantly higher levels at 15 min of reperfusion, in erythropoietin-treated hearts compared to controls. These findings suggest that the response of erythropoietin to injury is rapid, and sufficient to confer cardio-protection in the isolated, ischemic heart, and possibly mediated through the preservation of ATP.

## Effect of erythropoietin on exercise performance

Exercise integrates the physiologic response of multiple organ systems, that is, heart, lungs, muscles, and vasculature to meet the increased workload. Peak oxygen consumption is the product of cardiac output and the arteriovenous oxygen difference; thus, the oxygen carrying capacity of the blood has direct effect on our ability to exercise.

The impact of anemia on exercise performance has been studied in normal patients before and after transfusion [80]. The change in maximal oxygen consumption ($VO_2$) is proportional to the change in hemoglobin as would be expected from the Fick equation. Reinfusion of autologous erythrocytes (blood doping) has also been shown to enhance exercise performance [81]. Submaximal and maximal exercise adaptations to prolonged low doses of erythropoietin were studied in 21 recreational athletes randomized to erythropoietin plus intravenous iron, erythropoietin plus oral iron, or placebo for 8 weeks. Erythropoietin was given three times weekly at a dose of 50 IU/kg body mass for the first 3 weeks and then 20 IU/kg body mass for the next 5 weeks. Exercise testing was conducted at weeks 0 and 12. $VO_{2\,max}$ was 6–8% higher at week 12 for both erythropoietin groups [82].

The impact of recombinant human erythropoietin on exercise capacity has also been assessed in hemodialysis patients. The exercise capacity of patients with end stage renal disease is low, with $VO_{2\,max}$ reported to average 19.1 mL/kg/min, and had been assumed to be secondary to anemia [83]. However, several studies demonstrated that large increases in hemoglobin achieved with recombinant human erythropoietin were accompanied by modest increases in peak $VO_2$ in contrast to the findings in normal individuals [84–88]. The fractional change in $VO_{2\,max}$ per change in hemoglobin has been shown to range from to 0.03–0.45 in hemodialysis patients compared to 0.5–0.9 in normal patients [80,84–92]. Such findings suggest that in anemic hemodialysis patients exercise capacity is limited by central factors such as a reduced cardiac output from systolic or diastolic dysfunction and/or peripheral changes in the muscle or vasculature.

The impact of erythropoietin therapy on exercise capacity in anemic patients with CHF was recently studied in 26 patients with class III–IV CHF [10]. These patients were on a stable medical regimen for 4 weeks with hematocrit <35%, serum creatinine <2.5 mg/dL, erythropoietin level <100 mU/mL. The patients were randomized 2:1 to receive either erythropoietin or placebo for 3 months. Submaximal and maximal exercise capacity improved with erythropoietin therapy. Peak $VO_2$ increased significantly from 11 to 12.7 mL/kg/min in the treatment group, as did $VO_2$ at the anaerobic threshold. A positive linear correlation was observed between the change in plasma hemoglobin and the change in peak $VO_2$. Additionally, quality of life as assessed by the Minnesota Living with Heart Failure Questionnaire improved compared to controls. No effect on muscle oxidative metabolism or forearm vasodilatation was observed with erythropoietin. Taken together, the findings suggest that the mechanism for increased exercise capacity appears to be increased oxygen delivery secondary to increased hemoglobin concentration. Similar to patients on hemodialysis the improvement in peak $VO_2$ was less than predicted based on changes in hemoglobin again suggesting that central or other peripheral factors limit exercise capacity in these patients.

## The use of erythropoietin in heart failure patients

Several small studies have investigated the role of erythropoietin in treating the anemia associated with CHF. In 2000, Silverberg and colleagues reported the results of 26 anemic patients with class III to IV CHF treated with erythropoietin and IV iron [7]. All patients received weekly IV iron and subcutaneous erythropoietin at a starting dose of 2000 IU to achieve and maintain a target hemoglobin level of 12 g/%. The patients were studied for a mean duration of 7 months. Treatment of the anemia was associated with improved functional status (NYHA class 3.7 to 2.7), higher ejection fraction (28 to 35%) reduced hospitalizations (2.7 to 0.2), and reduced need for both oral and IV furosemide. While the results of the study looked promising and suggested that the treatment of anemia may be an important addition to the treatment of CHF the study was limited by its small sample size and open-label, uncontrolled study design.

In 2001, Silverberg went on to report the results from a randomized-controlled study using subcutaneous erythropoietin and IV iron in 32 anemic patients with moderate to severe CHF [9]. The patients were randomized to receive IV iron and subcutaneous erythropoietin weekly or no treatment for anemia. The findings were consistent with the previous open-label, uncontrolled trial of anemia treatment in CHF patients. Correction of anemia resulted in improvement in cardiac function and NYHA functional class with a reduced need for hospitalization and oral and IV furosemide. Small sample size and lack of blinding were the major limitations. In 2003, Silverberg and colleagues investigated the use of subcutaneous erythropoietin and IV iron to correct anemia in a larger cohort of 179 diabetics and nondiabetics with severe CHF and chronic renal failure [27]. The findings of the study were again consistent with the prior two trials and provided further evidence of the beneficial effect of erythropoietin therapy in anemic CHF patients.

Given this pilot data, the role of darbepoetin alfa is now being investigated in the Study of Anemia in Heart Failure Trial (STAMINA-HeFT). This large multicenter, randomized, double-blind, placebo-controlled study of anemic CHF patients sponsored by Amgen has exercise tolerance as its primary endpoint. Enrollment is complete and the results of this trial should be available in the coming year.

## Conclusion

Preliminary studies suggest that anemia is common in patients with CHF and is associated with worse outcomes. Small-scale studies have begun to address whether correction of anemia in CHF patients, particularly with erythropoietin, is beneficial. The data suggest that in patients with moderate to severe heart failure correction of anemia with erythropoietin improves cardiac function, exercise capacity, NYHA functional class, hospitalization rate, and quality of life. While the data are encouraging many significant questions remain such as optimal timing of erythropoietin treatment, dosage, target hemoglobin level, impact on mortality, and cost-benefit analysis. The mechanism of action for the beneficial effect of this drug remains unclear and may involve not only the correction of anemia but direct protective and even reparative cardiac effects. This interesting drug clearly deserves further clinical investigation.

## References

1 Anand I, McMurray JJV, Whitmore J et al. Anemia and its relationship to clinical outcome in heart failure. Circulation 2004;110:149–154.

2 Ezekowitz JA, McAlister FA, Armstrong, PW. Anemia is common in heart failure and is associated with poor outcomes. Circulation 2003;107:223–225.

3 Mozaffarian D, Nye R, Levy WC. Anemia predicts mortality in heart failure. J Am Coll Cardiology 2003;41:1933–1939.

4 Al-Ahmad A, Rand WM, Manjunath G et al. Reduced kidney function and anemia as risk factors for mortality in patients with left ventricular dysfunction. J Am Coll Cardiology 2001;38:955–962.

5 Horwich TB, Fonarow GC, Hamilton MA, MacLellan WR, Borenstein J. Anemia is associated with worse symptoms, greater impairment in functional capacity and a significant increase in mortality in patients with advanced heart failure. J Am Coll Cardiology 2002;39:1780–1786.

6 Kosiborod M, Smith GL, Radford MJ, Foody JM, Krumholz HM. The prognostic importance of anemia in patients with heart failure. Am J Med 2003;114:112–119.

7 Silverberg DS, Wexler D, Blum M et al. The use of subcutaneous erythropoietin and intravenous iron for the treatment of the anemia of severe, resistant congestive heart failure improves cardiac and renal function and functional cardiac class, and markedly reduces hospitalizations. J Am Coll Cardiol 2000;35:1737–1744.

8 Androne AS, Katz SD, Lund L et al. Hemodilution is common in patients with advanced heart failure. Circulation 2003;107:226–229.

9 Silverberg DS, Wexler D, Sheps D et al. The effect of correction of mild anemia in severe, resistant congestive heart failure using subcutaneous erythropoietin and intravenous iron: a randomized controlled study. J Am Coll Cardiol 2001;37:1775–1880.

10 Mancini DM, Katz SD, Lang CC, LaManca J, Hudaihed A, Androne AS. Effect of erythropoietin on exercise capacity in patients with moderate to severe chronic heart failure. Circulation 2003;107:294–299.

11 World Health Organization. Iron deficiency anaemia assessment, prevention, and control. Geneva, Switzerland, 2001.

12 Means RT Jr. Advances in the anemia of chronic disease. Int J Hematol 1999;70:7–12.

13 Mancini DM, Kunavarapu C. Effect of erythropoietin on exercise capacity in anemic patients with advance heart failure. Kidney Int 2003;87:48–52.

14 Means RT Jr. Pathogenesis of the anemia of chronic disease: a cytokine-mediated anemia. Stem Cells 1995;13:32–37.

15 Levine B, Kalman J, Mayer L, Fillit HM, Packer, M. Elevated circulating levels of tumor necrosis factor in severe chronic heart failure. N Engl J Med 1990;323:236–241.

16 Herrera-Garza EH, Stetson SJ, Cubillos-Garzon A, Vooletich MT, Farmer JA, Torre-Amione G. Tumor necrosis factor. A mediator of disease progression in the failing human heart. Chest 1999;115:1170–1174.

17 Goicoechea M, Martin J, De Sequera P et al. Role of cytokines in the response to erythropoietin in hemodialysis patients. Kidney Int 1998;54:1337–1343.

18 Volpe M, Tritto C, Testa U. Blood levels of erythropoietin in congestive heart failure and correlation with clinical, hemodynamic, and hormonal profiles. Am J Cardiol 1994;74:468–473.

19 Iverson PO, Woldbaek PR, Tonnessen T, Christensen G. Decreased hematopoiesis in bone marrow of mice with congestive heart failure. Am J Physiol: Regul Integr Comp Physiol 2002;282:166–172.

20 Witte KKA, Clark AL. Nutritional abnormalities contributing to cachexia in chronic illness. Int J Cardiol 2002;85:23–31.

21 Pittman J, Cohen P. The pathogenesis of cardiac cachexia. New Engl J Med 1964;271:403–409.

22 Ansari A. Syndromes of cardiac cachexia and the cachetic heart: current perspective. Prog Cardiovasc Dis 1987;30:45–60.

23 Anker SD, Ponikowski P, Varney S et al. Wasting as an independent risk factor for mortality in chronic heart failure. Lancet 1997;349:1050–1053.

24 Witte KKA, Desilva R, Chattopadhyay S, Ghosh J, Cleland JGF, Clark AL. Are hematinic deficiencies the cause of anemia in chronic heart failure? Am Heart J 2004;147:924–930.

25 Macdougall IC. The role of ACE inhibitors and angiotensin II receptor blockers in the response to epoetin. *Nephrol Dial Transplant* 1999;**14**:1836–1841.

26 Katz SD, Mancini DM, Androne AS, Hryniewicz K. Treatment of anemia in patients with chronic heart failure. *J Card Fail* 2004;**10**:S13–S16.

27 Silverberg DS, Wexler D, Blum B *et al.* The effect of correction of anaemia in diabetics and non-diabetics with severe resistant congestive heart failure and chronic renal failure by subcutaneous erythropoietin and intravenous iron. *Nephrol Dial Transplant* 2003;**18**:141–146.

28 Beckingham I, Woodrow G, Hinwood M *et al.* A randomized placebo-controlled study of enalapril in the treatment of erythrocytosis after renal transplantation. *Nephrol Dial Transplant* 1995;**10**:2316–2320.

29 Tsumamoto T, Wada A, Maeda K *et al.* Attenuation of compensation of endogenous cardiac natriuretic peptide system in chronic heart failure. *Circulation* 1997;**96**:509–516.

30 Maeda K, Tsumamoto T, Wada A *et al.* High levels of brain natriuretic peptide and interleukin-6 after optimized treatment for heart failure are independent risk factors for morbidity and mortality in patients with congestive heart failure. *J Am Coll Cardiol* 2000;**36**:1587–1593.

31 Van Cheng BS, Kanazegra R, Garcia A *et al.* A rapid bedside test for b-type peptide predicts treatment outcomes in patients admitted with decompensated heart failure: a pilot study. *J Am Coll Cardiol* 2001;**37**:386–391.

32 Stanek B, Frey B, Hulsmann M *et al.* Prognostic evaluation of neurohumoral plasma levels before and during beta-blocker therapy in advanced left ventricular dysfunction. *J Am Coll Cardiol* 2001;**38**:436–432.

33 Harrison A, Morrison LK, Krishnaswamy P *et al.* B-type natriuretic peptide predicts future cardiac events in patients presenting to the emergency department with dyspnea. *Ann Emerg Med* 2002;**39**:131–138.

34 Berger B, Huelsman M, Strecker K *et al.* B-type natriuretic peptide predicts sudden death in patients with chronic heart failure. *Circulation* 2002;**105**:2392–2397.

35 Maisel A. B-type natriuretic peptide levels: diagnostic and prognostic in congestive heart failure. *Circulation* 2002;**105**:2328–2331.

36 Duke M, Abelmann WH. The hemodynamic response to chronic anemia. *Circulation* 1969;**39**:503–515.

37 Varat MA, Adolph RJ, Fowler NO. Cardiovascular effects of anemia. *Am Heart J* 1972;**83**:415–426.

38 Gerry JL, Baird MG, Fortuin NJ. Evaluation of left ventricular function in patients with sickle cell anemia. *Am J Med* 1976;**60**:968–972.

39 Levin A, Thompson CR, Ethier J *et al.* Left ventricular mass index increase in early renal disease: impact of decline in hemoglobin. *Am J Kidney Dis* 1999;**34**:125–134.

40 Metivier F, Marchais SJ, Guerin AP, Pannier B, London GM. Pathophysiology of anaemia: focus on the heart and blood vessels. *Nephrol Dial Transplant* 2000;**15**:14–18.

41 Gibbons GH, Dzau VJ. The emerging concept of vascular remodeling. *N Engl J Med* 1994;**330**:1431–1438.

42 Sarnak MJ, Tighiouart H, Manjunath G *et al.* Anemia as a risk factor for cardiovascular disease in the atherosclerosis risk in communities study. *J Am Coll Cardiol* 2002;**40**:27–33.

43 Carson, JL. Morbidity risk assessment in the surgically anemic patient. *Am J Surg* 1995;**170**:32S–36S.

44 Carson JL, Duff A, Poses RM. Effect of anaemia and cardiovascular disease on surgical mortality and morbidity. *Lancet* 1996;**348**:1055–1060.

45 Wu WC, Rathore SS, Wang Y, Radford MJ, Krumholz HM. Blood transfusion in elderly patients with acute myocardial infarction. *N Engl J Med* 2001;**345**:1230–1236.

46 Smith KJ, Bleyer AJ, Little WC, Sane DC. The cardiovascular effects of erythropoietin. *Cardiovasc Res* 2003;**59**:538–548.

47 van der Meer P, Voors AA, Lipsic E, van Gilst WH, van Veldhuisen DJ. Erythropoietin in cardiovascular diseases. *Eur Heart J* 2004;**25**:285–291.

48 Ozaki K, Leonard WJ. Cytokine and cytokine receptor pleiotropy and redundancy. *J Biol Chem* 2002;**277**:29355–29358.

49 Winearls CG. Recombinant human erythropoietin: 10 years of clinical experience. *Nephrol Dial Transplant* 1988;**13**:3–8.

50 Besarab A, Bolton WK, Browne JK *et al.* The effects of normal as compared with low hematocrit values in patients with cardiac disease who are receiving hemodialysis and epoetin. *N Engl J Med* 1998;**339**:584–590.

51 Foley RN, Parfrey PS, Harnett JD, Kent GM, Murray DC, Barre PE. The impact on cardiomyopathy, morbidity, and mortality in end stage renal disease. *Am J Kidney Dis* 1996;**28**:53–61.

52 Levin A, Singer J, Thompson CR, Ross H, Lewis M. Prevalent left ventricular hypertrophy in the pre-dialysis population: identifying opportunities for intervention. *Am J Kidney Dis* 1996;**27**:347–354.

53 Silverberg JS, Rahal DP, Patton DR, Sniderman AD. Role of anemia in the pathogenesis of left ventricular hypertrophy in end-stage renal disease. *Am J Cardiol* 1989;**64**:222–224.

54 Canella G, La Canna G, Sandrini M. Reversal of left ventricular hypertrophy following recombinant human erythropoietin treatment of anaemic dialysed uraemic patients. *Nephrol Dial Transplant* 1991;**6**:31–37.

55 Collins A, Ma JZ, Ebben J. Impact of hematocrit on morbidity and mortality. *Semin Nephrol* 2000;**20**:345–349.

56 Pickett JL, Theberge DC, Brown WS, Schweitzer SU, Nissenson AR. Normalizing hematocrit in dialysis patients improves brain function. *Am J Kidney Dis* 1999;**33**:1122–1130.

57 Valderrabano F, Jofre R, Lopez-Gomez JM. Quality of disease in end-stage renal disease patients. *Am J Kidney Dis* 2001;**38**:443–464.

58 Product Information: Epogen, epoetin alfa. Amgen, Thousand Oaks, CA, 2004.

59 Eschbach JW, Egrie JC, Downing MR, Brown JK, Adamson JW. Correction of the anemia of end-stage renal disease with recombinant human erythropoietin. Results of a combined phase I and phase II clinical trial. *N Engl J Med* 1987;**316**:73–78.

60 Eschbach JW, Abdulhadi MH, Browne JK *et al.* Recombinant human erythropoietin in anemic patients with end-stage renal disease. Results of a phase III multicenter clinical trial. *Ann Int Med* 1989;**111**:992–1000.

61 Revised European best practice guidelines for the management of anaemia in patients with chronic renal failure. *Nephrol Dial Transplant* 2004;**19**:1–47.

62 Erslev, AJ. Erythropoietin. *N Engl J Med* 1991;**324**: 1339–1344.

63 Product Information: Aranesp, darbepoetin alfa. Amgen, Thousand Oaks, CA, 2003.

64 Macdougall IC, Gray SJ, Elston O *et al.* Pharmacokinetics of novel erythropoiesis stimulating protein compared with epoetin alfa in dialysis patients. *J Am Soc Nephrol* 1999;**10**:2392–2395.

65 Vanrenterghem Y, Barany P, Mann JFE *et al.* Randomized trial of darbepoetin alfa for treatment of renal anemia at a reduced dose frequency compared with rHuEPO in dialysis patients. *Kidney Int* 2002;**62**:2167–2175.

66 Nissenson AR, Swan SK, Lindberg JS *et al.* Randomized, controlled trial of darbepoetin alfa for the treatment of anemia in hemodialysis patients. *Am J Kidney Dis* 2002;**40**:1334–1335.

67 National Kidney Foundation. K/DOQI Clinical practice guidelines for anemia of chronic disease. *Am J Kidney Dis* 2000;**37**:S182–S238.

68 Silverstein SB, Rodgers GM. Parenteral iron therapy options. *Am J Hematol* 2004;**76**:74–78.

69 Macdougall IC. An overview of the efficacy and safety of novel erythropoiesis stimulating protein (NESP). *Nephrol Dial Transplant* 2001;**16**:14–21.

70 Erythropoietin (procrit; epogen) revisited. *Med Lett* 2001;**43**:40–41.

71 Brines ML, Ghezzi P, Keenan S *et al.* Erythropoietin crosses the blood-brain barrier to protect against experimental brain injury. *Proc Natl Acad Sci USA* 2000;**97**:10526–10531.

72 Ammarguellat F, Llovera M, Kelly PA, Goffin V. Low doses of EPO activate MAP kinases but not JAK2-STAT5 in rat vascular smooth muscle cells. *Biochem Biophys Res Comm* 2001;**284**:1031–1038.

73 Anagnostou A, Liu Z, Steiner M *et al.* Erythropoietin receptor mRNA expression in human endothelial cells. *Proc Natl Acad Sci USA* 1994;**91**:3974–3978.

74 Nagai T, Akizawa T, Kohjiro S *et al.* rHuEpo enhances the production of plasminogen activator inhibitor-1 in cultured endothelial cells. *Kidney Int* 1996;**50**: 102–107.

75 Anagnostou A, Lee ES, Kessimian N, Levinson R. Erythropoietin has a mitogenic and positive chemotactic effect on endothelial cells. *Proc Natl Acad Sci USA* 1990;**87**:5978–5982.

76 Wu H, Lee SH, Gao J, Liu X, Iruela-Arispe ML. Inactivation of erythropoietin leads to defects in cardiac morphogenesis. *Development* 1999;**126**:3597–3605.

77 Parsa CJ, Matsumoto A, Kim J *et al.* A novel protective effect of erythropoietin in the infarcted heart. *J Clin Invest* 2003;**112**:999–1007.

78 Parsa CJ, Kim J, Riel R *et al.* Cardioprotective effects of erythropoietin in the reperfused ischemic heart. *J Biol Chem* 2004;**279**:20655–20662.

79 Wright GL, Hanlon P, Amin K, Steenbergen C, Murphy E, Arcasoy MO. Erythropoietin receptor expression in adult rat cardiomyocytes associated with an acute cardioprotective effect for recombinant erythropoietin during ischemia-reperfusion injury. *Faseb J* 2004;**18**: 1031–1033.

80 Ekblom B, Goldbarg AN, Gullbring B. Response to exercise after blood loss and reinfusion. *J Appl Physiol* 1972;**33**:175–180.

81 Brien AJ, Simon TL. The effects of red cell infusion on 10 km race time. *JAMA* 1987;**257**:2761–2765.

82 Russell G, Gore CJ, Ashenden MJ, Parisotto R, Hahn AG. Effects of prolonged low doses of recombinant human erythropoietin during submaximal and maximal exercise. *Eur J App Physiol* 2002;**86**:442–449.

83 Painter P, Messer-Rehak D, Hanson P, Zimmerman SW, Glass NR. Exercise capacity in hemodialysis, CAPD, and renal transplant patients. *Nephron* 1986;**42**:47–51.

84 Painter P, Moore GE. The impact of recombinant human erythropoietin on exercise capacity in hemodialysis patients. *Adv Ren Replace Ther* 1994;**1**:55–65.

85 Mayer G, Thum J, Cada EM. Working capacity is increased following recombinant human erythropoietin treatment. *Kidney Int* 1988;**34**:525–528.

86 Lundin AP, Akerman MJ, Chesler RM *et al.* Exercise in hemodialysis patients after treatment with recombinant human erythropoietin. *Nephron* 1991;**58**:315–319.

87 Metra M, Cannella G, La Canna G *et al.* Improvement in exercise capacity after correction of anemia in patients with end-stage renal failure. *Am J Cardiol* 1991;**68**: 1060–1066.

88 Macdougall IC, Lewis NP, Saunders MJ *et al.* Long-term cardiorespiratory effects of amelioration of renal anaemia by erythropoietin. *Lancet* 1990;**335**:489–493.

89 Woodson RD, Wills RE, Lenfant C. Effect of acute and established anemia on oxygen transport at rest, sub-maximal and maximal work. *J Appl Physiol* 1978;**44**: 36–43.

90 Celsing F, Svedenhag J, Pihlstedt P, Ekblom B. Effects of anaemia and stepwise-induced polycythaemia on maximal aerobic power in individuals with high and low haemoglobin concentrations. *Acta Physiol Scand* 1987;**129**:47–54.

91 Buick FJ, Gledhill N, Froese AB, Spriet L, Meyers EC. Effect of induced erythrocythemia on aerobic work capacity. *J Appl Physiol* 1978;**48**: 636–642.

92 Robertson RJ, Gilcher R, Metz KF *et al.* Effect of induced erythrocythemia on hypoxia tolerance during physical exercise. *J Appl Physiol* 1982;**53**:490–495.

# CHAPTER 15

# Endothelin antagonism in cardiovascular disease

*Srinivas Murali,* MD

## Introduction

Endothelin (ET) is a family of three 21 amino acid peptides, ET-1, ET-2, and ET-3 produced by the endothelial cells that was first identified in 1988 [1]. It is homologous to the snake venom sarafotoxin that is produced by a viper snake called the Israeli burrowing asp. ET-1 is the main isoform produced in the cardiovascular system, ET-2 is mainly produced in the kidney and small intestine, and ET-3 predominantly in the central nervous system [2]. ET-1 is physiologically the most significant and the most potent endogenous vasoconstrictor peptide in the human body. It induces a more potent and long-lasting vasoconstriction compared to angiotensin II. In addition, it stimulates the sympathetic nervous system and cell proliferation [3]. Because of these important biologic actions regulation of ET-1 is thought to play a critical role in the pathophysiology of several cardiovascular diseases, including systemic and pulmonary hypertension and heart failure. Disruption of the biologic effects of ET-1 has emerged as an intriguing therapeutic target in these conditions. The roles of ET-2 and ET-3 in human physiology are however unclear.

## Biology of the ET system

### Synthesis and release

Endothelin-1 is synthesized and released not only by the endothelial cell but also by other cell types such as leukocytes, macrophages, cardiomyocytes, vascular and airway smooth muscle cells, and mesangial cells (Figure 15.1). Physico-chemical factors such as hypoxemia, pulsatile stretch, low shear stress, pH, and osmolarity promote endothelin synthesis and release [4,5]. Other factors including pro-inflammatory cytokines (interleukin-1 and -2, tumor necrosis factor-$\alpha$), transforming growth factor $\beta$, endotoxin, oxidized low density lipoprotein particles, thrombin, circulating hormones such as epinephrine, angiotensin II, vasopressin, bradykinin, insulin, and cortisol also promote the endothelin message [6–8]. Nitric oxide, prostacyclin, estrogens, and atrial natriuretic peptides inhibit ET synthesis. The message for ET synthesis from the nucleus results in the release of an inactive precursor prepro-ET into the cytoplasm [2]. This precursor is then cleaved by a furin-like enzyme into an inactive intermediate called big ET. There are three subtypes of big ET (big ET-1, big ET-2, big ET-3) all of which are further cleaved by the ET-converting enzyme (ECE) to active ET (ET-1, ET-2, ET-3). There are four sub iso-forms of ECE but the physiologic relevance of the different forms is not well understood. ECE independent pathways of ET-1 synthesis that involves tissue chymases have also been described.

## ET receptors

Following release, ET-1 mediates its effects through interaction with two classes of cell surface receptors both of which are G protein coupled transmembrane proteins with different molecular and physiologic functions [9]. ET-1 binding to these receptors activates the phosphatidyl inositol phospholipase C pathway, which in turn signals several key cell-specific events. The ET type A (ET-A) receptors are located mainly on the vascular smooth muscle cells and mediate vasoconstriction and cell proliferation. They are also present on the cardiac

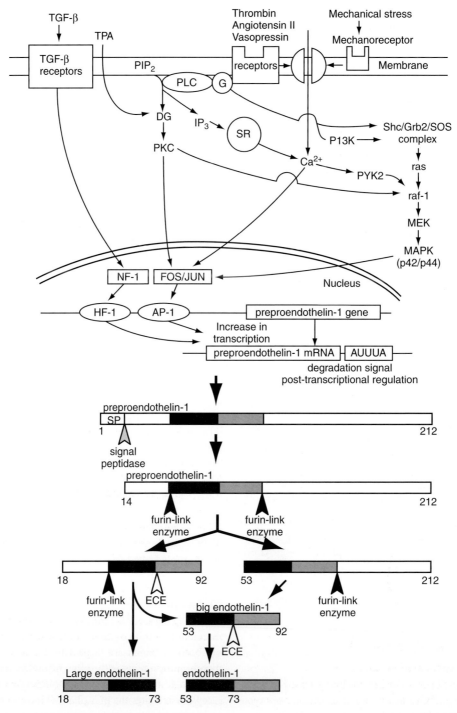

**Figure 15.1** Synthesis of ET-1. (Adapted from [11].)

myocyte, cardiac fibroblast, lung, kidney, and the brain. The ET type B (ET-B) receptors are present predominantly on endothelial cells but are also located on the vascular smooth muscle cells, and other organs such as the heart, kidney, brain, intestine, and melanocytes. Activation of these receptors on endothelial cells mediates nitric oxide-dependent vasodilation and prostacyclin release as well as ET-1 clearance particularly in the pulmonary and renal vascular beds, while those on the smooth muscle cells mediates vasoconstriction. The net biologic effect of ET-1 depends on the density of ET-A receptors on the vascular smooth muscle cell and the ET-B receptors on the endothelial cell. ET-B receptors are also important for sodium and water absorption in the distal renal tubules. ET-2 also binds to the ET-A receptors on the vascular smooth muscle cell and ET-3 binds exclusively to the ET-B receptors located both on the endothelial cell and the smooth muscle cell. In health, ET-A receptors constitute up to 80% of the total ET receptor density [10].

## Biologic actions of ET-1

Under physiologic conditions, ET-1 causes vasoconstriction, cell proliferation, and differentiation determined by a complex interplay between its effects on ET-A and ET-B receptors. The biologic actions of ET-1 that are relevant to cardiovascular physiology are listed in Table 15.1. ET-1 is important for maintenance of basal tone in many vascular beds [11]. Systemic infusion of ET-1 produces a slow onset, dose-dependent vasoconstriction that is sustained for about 2 h. This effect is abolished with an ET-A receptor antagonist indicating that this is predominantly ET-A receptor mediated. Other effects of ET-1 include a reduction in heart rate, decrease in coronary blood flow, and coronary sinus oxygen saturation suggesting its potential role in regulating coronary vascular tone. Cardiac contractility is increased by ET-1 in normal subjects, but this effect is not seen in patient with dilated cardiomyopathy. In fact, in animal models of heart failure ET-1 has been shown to depress left ventricular contractility and slow relaxation.

In pathological states, the ET receptors are regulated differently, which results in different acute and chronic biologic effects. The acute effects involve vasoconstriction and inflammation by increasing vascular permeability, induction of cytokine release, stimulating lipo-oxygenase activity, and increasing production of monocyte chemoattractant protein-1 and several adhesion molecules. The chronic effects include fibroblast proliferation, synthesis of extracellular matrix components (fibronectin, collagen, and laminin), hypertrophy of cardiac myocytes, neurohormonal secretion, and cell proliferation. ET-1 interacts with other neurohormonal pathways both in health and in disease. It increases plasma renin activity, enhances conversion of angiotensin I to angiotensin II, and augments the synthesis and release of aldosterone from the adrenal glands [12,13].

There is a wealth of experimental evidence indicating a critical role for ET-1 in pulmonary vascular biology [14–17]. In isolated perfused rat lungs, ET-1 causes a concentration-dependent pulmonary vasoconstriction. This effect is reversed by dual

**Table 15.1** Biologic effects of ET-1 relevant to cardiovascular physiology.

Vasoconstriction: Most potent known vasoconstrictor
  Systemic
  Pulmonary
  Renal
  Coronary

Neurohormonal activation
  Increases plasma levels of aldosterone, norepinephrine, and angiotensin II
  Synergistic with effects of angiotensin II, norepinephrine
  Induces release of pro-inflammatory cytokines

Cardiac Remodeling
  Myocyte hypertrophy
  Fibroblast proliferation
  Extracellular matrix deposition
  Adhesion molecule expression

Vascular Remodeling
  Vascular smooth muscle cell hyperplasia
  Fibroblast proliferation
  Extracellular matrix deposition
  Adhesion molecule expression
  Glomerular mesangial proliferation

Pro-arrhythmic
  Implicated in reperfusion ventricular arrhythmias
  Causes atrial arrhythmias

ET-A and ET-B inhibition. Incubation of normal human dermal fibroblasts with ET-1 for 48 h results in a significant induction of type I collagen synthesis and a significant decrease in interstitial collagenase (MMP-1) expression. ET-1 stimulates fibroblast proliferation and fibroblast production of collagen type III in a concentration-dependent manner. Since both ET-A and ET-B receptor subtypes are expressed on fibroblasts dual blockade of these receptors abolishes these effects. In a rat model of hypoxic pulmonary vasoconstriction the increase in pulmonary arterial wall thickness is both prevented and reversed by exposure to dual ET-1 antagonism. Further, in the experimental overcirculation pig model, pretreatment with dual ET-1 antagonists prevents both pulmonary vascular remodeling and right ventricular dysfunction. Transgenic mice overexpressing the human ET-1 gene develop significant pulmonary fibrosis when compared to age matched littermates. This fibrosis is predominantly seen in the peri-vascular and peri-bronchial space around the medium and large sized pulmonary arteries. Bleomycin-induced pulmonary fibrosis in rats is associated with elevated ET-1 levels and attenuated by dual ET-1 receptor antagonism. ET-1 promotes collagen deposition in cardiac and renal tissue as well, and these biologic effects are also attenuated by dual ET-1 antagonism.

## ET-1 in pathologic states

Both ET-1 and ECE expression are increased in the endothelial cells and cardiac myocytes in experimental models of acute myocarditis and dilated cardiomyopathy. In patients with chronic heart failure, plasma ET-1 levels are increased and correlate directly with functional impairment and inversely with left ventricular ejection fraction. There is activation of the cardiac ET system with increased tissue ET-1 concentrations in the failing myocardium. The cellular effects of ET-1 promote progressive cardiac and vascular remodeling, while the effects on central and autonomic nervous system, baroreceptor function, and renal sodium excretion are associated with the clinical manifestations of heart failure. There is a direct correlation between plasma ET-1 levels and left ventricular filling pressures and an indirect correlation with survival and need for transplantation

in chronic heart failure patients. Unlike other neurohormones, however, plasma ET-1 also correlates with the severity of pulmonary hypertension in chronic heart failure patients [18–22].

Endothelin-1 expression in the pulmonary vasculature is increased in patients with pulmonary arterial hypertension and plays a critical role in the progressive pulmonary vascular remodeling that occurs in this disorder. Plasma ET-1 levels are elevated not only in patients with idiopathic pulmonary hypertension, but also in pulmonary hypertension associated with connective tissue diseases and congenital heart disease [16,23].

The ET-receptor expression distribution in experimental models and chronic heart failure patients is changed, with a proportionately greater increase in the ET-A receptor population. The high plasma levels of ET-1 in chronic heart failure and pulmonary hypertension may not only be from increased synthesis but also from reduced clearance. The lung is an important site for both synthesis and clearance of ET-1. In patients with pulmonary arterial hypertension and heart failure due to myocardial infarction the clearance of ET-1 in the lung is reduced [24–26].

## Antagonism of the ET system

Antagonism of the ET system can be achieved either by ECE inhibition or by blocking ET-A and ET-B receptors. Most ECE inhibitors also inhibit neutral endopeptidase (NEP), and so they not only inhibit ET-1 production but also prevent the metabolism of vasodilating mediators such as atrial natriuretic peptide and bradykinin. The net effect is profound vasodilation with reduction in systemic blood pressure. The effectiveness of ECE inhibitors may be limited by non-ECE mediated conversion of big ET-1 to ET-1 (ECE escape). So far not much progress has been made with the clinical development of ECE inhibitors [27,28]. ET-receptor antagonists either selectively block ET-A or ET-B receptor or both. Most ET-receptor antagonists in clinical development are nonpeptides and thus not subject to hydrolyzation by peptidases in the gastrointestinal tract. The affinity of these drugs to the ET-A and ET-B receptors is different. There are 'mixed' or 'dual' or nonselective ET-receptor antagonists that block both ET-A and ET-B receptors and selective ET-A receptor antagonists that predominantly block ET-A receptors.

Bosentan is the prototype nonselective ET receptor antagonist (20-fold ET-A selective over ET-B). In a rat model of heart failure, bosentan causes vasodilation and reduces mean arterial blood pressure. This effect is synergistic to that seen with angiotensin-converting enzyme inhibition. It reduces significantly cardiac hypertrophy induced by norepinephrine and cardiac fibrosis induced by angiotensin II or aldosterone. Bosentan treatment also improves survival. It also reverses endothelial dysfunction in other animal models. In hamsters fed with cholesterol rich diet treatment with bosentan decreases early atherosclerosis and restores nitric oxide mediated vasodilation. Atherosclerosis that spontaneously develops in apolipoprotein E deficient mice is inhibited by bosentan exposure. In other experimental hypercholesterolemia models, bosentan has been shown to preserve coronary endothelial function [29–32].

In pilot studies in heart failure patients, besides causing vasodilation and restoring the integrity of endothelial function, bosentan induces favorable hemodynamic effects. Bosentan administration causes reduction of systolic, diastolic and mean pulmonary artery pressures, right atrial and pulmonary capillary wedge pressures, and both pulmonary and systemic vascular resistances. These salutary hemodynamic effects are associated with an increase in both cardiac index and stroke volume index and no change or a decrease in heart rate. These hemodynamic changes are seen within hours of drug administration and persist through a 2-week treatment period [21].

Tezosentan is also a nonselective ET-1 antagonist (65-fold ET-A selective over ET-B), where as ambrisentan (100-fold ET-A selective), darusentan (250-fold ET-A selective), and sitaxsentan (6500-fold ET-A selective) are ET-A selective agents. Selective ET-A antagonism has very similar effects to nonselective ET-1 antagonism in animal models [33–35]. Hemodynamic effects are similar, as are the effects on left ventricular measures of remodeling, cardiac fibrosis, and survival. In *in vitro* preparations of rat adrenal cortical tissue the addition of an ET-A selective antagonist does not affect the production of aldosterone but the application of an ET-B antagonist decreases aldosterone

production, similar to that seen with nonselective ET-1 antagonism. Thus the endothelin-induced production of aldosterone appears to be mediated by ET-B receptors. The acute effects of selective ET-A and selective ET-B antagonism in chronic heart failure patients have been compared [36,37]. Infusion of BQ-123, an intravenous ET-A antagonist, decreases mean arterial pressure, cardiac filling pressures, and systemic vascular resistance while increasing cardiac index. Intravenous BQ-788 infusion, a selective ET-B antagonist, on the other hand raises mean arterial pressure, cardiac filling pressures, and systemic vascular resistance while lowering cardiac index. The addition of BQ-123 to BQ-788 infusion or dual ET-A and ET-B receptor antagonism reverses the vasoconstriction seen with BQ-788 infusion by causing systemic and pulmonary vasodilation. Infusion of BQ-123 does not change plasma ET-1 concentrations, whereas BQ-788 infusion raises plasma ET-1 levels. Combination of BQ-123 and BQ-788 has no effect on plasma ET-1 levels. Selective ET-B antagonism therefore raises plasma ET-1 levels and causes adverse hemodynamic effects; thus confirming that ET-B receptors mediate clearance of ET-1 in man and their blockade may not have therapeutic benefit. Both selective ET-A antagonism and nonselective ET-1 antagonism, on the other hand, have potential for therapeutic benefit in both heart failure and pulmonary hypertension patients [36,37].

## ET-1 receptor antagonism in heart failure

### Acute decompensated heart failure

Tezosentan, which is a nonselective ET-1 receptor antagonist, is ideally suited for intravenous use in acute heart failure because of high water solubility, rapid onset of action, and a short half-life of 10 min [37]. Acute short-term hemodynamic effects of tezosentan was evaluated in two separate prospective, double-blind, randomized, placebo-controlled phase II studies [38–41]. In the first study, 38 patients with acute decompensated heart failure received progressively increasing doses of tezosentan (from 20 to 100 mg/h) for a maximum of 6 h. In the second study, 61 patients with acute decompensated heart failure were randomly assigned to placebo or one of four different doses of tezosentan (5, 20, 50, 100 mg/h) for 6 h. In both of these studies, tezosentan significantly increased cardiac index, while decreasing pulmonary pressures, pulmonary capillary wedge pressure, and systemic vascular resistance. There was no effect on heart rate and no hypotension or arrhythmia was noted. In another study, tezosentan was both safe and tolerable over a 48-h infusion period. These favorable data led to the phase IIIRandomized Intravenous TeZosentan (RITZ) clinical trial program. The RITZ-1 trial randomized 675 patients with acute decompensated heart failure and failed to show an improvement from baseline in the primary endpoint of dyspnea after a 6-h infusion of Tezosentan at a dose of 50 mg/h [42]. The RITZ-2 trial, on the other hand, showed a significant improvement from baseline in cardiac index at 6 and 24 h (primary endpoint) following tezosentan infusions (50 mg and 100 mg/h) in 285 randomized patients with acute decompensated heart failure [43]. In addition, the pulmonary capillary wedge pressures decreased and dyspnea scores improved. The effect on cardiac index was sustained for 6 h after discontinuation of tezosentan therapy. These contrasting results in these two trials highlighted the discordance between clinical and hemodynamic improvement that is sometimes seen in patients with acute decompensated heart failure. In the RITZ-4 trial the effect of tezosentan was evaluated in 192 patients admitted with acute decompensated heart failure associated with an acute coronary syndrome. No significant differences were observed in the primary endpoint (which was a composite of death, worsening heart failure, recurrent ischemia, and recurrent or new myocardial infarction within 72 h) between placebo and tezosentan 50 mg/h. In the RITZ-5 trial, 84 patients with acute pulmonary edema were randomized to tezosentan (50 or 100 mg/h) or placebo for up to 24 h. The primary endpoint, the change in oxygen saturation from baseline to 1 h, was $9.1 \pm 6.3\%$ in the placebo arm versus $7.6 \pm 10\%$ in the tezosentan group ($p =$ NS). The incidence of death, recurrent pulmonary edema, mechanical ventilation, and myocardial infarction during the first 24 h of treatment was 19% in both groups [43].

The VERITAS program (Value of Endothelin Receptor Inhibition with Tezosentan in Acute heart failure Studies) consisted of two, double-blind, randomized, placebo-controlled, concurrently conducted trials performed in 150 centers in Europe, Israel, Australia, and North America [44]. The aim of the study was to evaluate the effect of tezosentan on dyspnea over 24 h and the incidence of death or worsening heart failure at 7 and 30 days in patients presenting with acute decompensated heart failure. The study was stopped by the Data Safety and Monitoring Board after 1435 patients had been enrolled, based on an interim analysis that indicated that the chance of meeting the efficacy endpoints was too remote. Though dyspnea improved rapidly and similarly over 24 h in both the tezosentan and placebo groups there was no difference in the incidence of death or worsening heart failure or adverse events between the treatment groups at either 7 or 30 days. Based on these findings, it was concluded that tezosentan was safe but showed no significant clinical benefit in the treatment of acute decompensated heart failure. The effects of selective ET-A receptor antagonism has not been evaluated in a prospective, randomized, multicenter clinical trial in patients with acute decompensated heart failure [45].

## Chronic heart failure

The long-term effects of the nonselective ET-receptor antagonist, Bosentan, was investigated in a multicenter pilot study called the Research on Endothelin Antagonism in Chronic Heart Failure (REACH-1) trial in which 370 patients with New York Heart Association class III or IV symptoms and left ventricular ejection fraction <35% were randomized [46]. The primary endpoint in this trial was the change in clinical status after 26 weeks of therapy. Clinical status took into consideration death, hospitalization for worsening heart failure, and change in New York Heart Association class. Patients were randomized (1:2) to placebo or bosentan 500 mg twice daily optimal dosing was achieved either by slow titration over 3 weeks or by rapid titration over 2 weeks. There was no significant difference in the distribution of changes in clinical status between the two groups. However, in a subgroup analysis of randomized patients who were followed for at least 26 weeks patients treated with bosentan were significantly

($p$ = 0.045) more likely to improve (26% on bosentan versus 19% on placebo) and less likely to worsen (28% on bosentan versus 43% on placebo) their clinical status. There was also a biphasic response to treatment with bosentan. Compared to placebo, bosentan-treated patients had an increased risk of worsening heart failure during the first month of treatment, though this risk was higher in the placebo group during the latter half of the trial. There were no differences between the groups in the combined secondary endpoint of all-cause mortality and worsening heart failure. The increased early risk of worsening heart failure with bosentan is an interesting phenomenon and not due to reduction in cardiac contractility or sodium retention. It may be related to the vasodilating action of bosentan on pulmonary arterioles, which in turn acutely removes the 'protective' restraint that pulmonary vasoconstriction exerts on blood flow into the pulmonary capillaries and consequent transudation of fluid into the alveoli in patients with high pulmonary venous pressures. A similar effect has been previously observed with other drugs that exert potent pulmonary arteriolar dilation in patients with increased pulmonary venous pressures. The major adverse effect of bosentan was a significant increase in hepatic transaminases to more than three times the upper limit of normal (in 15.6% of patients) and a decrease in serum hemoglobin concentrations of $\geq 1$ g/dL. There was no evidence for bone marrow suppression, hemolysis, or bleeding with bosentan. Possibly this effect on hemoglobin is related to an increase in blood volume or a decrease in erythropoietin production. The elevations in hepatic transaminases were not accompanied by increases in serum bilirubin and resolved after discontinuation of bosentan therapy. Bosentan is predominantly metabolized in the liver by cytochrome P450 (CYP) oxidases, CYP3A4 and CYP2C9, and excreted into the bile using the bile acid export pump. Bosentan increases activity of these enzymes that may impair efficacy of other drugs such as hormonal contraceptives and oral anticoagulants. Competition with transport of bile acids in turn results in local inflammation from intrahepatic accumulation of bile acids; thus raising the liver aminotransferases. This explains the dose dependence of this effect and the observed increased frequency when bosentan is

administered concomitantly with other drugs such as glyburide and cyclosporine that either inhibit the bile acid export pump or also use this transport system [47,48].

The time-dependent favorable effects of bosentan treatment in chronic heart failure noted in the REACH-1 pilot trial were evaluated in an international, long-term morbidity and mortality, multicenter, placebo-controlled trial. The Endothelin Antagonist Bosentan for Lowering cardiac Events in chronic heart failure (ENABLE) trial randomized 1613 patients with New York Heart Association class III or IV chronic heart failure associated with a left ventricular ejection fraction of <30% to bosentan (initial dose 62.5 mg bid for 4 weeks with uptitration to 125 mg bid thereafter) or placebo in addition to background therapy with diuretics, ACE inhibitors, and β-blockers [49]. The primary endpoint was a composite of death and hospitalization for worsening heart failure. During a mean follow-up of 18 months there was no significant difference observed between bosentan and placebo either in the primary endpoint or all-cause mortality. There was no improvement in clinical status at 9 months in the bosentan group. Patients randomized to bosentan had early weight gain accompanied by peripheral edema and a fall in serum hemoglobin levels. The incidence of elevated hepatic aminotransferases was 9.5% in the bosentan group compared to 2.7% in the placebo group ($p$ < 0.05). These results were disappointing and questioned the merits of nonselective or dual endothelin receptor blockade in chronic heart failure [49].

The short-term hemodynamic effects of selective ET-A antagonism was evaluated in the Heart Failure ET-A Receptor Blockade Trial (HEAT). In this trial, 157 patients with New York Heart Association class III chronic heart failure were randomly assigned in a double blind fashion to placebo or darusentan (30, 100, or 300 mg/day). Acutely over a period of 6 h darusentan increased cardiac index in a dose-dependent manner, though this did not reach statistical significance. However, cardiac index increased and systemic vascular resistance decreased significantly after 3 weeks of darusentan treatment. There was no effect noted in the cardiac filling pressures, systemic blood pressure, or heart rate. Higher dosages were associated

**Table 15.2** Placebo-controlled clinical trials with ET-1 antagonists in acute and chronic heart failure.

| Trial | Condition | Drug studied | N | Effect on primary endpoint |
|-------|-----------|--------------|---|----------------------------|
| RITZ-1 | Acute heart failure | Tezosentan 50 mg/h infusion | 675 | No change in dyspnea after 6 h |
| RITZ-2 | Acute heart failure | Tezosentan 50 and 100 mg/h | 285 | Significant increase in cardiac index at 6 and 24 h |
| RITZ-4 | Acute coronary syndrome | Tezosentan 50 mg/h | 192 | No change in composite of death, worsening heart failure, recurrent ischemia, or infarction |
| RITZ-5 | Acute pulmonary edema | Tezosentan 50 and 100 mg/h | 50 | No change in $O_2$ saturation at 60 min |
| VERITAS | Acute heart failure | Tezosentan 5 mg/h for 30 min and 1 mg/h for 24–72 h | 1435 | No change in incidence of death or worsening heart failure at 7 and 30 days |
| REACH-1 | Chronic heart failure | Bosentan 500 mg bid for 26 weeks | 370 | No change in clinical status |
| ENABLE | Chronic heart failure | Bosentan 125 mg bid for 18 months | 1613 | No change in all-cause mortality |
| HEAT | Chronic heart failure | Darusentan 30, 100, or 300 mg/day for 3 weeks | 157 | Significant increase in cardiac index and decrease in systemic vascular resistance |
| EARTH | Chronic heart failure | Darusentan 10, 25, 50, 100, or 300 mg/day | 642 | No change in left ventricular end-systolic volume by MRI |

with a higher frequency of adverse events including death and worsening heart failure [50]. These findings led to further investigation of the long-term effects of darusentan on left ventricular remodeling and clinical outcomes in the Endothelin-A Receptor antagonist Trial in Heart failure (EARTH). In this study, 642 patients with chronic heart failure on background therapy with angiotensin converting enzyme inhibitor, β-blocker, and aldosterone antagonist were randomized in a double blind fashion to darusentan at 10, 25, 50, 100, or 300 mg daily or placebo for 24 weeks. The primary endpoint was the change in left ventricular end-systolic volume as measured by magnetic resonance imaging. There was no significant observed change in left ventricular end-systolic volume between the different doses of darusentan and placebo. The frequency of worsening heart failure and death was similar in the darusentan and placebo groups. No differences were observed in 6-min walking distance, global assessment, Minnesota living with Heart failure Questionnaire, concentrations of A-type and B-type natriuretic peptides, norepinephrine, epinephrine, and

aldosterone between the darusentan and placebo groups [51].

All the placebo controlled clinical trials with ET-1 antagonists in acute and chronic heart failure are summarized in Table 15.2. Based on evidence available at this time neither selective ET-A nor nonselective ET-1 antagonism is likely to have an important role in the management of patients with acute decompensated heart failure or chronic heart failure receiving standard therapy [52–54].

**Pulmonary arterial hypertension**

The role of ET-1 in the pathobiology of pulmonary arterial hypertension is well-documented. ET-1 expression in the pulmonary blood vessels is increased in patients with idiopathic pulmonary arterial hypertension, and pulmonary hypertension associated with connective tissue disease and congenital heart disease. Further, the vasodilating, antiproliferative, antifibrotic, and anti-inflammatory effects of ET-1 antagonism in experimental studies validates the rationale for this therapeutic strategy [55–58].

A pilot, randomized, placebo-controlled trial of the dual, nonselective ET-1 antagonist bosentan in 32 ambulatory patients with idiopathic or pulmonary arterial hypertension associated with systemic sclerosis and WHO class III symptoms demonstrated a significant improvement in 6-min walk distance over a 12-week period. Bosentan-treated patients increased the walk distance by $70.3 \pm 12.3$ m compared to a small decrease of $-5.8 \pm 36.3$ m in the placebo group ($p = 0.02$). The mean pulmonary artery pressure and pulmonary vascular resistance decreased and the cardiac index increased significantly in the bosentan group compared to placebo-treated patients. Among bosentan-treated patients 43% improved to WHO class II while this occurred in only 9.1% of the placebo group. More placebo-treated patients had clinical worsening during 28 weeks of follow-up. In 29 patients who received open-label bosentan upto a year improvement in hemodynamics and WHO class persisted. Bosentan was well-tolerated by the patients in this study [59].

These encouraging preliminary results led to a subsequent double-blind, placebo-controlled, multicenter Bosentan Randomized trial of Endothelin receptor Antagonist THERapy for pulmonary hypertension (BREATHE-1) (Figure 15.2). In this study, 213 patients with idiopathic or pulmonary hypertension associated with systemic sclerosis or systemic lupus erythematosus and WHO class III or IV symptoms were randomly assigned $1:1:1$ to placebo or bosentan 125 or 250 mg twice daily for 16 weeks. Bosentan therapy significantly improved the primary endpoint, which was 6-min walk distance at 16 weeks (net placebo corrected benefit 44 m, $p = 0.0002$). There were no differences in the effects of the two doses of bosentan. A treatment effect was seen in the bosentan group as early as 4 weeks into the trial. The improvement was persistent over 28 weeks of therapy. Time from randomization to clinical worsening, which was the main secondary endpoint, was defined as the shortest time to either death, lung transplantation, hospitalization due to worsening pulmonary hypertension symptoms, lack of clinical improvement, or worsening leading to discontinuation, initiation of epoprostenol therapy, or atrial septostomy. During the 16 weeks of the study the risk of clinical worsening was significantly less in the bosentan-treated patients ($p = 0.0038$). This trend continued during 28 weeks of therapy. Additional observations included a significant decrease in the Borg dyspnea score (the patients' perception of dyspnea immediately at the end of the 6-min walk test) in the bosentan group, and improvement in WHO functional class. Overall, 42% of the bosentan-treated patients and 30% of the placebo-treated patients were in a better functional class at week 16 than at baseline, resulting in a mean treatment effect of 12% in favor of bosentan (95% confidence interval, $-3–25\%$). In a subgroup echocardiogram analysis, bosentan-treated patients had a smaller increase from baseline in diastolic right ventricular remodeling index (ratio of minor and major axis in diastole), greater increase in right ventricular ejection time, and a greater reduction in right ventricular Tei index compared to the placebo group.

Bosentan was generally well-tolerated, but increase in hepatic aminotransferases were seen in 4% of patients receiving 125 mg bid and 14% of patients receiving 250 mg bid. When the safety data from both studies in pulmonary arterial hypertension with bosentan were combined 12.7% of patients experienced elevations in hepatic aminotransferases to greater than three times the upper limit of normal. These elevations were seen during the first 16 weeks of treatment in over 90% of the patients. They were dose dependent and usually reversible with dose reduction, though discontinuation of bosentan therapy was necessary in 1.8% of patients [60,61].

In the aforementioned trials, 169 patients who received bosentan were followed for a mean period of $2.1 \pm 0.5$ years (range 0.1–3.3). There were 20 (12%) deaths, 3 pulmonary transplantations and 1 patient was lost to follow-up. The observed survival was 96% at 1 year, 89% at 2 years, and 86% at 3 years. This was better than the predicted survival as determined by the National Institutes of Health Registry formula, which was 69% at 1 year, 57% at 2 years, and 44% at 3 years. However, it must be noted that 39 (23%) of patients required addition of or transition to a parenteral prostanoid drug during follow-up. In another retrospective analysis of WHO class III pulmonary arterial hypertension patients only first-line therapy with bosentan had a 1 and 2-year survival (97% and 91% respectively)

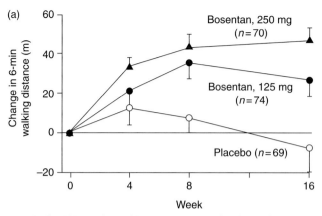

(a)

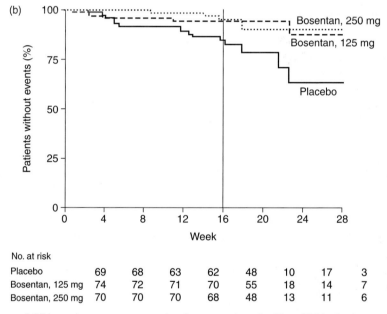

(b)

$p < 0.01$ for 125-mg dose of bosentan versus placebo and $p < 0.001$ for 250-mg bosentan dose versus placebo by the Mann–Whitney U test. There was no significant difference between the two bosentan groups ($p = 0.18$ by the Mann–Whitney U test).

No. at risk

| | | | | | | | | |
|---|---|---|---|---|---|---|---|---|
| Placebo | | 69 | 68 | 63 | 62 | 48 | 10 | 17 | 3 |
| Bosentan, 125 mg | 74 | 72 | 71 | 70 | 55 | 18 | 14 | 7 |
| Bosentan, 250 mg | 70 | 70 | 70 | 68 | 48 | 13 | 11 | 6 |

$p < 0.05$ bosentan groups versus placebo group at weeks 16 and 28 by the log-rank test. There was no significant difference between the two bosentan groups at weeks 16 and 18 ($p = 0.87$)

**Figure 15.2** Continued.

comparable to that observed with first line epoprostenol therapy (91% and 84% respectively). Based upon these positive findings bosentan was approved by the FDA for the treatment of pulmonary arterial hypertension and WHO class III and IV symptoms. Bosentan is prescribed at a starting dose of 62.5 mg bid, with uptitration to 125 mg bid in 4 weeks. It is recommended that hepatic aminotransferases be checked at baseline and monthly on bosentan therapy. If the enzymes increase to greater than three times upper limit of normal the dose should be reduced and if the enzymes increase to greater than eight times the upper limit of normal therapy must be discontinued. Uncontrolled data indicate that bosentan may also be effective in pulmonary arterial hypertension associated with congenital

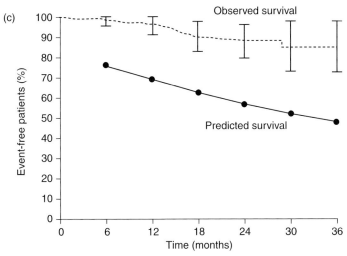

Kaplan–Meier estimates with 99.9% confidence intervals and predicted survival using the D'Alonzo equation. There was significant difference between the two curves at each 6-month interval.

**Figure 15.2** Bosentan therapy for pulmonary arterial hypertension. (a) Mean (±SE) change in 6-min walk distance from baseline to week 16. (b) Kaplan–Meier estimates of the proportion of patients with clinical worsening. (c) Observed survival on bosentan therapy versus predicted survival in IPAH patients only.

right to left intracardiac shunts and human immunodeficiency virus infection [62–64].

The selective ET-A antagonist, sitaxsentan has been evaluated in pulmonary arterial hypertension in the Sitaxsentan To Relieve ImpaireD Exercise (STRIDE) clinical trials program. The STRIDE-1 trial was a multicenter, double-blind, placebo-controlled study where 178 patients with idiopathic pulmonary arterial hypertension and pulmonary hypertension associated with connective tissue disease or congenital right to left intracardiac shunts and WHO class II, III, or IV symptoms were randomized 1:1:1 to either placebo, 100 mg, or 300 mg once daily of sitaxsentan for 12 weeks. Only the 300 mg dose of sitaxsentan significantly improved the primary endpoint of % predicted peak exercise oxygen consumption (+3%; $p < 0.01$). Both sitaxsentan dosages significantly improved 6-min walk distance at 12 weeks compared to placebo (100 mg: +35 m; 300 mg: +33 m). The mean pulmonary artery pressure and pulmonary vascular resistance decreased and cardiac index increased significantly with both doses of sitaxsentan. Functional class also improved in both sitaxsentan groups. Liver aminotransferase elevations to greater than three times upper limit of normal was not observed in the 100 mg sitaxsentan group, but was present in 10% of patients in the 300 mg group. Unlike bosentan, sitaxsentan inhibits cytochrome P450 (CYP) oxidases CYP2C9, CYP3A4, and CYP2C19; thus inhibiting the metabolism of warfarin. Significant increases in international normalized ratio (INR) was observed in 14% of patients in the 100 mg sitaxsentan group and 24% receiving 300 mg. Based on these results it was decided to further evaluate 100 mg and lower doses of sitaxsentan to determine the ideal dose for chronic therapy [65]. The recently completed STRIDE-2 trial compared the safety and efficacy of 50 and 100 mg of sitaxsentan once daily to placebo once daily and bosentan 125 mg twice daily in pulmonary arterial hypertension. This phase III trial enrolled 246 patients with idiopathic pulmonary arterial hypertension, pulmonary hypertension associated with connective tissue disease, or congenital right to left intracardiac shunts and WHO class II–IV symptoms for 18 weeks. Sitaxsentan 100 mg daily increased the primary endpoint of 6-min walk distance by 31.4 m over placebo ($p = 0.03$), while bosentan increased by 29.5 m ($p = 0.05$). Sitaxsentan 50 mg daily increased 6-min walk distance by 24.2 m over placebo, which was not statistically significant. Sitaxsentan 100 mg daily improved WHO functional class, but both bosentan and sitaxsentan 50 mg daily did not. Interestingly, there were five (6.5%) clinical worsening events in the sitaxsentan 100 mg daily group, seven (8.1%) in the sitaxsentan 50 mg group, 13 (14.6%) in the placebo group and 15 (16.3%) in the bosentan group. Elevated hepatic aminotransferases were seen in 3% of patients receiving sitaxsentan 100 mg daily, 5% receiving sitaxsentan 50 mg daily, 6% receiving placebo, and 11% receiving bosentan.

The STRIDE-4 trial compared the effects of sitaxsentan 50 mg daily and 100 mg daily for 12 weeks to placebo in 98 patients enrolled in Latin America, Poland, and Spain. The primary endpoint of 6-min walk distance improved by 22 m in the sitaxsentan 50 mg daily group and 58 m in the 100 mg daily group ($p = 0.014$). Interestingly, the primary endpoint also improved in the placebo group by 34 m ($p = 0.2$ versus 100 mg daily dose). The improvement noted in the placebo group was unexpected and contrary to that observed in all other placebo-controlled trials in pulmonary arterial hypertension. It was speculated that the improvement in the placebo group reflected the benefit of participation in a clinical trial for the enrolled patients. The other efficacy parameters like improvement in WHO class and Borg dyspnea score trended towards significance in the 100 mg dose group. The safety profile of sitaxsentan was favorable. The STRIDE-6 trial evaluated the effects of sitaxsentan 50 mg daily or 100 mg daily for 12 weeks in 48 patients with pulmonary arterial hypertension who discontinued bosentan either for safety reasons or lack of clinical benefit. The mean duration of bosentan treatment prior to discontinuation was 13.4 months (0.1–39). In the 35 patients who discontinued bosentan for lack of clinical benefit, improvement defined as ≥15% increase in 6-min walk distance occurred in 10% of patients receiving sitaxsentan 50 mg daily and 33% of patients receiving 100 mg daily. Among 13 patients who discontinued bosentan for safety reasons, only one patient needed to discontinue sitaxsentan because of an increase in hepatic aminotransferase. Collectively, these trials demonstrate that sitaxsentan at a dose of 100 mg daily is safe and effective in patients with pulmonary arterial hypertension. Sitaxsentan is not yet approved by the FDA [61,66].

Ambrisentan is also a selective ET-A receptor antagonist that is under evaluation for treatment of pulmonary arterial hypertension. It has 80% bioavailability and no relevant interactions with the cytochrome P450 (CYP) oxidases. In a phase II randomized, placebo-controlled trial of ambrisentan for 12 weeks in 64 patients with idiopathic and pulmonary hypertension associated with connective tissue disease, HIV infection, or anorexigen use and WHO class II or III symptoms, 6-min walk distance improved by 36.1 m ($p < 0.0001$), with similar significant improvements (range 33.9–38.1 m) for each dose group (1, 2.5, 5, or 10 mg daily). WHO class and Borg dyspnea score also improved with ambrisentan therapy. A significant decrease in mean pulmonary artery pressure and an increase in cardiac index was seen after 12 weeks of treatment. Both WHO class II and III patients and both idiopathic and associated pulmonary hypertension patients showed similar improvements with ambrisentan therapy. Ambrisentan was well-tolerated and hepatic aminotransferase elevation to greater than three times the upper limit of normal was noted in 3.1% of patients. The 1-year follow-up data showed that there was a progressive improvement with ambrisentan. At week 24 the increase in 6-min walk distance was 54.2 m and at week 48 it was 54.5 m. Functional class and Borg dyspnea score also showed progressive and sustained improvement with ambrisentan therapy. One year survival was 92% for patients with idiopathic pulmonary arterial hypertension and 95% for associated pulmonary hypertension. The adverse event profile was unchanged during long-term follow-up. Phase III trials with ambrisentan are currently in progress (ARIES trials). The ARIES trials are randomized, double-blind, placebo-controlled trials of identical design except for the doses of ambrisentan and the geographic locations of the investigative sites. The studies anticipate enrolling 186 patients (62 patients per dose group) in each trial. ARIES-1 will evaluate 5 and 10 mg once daily doses and ARIES-2 will evaluate 2.5 and 5 mg once daily doses of ambrisentan for 12 weeks. The primary efficacy endpoint is exercise capacity, measured as the change from baseline in the 6-min walk test distance compared to placebo. Secondary endpoints include Borg dyspnea score, WHO functional class,

**Table 15.3** Placebo-controlled clinical trials with ET-1 antagonists in pulmonary arterial hypertension.

| Trial | Condition | Drug studied | N | Effect on primary endpoint |
|-------|-----------|--------------|---|----------------------------|
| Bosentan pilot | IPAH, PAH associated with CTD | Bosentan 125 mg bid for 12 weeks | 32 | Significant increase in 6-min walk distance |
| BREATHE-1 | IPAH, PAH associated with CTD | Bosentan 125 or 250 mg bid for 16 weeks | 213 | Significant increase in 6-min walk distance |
| STRIDE-1 | IPAH, PAH associated with CTD or CHD | Sitaxsentan 100 or 300 mg daily for 12 weeks | 178 | Significant increase in % predicted peak exercise VO2 (300 mg dose only) and 6-min walk distance |
| STRIDE-2 | IPAH, PAH associated with CTD or CHD | Sitaxsentan 50 or 100 mg daily or bosentan 125 mg bid for 18 weeks | 246 | Significant increase in 6-min walk distance with 100 mg daily of sitaxsentan and bosentan |
| Ambrisentan pilot | IPAH, PAH associated with CTD or HIV or anorexinogen use | Ambrisentan 1, 2.5, 5, or 10 mg daily for 12 weeks | 64 | Significant increase in 6-min walk distance |

IPAH = idiopathic pulmonary arterial hypertension; CTD = connective tissue disease; CHD = congenital right to left intracardiac shunt; HIV = human immuno-deficiency virus.

quality of life assessment, and time to clinical worsening [67].

All the placebo controlled clinical trials with ET-1 antagonists in pulmonary arterial hypertension are summarized in Table 15.3. Based on available evidence it does not appear that selective ET-A receptor antagonism with sitaxsentan or ambrisentan has greater clinical benefit than nonselective ET-1 antagonism with bosentan in pulmonary arterial hypertension [61,68].

## Systemic arterial hypertension

There is a wealth of experimental evidence that suggests that ET-1 plays a possible role in systemic arterial hypertension. ET system is activated and the circulating levels of ET-1 are elevated in salt-dependent animal models of hypertension, such as deoxycorticosterone acetate (DOCA) salt treated rats and Dahl salt sensitive rats. Consistent with these findings, ET-receptor antagonists have been shown to lower blood pressure in these models. In transgenic rats that develop systemic hypertension due to endogenous activation of the renin–angiotensin system administration of the nonselective ET-1 antagonist, bosentan, decreases end-organ damage and increases survival. Vascular ET-1 activity is increased in hypertensive patients as well as evidenced by greater vasodilation of the forearm vasculature following infusion of ET-1

blockers in these patients compared to normotensive subjects [69–71]. The effect of ET-1 antagonism on blood pressure control was evaluated in a randomized, clinical trial where 293 patients with mild-moderate systemic hypertension were randomized to placebo, one of four oral doses of bosentan (100, 500, 1000 mg once daily or 1000 mg twice daily), or the angiotensin converting enzyme inhibitor, enalapril (20 mg daily) for 4 weeks. As compared to placebo, two doses of bosentan (500 mg daily and 1000 mg twice daily) significantly reduced diastolic blood pressure, similar to that seen with enalapril. There were no significant changes in heart rate with bosentan therapy. Bosentan treatment did not increase plasma norepinephrine, renin activity, or angiotensin II levels; thus demonstrating that it does not cause reflexive neuro-hormonal stimulation. Bosentan therapy increased plasma ET-1 levels in a dose-dependent fashion, possibly from ET-B receptor antagonism. The drug was well-tolerated during the 4-week treatment period [72]. The selective ET-A receptor antagonist, darusentan, was evaluated in a multicenter, randomized clinical trial of 392 patients with moderate systemic hypertension. Patients were randomized to either 10 or 30 or 100 mg of darusentan daily or placebo for 6 weeks. Darusentan therapy decreased both systolic and diastolic blood pressure compared to placebo in a dose-dependent manner without affecting heart rate. The 10 and 30 mg dosage groups had a similar adverse event profile to the placebo group, but there was a higher incidence of adverse events in the 100 mg dosage group [73].

Endothelin-1 may have a role in the pathogenesis of cyclosporine (CyA) or tacrolimus-induced hypertension in solid organ transplant recipients. Plasma ET-1 levels are increased in transplant recipients taking chronic CyA therapy and these patients have a blunted response to ET-A receptor blockade. Certain other groups of systemic hypertensives may also have ET-1 dependent hypertension, notably African Americans, salt-sensitive hypertensives, patients with low renin hypertension, and those with obesity and insulin resistance. ET-1 levels are elevated four–eightfold higher in African American hypertensives, compared to Caucasians. In response to stress, ET-1 levels are increased more in African Americans compared to Caucasians. The ET-B receptor density is lower in the peripheral vasculature of African Americans and these patients have a higher ET-A dependent vasoconstrictor tone, than Caucasians. Since, ET-1 induces sustained vasoconstriction and modulates sympathetic nervous system mediated contractility it appears that ET-1 may significantly contribute to the abnormal vascular reactivity in African American hypertensives. Therefore, though ET-1 antagonists are unlikely to become first-line therapy for systemic hypertension they may have a role in the future treatment of select hypertensive populations such as African Americans. Longitudinal multicenter, clinical trials with both selective and nonselective ET-1 antagonists are warranted in large numbers of select hypertensive populations such as African Americans to provide an accurate risk/benefit assessment [74,75].

## Atherosclerosis

Atherosclerosis accounts for the majority of cardiovascular morbidity and mortality in industrialized countries and its incidence is increasing in developing countries. It is characterized by endothelial cell dysfunction and inflammation that leads to progressive vascular remodeling. Endothelium-dependent relaxation is reduced in part due to decreased bioavailability of nitric oxide and increased release of oxygen-derived free radicals. There is increased production of vasoconstrictors and growth factors, adhesion of leukocytes, thrombosis, inflammation, cell proliferation, along with an increase in vascular tone. ET-1 is important for the maintenance of basal vascular tone. Since endothelial dysfunction occurs early on in atherosclerosis and ET-1 expression is increased in endothelial dysfunction it is apparent that the ET system plays a role in the progression of atherosclerosis. Plasma ET-1 levels are increased in children and adolescents with risk factors such as hypertension, hypercholesterolemia, and diabetes mellitus. Serum cholesterol, serum triglyceride levels, and body mass index have a direct correlation with plasma ET-1 levels. Within the atherosclerotic plaque, ET-1 expression and ET-A and ET-B-receptor density are increased not only on the endothelial cell but also on the vascular smooth muscle cell and foamy macrophages. ET-1 levels are also increased in patients with coronary artery disease and both ECE and ET-1 immune-reactivity are increased in active coronary lesions compared to nonactive lesions. Plasma nitric oxide to ET-1 ratio is a useful biological marker for predicting coronary artery disease. After myocardial infarction plasma ET-1 levels increase and inversely correlate with survival. In animal models, ET-A receptor antagonism prolongs survival after myocardial infarction. In patients with diabetes mellitus the vascular ET-1 activity is enhanced in resistance vessels, suggesting that ET-1 based vasoconstriction is important in the pathophysiology of vascular complications of diabetes. In animal models of hypercholesterolemia and atherosclerosis ET-1 antagonism increases nitric oxide synthase activity, nitric oxide-mediated vasodilation, and inhibits progression of atherosclerosis. Its well-established that pharmacological inhibition of the renin–angiotensin system and statin therapy have therapeutic benefit both for patients with overt atherosclerosis and for those at risk. Whether ET receptor antagonism will have a similar therapeutic role in atherosclerosis is not known at this time [76–80].

## Chronic renal failure

Endothelin-1 is involved in the pathophysiology of both acute and chronic renal failure. In patients with minimal change nephropathy ET-1 expression in blood vessels, tubules, and glomeruli are increased when acute renal failure occurs. In a randomized, placebo-controlled, double-blind, four-way crossover trial, selective ET-A antagonism alone and in combination with ET-B antagonism decreased blood pressure in patients with chronic renal failure. However, only ET-A antagonism reduced renal vascular resistance, increased renal blood flow, and reduced effective filtration fraction. Neither ET-A antagonism nor the combination of ET-A and ET-B antagonism had any effect on normal control subjects. ET-B antagonism alone produced renal and systemic vasoconstriction in both patients with renal failure and healthy controls. These findings suggest a role for selective ET-A antagonism in the treatment of hypertensive patients with chronic renal failure. ET-1 is thought to have a role in the development of contrast-induced nephropathy in patients with renal insufficiency. Whether ET-1 antagonism can protect against contrast-induced renal dysfunction is not known. In patients with chronic renal failure, ET-1 may be responsible for parathyroid cell proliferation and thus influence the development of secondary hyperparathyroidism. In a rat model of renal failure treatment with bosentan prevented proliferation of parathyroid cells. Finally, the combination of selective ET-A receptor antagonism and angiotensin-converting enzyme inhibition has synergistic effects on natriuresis, reduction of blood pressure, and renal vascular resistance, which makes it a potentially attractive therapeutic combination in chronic renal failure patients. Prospective, randomized clinical trials are needed to systematically evaluate the long-term benefits of selective ET-A and nonselective ET-1 receptor antagonist therapy in both acute and chronic renal failure. Renal ET-1 is known to be activated in heart failure patients. Urinary excretion of ET-1 is increased proportional to plasma ET-1 levels, which is inversely related to New York Heart Association Class. Urine sodium excretion is also inversely related to urinary ET-1 levels in heart failure patients. This suggests that during the clinical course of heart failure there is increased renal expression of ET-1 with an early increase in urine ET-1 that accompanies sodium retention. Renal ET-1 antagonism may be important for promoting urinary sodium excretion in heart failure patients [81–85].

## Summary

The ET system is an important regulator of vascular tone in humans. The main isoform ET-1 is produced predominantly by the endothelial cells and acts as an important local endocrine, autocrine, and paracrine factor with biological activities such as vasoconstriction, mitogenesis, fibrosis, inflammation, and inotropic effects on the heart. The biologic effects of ET-1 are through interaction with two cell surface receptors: ET-A that is mainly located on the vascular smooth muscle cell and mediates vasoconstriction, cell proliferation, fibrosis, and inflammation and ET-B that is predominantly on the endothelial cell and mediates vasodilatation (via nitric oxide and prostacyclin release) and ET-1 clearance. The net biologic activity of ET-1 in health and disease is therefore determined by the density of the ET-A and ET-B receptors, which is altered particularly in pathological states. ET-1 plays an important role in the genesis and pathophysiology of a number of disease states including heart failure, systemic hypertension, atherosclerosis, pulmonary arterial hypertension, renal failure, and coronary artery disease. Antagonism of the ET system therefore in theory is a potential therapeutic target in all these conditions. The limited number of clinical trials with both selective ET-A and nonselective ET antagonists have, however, so far yielded inconsistent results.

The clinical effectiveness of ET antagonism is well-established in patients with pulmonary arterial hypertension. The nonselective ET antagonist, bosentan, not only improves symptoms, hemodynamics, exercise tolerance, and quality of life but also prevents clinical worsening and disease progression. Preliminary results with selective ET-A receptor antagonists, sitaxsentan and ambrisentan, are also very encouraging. In acute decompensated heart failure treatment with nonselective ET antagonist tezosentan is safe, but without consistent clinical benefit. Another nonselective ET antagonist, bosentan, does not improve outcomes in patients with chronic heart failure. Selective ET-A antagonism with darusentan improves hemodynamics in acute decompensated heart failure, but does not attenuate ventricular remodeling in chronic heart failure. This observed discordance between theory and clinical trial findings may be related to dosage of drugs evaluated, choice of endpoints assessed, and our incomplete understanding of the complex interactions between the ET system and other biological systems in heart failure patients. In systemic hypertension clinical data suggests that ET-1 antagonists may have benefit in select populations, such as African Americans, salt-sensitive low renin hypertensives, obese hypertensives with insulin resistance, hypertensives with renal failure, and hypertensive solid organ transplant recipients. Large clinical trials have not yet been done to establish these observations. The benefit of ET antagonists in the development and progression of atherosclerosis and coronary artery disease is unknown at this time. Likewise the role of ET antagonists in attenuating progression of renal failure in patients with renal disease requires further study. Though much experimental and clinical data have been accumulated over the last 15 years defining the role of ET system in several disorders additional studies are needed so that the full therapeutic potential of ET antagonists in clinical medicine can be exploited.

## References

1 Yanagisawa M, Kurihara H, Kimura S et al. A novel potent vasoconstrictor peptide produced by vascular endothelial cells. Nature 1988;**332**:411–415.

2 Inuoe A, Yanagisawa M, Kimura S et al. The human endothelin family: three structurally distinct isopeptides predicted by three separate genes. Proc Natl Acad Sci USA 1989;**86**:2863–2867.

3 Levin ER. Endothelins. N Engl J Med 1995;**333**:356–363.

4 Inoue A, Yanagisawa M, Takuwa Y et al. The human preproendothelin-1 gene: complete nucleotide sequence and regulation of expression. J Biol Chem 1989;**264**:14954–14959.

5 Yoshizumi M, Kurihara H, Sugiyama T et al. Hemodynamic shear stress stimulates endothelin production by cultured endothelial cells. Biochem Biophys Res Commun 1989;**161**:859–864.

6 MaCarthur H, Warner TD, Wood EG et al. Endothelin-1 release from endothelial cells in culture is elevated both acutely and chronically by short periods of mechanical stretch. Biochem Biophys Res Commun 1994;**200**:395–400.

7 Boulanger CM, Tanner FC, Bea ML et al. Oxidized low density lipoproteins induce mRNA expression and release of endothelin from human and porcine endothelium. Circ Res 1992;**70**:1191–1197.

8 Kourembanas S, Marsden PA, McQuillan LP et al. Hypoxia induces endothelin gene expression and secretion in cultured human endothelium. J Clin Invest 1991;**88**:1054–1057.

9 Haynes WG, Webb DJ. The endothelin family of peptides: local hormones with diverse role in health and disease? Clin Sci 1993;**84**:485–500.

10 Nakao K, Arai H, Hosoda K et al. Molecular cloning of two subtypes of human endothelin receptor. J Vascular Med Bio 1991;**3**:303–307.

11 Miyauchi T, Masaki T. Pathophysiology of endothelin in the cardiovascular system. Annu Rev Physiol 1999;**61**:391–415.

12 Masaki T. The discovery of endothelins. Cardiovasc Res 1998;**39**:530–533.

13 Masaki T, Miwa S, Sawamura T, Ninomiya H, Okamoto Y. Subcellular mechanisms of endothelin action in vascular system. Eur J Pharmacol 1999;**375**:133–138.

14 Giaid A, Yanagisawa M, Langleben D et al. Expression of endothelin-1 in the lungs of patients with pulmonary hypertension. N Engl J Med 1993;**328**:1732–1739.

15 Miyauchi T, Yorikane R, Sakai S et al. Contribution of endogenous endothelin-1 to the progression of cardiopulmonary alterations in rats with monocrotaline-induced pulmonary hypertension. Circ Res 1993;**73**:887–897.

16 Galie N, Manes A, Branzi A. The endothelin system in pulmonary arterial hypertension. Cardiovasc Res 2004;**61**:227–237.

17 Rubin LJ. Current concepts: primary pulmonary hypertension. N Engl J Med 1997;**336**:111–117.

18 Pacher R, Bergler-Klein J, Globits S et al. Plasma big endothelin-1 concentrations in congestive heart failure patients with or without systematic hypertension. Am J Cardiol 1993;**71**:1293–1299.

19 Sakai S, Miyauchi T, Sakurai T et al. Pulmonary hypertension caused by congestive heart failure is ameliorated by long-term application of an endothelin receptor antagonist. J Am Coll Cardiol 1996;**28**:1580–1588.

20 Kobayashi T, Miyauchi T, Sakai S et al. Expression of endothelin-1, ET-A and ET-B receptors, and ECE and distribution of endothelin-1 in failing rat heart. Am J Physiol 1999;**276**:H1197–H1206.

21 Mulder P, Richard V, Derumeaux G et al. Role of endogenous endothelin in chronic heart failure: effect of long-term treatment with an endothelin antagonist on survival, hemodynamics and cardiac remodeling. Circulation 1997;**96**:1976–1982.

22 Sakai S, Miyauchi T, Kobayashi M, Yamaguchi I, Goto K, Sugishita Y. Inhibition of myocardial endo thelin pathway improves long-term survival in heart failure. *Nature* 1996;**384**:353–355.

23 Farber HW, Loscalzo J. Pulmonary arterial hypertension. *N Engl J Med* 2004;**351**:1655–1665.

24 Tonnessen T, Christensen C, Oie F, Holt E, KjekshusII, Smisell OA. Increased cardiac expression of endothelin-1 mRNA in ischemic heart failure in rats. *Cardiovas Res* 1997;**33**:601–610.

25 Picard P, Smith PJ, Monge JC *et al.* Coordinated upregulation of the cardiac endothelin system in a rat model of heart failure. *J Cardiovasc Pharmacol* 1983;**31**: S294–S297.

26 Kiowski W, Sutsch G, Ilunziker P *et al.* Evidence for endothelin-1 mediated vasoconstriction in severe chronic heart failure. *Lancet* 1995;**346**:732–736.

27 Xu D, Emoto N, Giaid A *et al.* ECE 1: a membrane-bond metalloproteinase that catalyzes the proteolytic activation of big endothelin-1. *Cell* 1994;**78**:473–485.

28 Mellin V, Jeng, AY, Monteil C *et al.* Triple ACE-ECE-NEP inhibition in heart failure: a comparison with ACE and dual ECE-NEP inhibition. *J Cardiovasc Pharmacol* 2005;**46**:390–397.

29 Guarda E, Katwa L, Myers P *et al.* Effects of endothelins on collagen turnover in cardiac fibroblasts. *Cardiovasc Res* 1993;**27**:2130–2134.

30 Bogoyevitch M, Glennoin P, Andersson M *et al.* Endothelin-1 and fibroblast growth factors stimulate the mitogen-activated protein kinase signaling cascade in cardiac myocytes. *J Bio Chem* 1994;**269**: 1110–1119.

31 Teerlink JR, Loffler BM, Hess P, Maire JP, Clozel M, Clozel JP. Role of endothelin in the maintainance of blood pressure in conscious rats with chronic heart failure. Acute effects of the endothelin receptor antagonist. Ro 47-0203 (Bosentan). *Circulation* 1994;**90**: 2510–2518.

32 Inada T, Fujiwara H, Hasegawa K *et al.* Upregulated expression of cardiac endothelin-01 participates in myocardial cell growth in Bio14.6 syrian cardiomyopathic hamsters. *J Am Coll Cardiol* 1999;**33**:565–571.

33 Ito H, Hiroe M, Hirata Y *et al.* Endothelin ET-A receptor antagonist blocks cardiac hypertrophy provoked by hemodynamic overload. *Circulation* 1994;**89**:2198–2203.

34 Saad D, Mukherjee R, Thomas P *et al.* The effects of endothelin-A receptor blockade during the progression of pacing-induced congestive heart failure. *J Am Coll Cardiol* 1998;**32**:1779–1786.

35 Cowburn PJ, Cleland JG, McArthur JD *et al.* Short-term hemodynamic effects of BQ-123, a selective endothelin ET(A)-receptor antagonist, in chronic heart failure (letter). *Lancet* 1998;**352**:201–202.

36 Psieker LE, Mitrovic V, Noll G *et al.* Acute hemodynamic and neurohumoral effects of selective ET(A)-receptor blockade in patients with congestive heart failure. *J Am Coll Cardiol* 2000;**35**:1745–1752.

37 Torre-Amione G, Young JB, Durnad JB *et al.* Hemodynamic effects of tezosentan, an intravenous duel endothelin receptor antagonist, in patients with class III to IV congestive heart failure. *Circulation* 2001;**103**:973–980.

38 Gattis WA, O'Connor CM, Hasselblad V, Adams KF Jr., Kobrin I, Gheorghiade M. Usefulness of an elevated troponin-I in predicting clinical events in patients admitted with acute heart failure and acute coronary syndrome (from the RITZ-4 trial). *Am J Cardiol* 2004;**93**:1436–1437.

39 Tovar JM, Gums JG. Tezosentan in the treatment of acute heart failure. *Ann Pharmacother* 2003;**37**: 1877–1883.

40 Torre-Amione G, Young JB, Colucci WS *et al.* Hemodynamic and clinical effects of tezosentan, an intravenous dual endothelin receptor antagonist, in patients hospitalized for acute decompensated heart failure. *J Am Coll Cardiol* 2003;**42**:140–147.

41 Kaluski E, Kobrin I, Zimlichman R *et al.* and RITZ-5 Investigators. RITZ-5: randomized intravenous TeZosentan (an endothelin-A/B antagonist) for the treatment of pulmonary edema: a prospective, multicenter, double-blind, placebo-controlled study. *J Am Coll Cardiol* 2003;**41**:204–210.

42 Coletta AP, Cleland JGF. Clinical trials update: highlights of the scientific sessions of the XXIII Congress of the European Society of Cardiology – WARIS II, ESCAMI, PAFAC, RITZ-1 and TIME. *Eur J Heart Fail* 2001;**3**: 747–750.

43 Louis A, Cleland JGF, Crabbe S *et al.* Clinical Trials Update: CAPRICORN, COPERNICUS, MIRACLE, STAF, RITZ-2, RECOVER and RENAISSANCE and cachexia and cholesterol in heart failure. Highlights of the Scientific Sessions of the American College of Cardiology, 2001. *Eur J Heart Fail* 2001;**3**:381–387.

44 Cleland JGF, Coletta AP, Freemantle N, Velavan P, Tin L, Clark AL. Clinical trials update from the American College of Cardiology meeting: CARE-HF and the Remission of Heart Failure, Women's Health Study, TNT, COMPASS-HF, VERITAS, CANPAP, PEECH and PREMIER. *Eur J Heart Fail* 2005;**5**:931–936.

45 Teerlink J, McMurray J, Bourge R *et al.* Tezosentan in patients with acute heart failure: design of the Value of Endothelin Receptor Inhibition with Tezosentan in Acute heart failure Study (VERITAS). *Am Heart J* 2005;**150**: 46–53.

46 Packer M, Caspi A, Charlton V *et al.* Multicenter, double-blind placebo-controlled study of long-term endothelin blockade with bosentan in chronic heart failure-results of the REACH-1 trial. *Circulation* 1998;**98**:12.

47 Packer M, McMurray J, Massie BM *et al*. For the REACH-1 study group. Clinical effects of endothelin receptor antagonism with Bosentan in patients with severe chronic heart failure: results of a pilot study. *J Card Fail* 2005;**11**:12–20.

48 Cowburn PJ, Cleland JGF. Endothelin antagonists for chronic heart failure: do they have a role? *Eur Heart J* 2001;**22**:1772–1784.

49 Coletta A, Thackray S, Nikitin N, Cleland JGF. Clinical trials update: highlights of the scientific sessions of the American College of Cardiology 2002: LIFE, DANAMI 2, MADIT-2, MIRACLE-ICD, OVERTURE, OCTAVE, ENABLE 1&2, CHRISTMAS, AFFIRM, RACE, WIZARD, AZACS, REMATCH, BNP trial, and HARDBALL. *Eur J Heart Fail* 2002;**4**:381–388.

50 Luscher TF, Enseleit F, Pacher R *et al*. Hemodynamic and neurohumoral effects of selective endothelin A (ET-A) receptor blockade in chronic heart failure: the heart failure ET-A receptor blockade trial (HEAT). *Circulation* 2002;**106**:2666–2672.

51 Anand I, McMurray J, Cohn JN *et al*. on behalf of the EARTH Investigators. Long-term effects of darusentan on left ventricular remodeling and clinical outcomes in the endothelin A receptor antagonist trial in heart failure (EARTH): randomized, double-blind, placebo-controlled trial. *Lancet* 2004;**364**:347–354.

52 Ergul A. Endothelin-1 and endothelin receptor antagonists as potential cardiovascular therapeutic agents. *Pharmacotherapy* 2002;**22**:54–65.

53 Jessup M, Brozena S. Heart failure. *N Engl J Med* 2003;**348**:2007–2018.

54 Cowburn PJ, Cleland JGF, McDonagh TA *et al*. Comparison of selective ET-A and ET-B receptor antagonists in patients with chronic heart failure. *Eur J Heart Fail* 2005;**7**:37–42.

55 Stewart DJ, Levy RD, Cernacek P, Langleben D. Increased plasma endothelin-1 in pulmonary hypertension marker or mediator of disease? *Ann Intern Med* 1991;**114**: 464–469.

56 Morelli S, Ferri C, Polettini E *et al*. Plasma endothelin-1 levels, pulmonary hypertension, and lung fibrosis in patients with systemic sclerosis. *Am J Med* 1995;**99**: 255–260.

57 Davie N, Haleen SJ, Upton PD *et al*. ET-A and ET-B receptors modulate the proliferation of human pulmonary artery smooth muscle cells. *Am J Respir Crit Care Med* 2002;**165**:398–405.

58 Park SH, Saleh D, Giaid A, Michel RP. Increased endothelin-1 in bleomycin induced pulmonary fibrosis and the effect of an endothelin receptor antagonist. *Am J Respir Crit Care Med* 1997;**156**:600–608.

59 Channick RN, Simonneau G, Sitbon O *et al*. Effects of the dual endothelin-receptor antagonist bosentan in patients with pulmonary hypertension a randomised placebo-controlled study. *Lancet* 2001;**358**:1119–1123.

60 Rubin LJ, Badesch DB, Barst RJ *et al*. Bosentan therapy for pulmonary arterial hypertension. *N Engl J Med* 2002;**346**:896–903.

61 Hoeper MM. Drug treatment of pulmonary arterial hypertension: current and future agents. *Drugs* 2005;**65**:1337–1354.

62 Sitbon O, Badesch DB, Channick RN *et al*. Effects of the dual endothelin receptor antagonist bosentan in patients with pulmonary arterial hypertension a 1-year follow-up study. *Chest* 2003;**124**:247–254.

63 Sitbon O, McLaughlin VV, Badesch DB *et al*. Survival in patients with class III idiopathic pulmonary arterial hypertension treated with first-line oral bosentan compared with an historical cohort of patients started on i.v. epoprostenol. *Thorax* 2005; doi: 10.1136/thx.2005.040618.

64 McLaughlin VV, Sitbon O, Badesch DB *et al*. Survival with first-line bosentan in patients with primary pulmonary hypertension. *Eur Respir J* 2005;**25**:244–249.

65 Barst RJ, Langleben D, Frost A *et al*. Sitaxsentan therapy for pulmonary arterial hypertension. *Am J Respir Crit Care Med* 2004;**169**:441–447.

66 Humbert M, Sitbon O, Simonneau G. Treatment of pulmonary arterial hypertension. *N Engl J Med* 2004;**351**:1425–1436.

67 Galié N, Badesch D, Oudiz R, Simonneau G *et al*. Ambrisentan therapy for pulmonary arterial hypertension. *J Am Coll Cardiol* 2005;**46**:529–535.

68 Attina T, Camidge R, Newby DE, Webb DJ. Endothelin antagonism in pulmonary hypertension, heart failure, and beyond. *Heart* 2005;**91**:825–831.

69 Taddei S, Virdis A, Ghiadoni L *et al*. Vasoconstriction to endogenous endothelin-1 is increased in the peripheral circulation of patients with essential hypertension. *Circulation* 1999;**100**:1680–1683.

70 Seo B, Oemar BS, Siebenmann R *et al*. Both ETA and ETB receptors mediate contraction to endothelin-1 in human blood vessels. *Circulation* 1994;**89**:1203–1208.

71 Haynes WG, Webb DJ. Endothelin as a regulator of cardiovascular function in health and disease. *J Hypertens* 1998;**16**:1081–1098.

72 Krum H, Viskoper RJ, Lacourciere Y, Budde M, Charlon V. The effect of an endothelin-receptor antagonist, bosentan, on blood pressure in patients with essential hypertension. Bosentan Hypertension Investigators. *N Engl J Med* 1998;**338**:784–790.

73 Nakov R, Pfarr E, Eberle S. HEAT Investigators. Darusentan: an effective endothelin A receptor antagonist for treatment of hypertension. *Am J Hypertens* 2002;**15**:583–589.

74 Campia U, Cardillo C, Panza JA. Ethnic differences in the vasoconstrictor activity of endogenous endothelin-1 in hypertensive patients. *Circulation* 2004;**109**:3191–3195.

75 Ergul A. Hypertension in black patients: an emerging role of the endothelin system in salt-sensitive hypertension. *Hypertension* 2000;**36**:62–67.

76 Gonon AT, Bulhak A, Bröijersén A, Pernow J. Cardioprotective effect of an endothelin receptor antagonist during ischaemia/reperfusion in the severely atherosclerotic mouse heart. *Br J Pharmacol* 2005;**144**:860–866.

77 Clozel M, Clozel JP. Effects of endothelin on regional blood flows in squirrel monkeys. *J Pharmacol Exp Ther* 1989;**250**:1125–1131.

78 Ihling C, Bohrmann B, Schaefer HE, Technau-Ihling K, Loeffler BM. Endothelin-1 and endothelin converting enzyme-1 in human atherosclerosis – novel targets for pharmacotherapy in atherosclerosis. *Curr Vasc Pharmacol* 2004;**2**:249–258.

79 Cardillo C, Kilcoyne CM, CannonIII RO *et al.* Increased activity of endogenous endothelin in patients with hypercholesterolemia. *J Am Coll Cardiol* 2000;**36**:753–758.

80 Kurita A, Matsui T, Ishizuka T *et al.* Significance of plasma nitric oxide/endothelial-1 ratio for prediction of coronary artery disease. *Angiology* 2005;**56**:259–264.

81 Goddard J, Johnston NR, Hand MF *et al.* Endothelin-A receptor antagonism reduces blood pressure and increases renal blood flow in hypertensive patients with chronic renal failure: a comparison of selective and combined endothelin receptor blockade. *Circulation* 2004;**109**:1186–1193.

82 Sarman B, Toth M, Somogyi A. Role of endothelin in diabetes mellitus. *Diabetes Metab Rev* 1998;**14**:171–175.

83 Cardillo C, Campia U, Bryant MB, Panza JA. Increased activity of endogenous endothelin in patients with type II diabetes mellitus. *Circulation* 2002;**106**:1783–1787.

84 Modesti PA, Cecioni I, Costoli A *et al.* Renal endothelin in heart failure and its relation to sodium excretion. *Am Heart J* 2000;**140**:617–623.

85 Boffa JJ, Tharaux PL, Dussaule JC, Chatziantoniou C. Regression of renal vascular fibrosis by endothelin receptor antagonism. *Hypertension* 2001;**37**:490–496.

# CHAPTER 16

# Pharmacogenetics

## *Richard Sheppard,* MD *& Dennis M. McNamara,* MD, FACC

Predictions in acute diseases, whether favorable or unfavorable, are not absolutely certain [1].
Hard and fast lines cannot be drawn in the question of prognosis . . . Every case must be judged
separately [2].

## Introduction

For subjects with heart failure, the marked variability of clinical outcomes has always limited the ability of practitioners, from Hippocrates [1] to Osler [2], to predict prognosis for an individual patient. Heart failure pathogenesis is driven by a complex systemic response to myocardial injury, collectively termed neurohormonal activation, and the magnitude of this systemic response likely determines the rate of progression of the clinical syndrome. Clinical heterogeneity is to a great extent genetically based, as an individual's genetic background is a major determinant of the degree of neurohormonal activation. The advances of the human genome project have led to increased recognition of the inherent variation of important disease modifiers and the potential medical implications [3]. A more complete understanding of the impact of genetic background on heart failure progression and therapeutics should provide future clinicians with tools not accessible to their predecessors.

With increasing evidence that genetic variability of disease modifiers alters clinical outcomes we stand at the brink of a revolution in the medical therapy of heart failure. Through modulating the neurohormonal response genetic background not only influences the rate of heart failure progression but will also alter the impact of the pharmacologic inhibitors of neurohormonal activation. Heart failure is clearly a polygenic disorder and multiple loci will influence prognosis and the effectiveness of therapy. As with polygenic disorders, such as hypertension and diabetes, several critical genetic loci will function as major drivers of

this "background effect", and knowledge of their pharmacogenetic interactions should form the foundation of individualized treatment decisions. Significant functional variation exists in the two central targets of heart failure pharmacotherapy: the angiotensin converting enzyme (ACE) and the cardiac beta-adrenergic receptor, and these critical loci will remain important "drivers" of heart failure pharmacogenetics. However, additional candidates are increasingly recognized that impact on left ventricular remodeling (matrix metalloproteinases) or on the vascular response to heart failure (genes central to nitric oxide and adenosine metabolism). This chapter reviews genetic modulators of neurohormonal activation and the systemic response to heart failure and potential clinical implications for individualized therapies.

## Renin–angiotensin–aldosterone system

### ACE D/I polymorphism and heart failure outcomes

The ACE deletion/insertion biallelic polymorphism of intron 16 has been the subject of hundreds of investigations since its initial discovery [4,5]. The physiologic association of the ACE D/I polymorphism with enzymatic activity has been consistent, as the D allele has been linked in nearly every clinical study to increased activity of the ACE enzyme and higher levels of the product of ACE activity the peptide mediator angiotensin 2 (a2) [6]. The cellular mechanism remains to be elucidated but this linkage of genotype with ACE activity is evident across multiple different clinical paradigms from hypertension to myocardial infarction [7–9] and demonstrates a D allele "dose effect" for a2 levels. Subjects with the DD genotype have the highest levels of a2, heterozygotes are intermediate, and those homozygous for I allele have the lowest levels. Given the role of angiotensin II in heart failure progression the potential implications of this genetically "ordered" ACE activity for this disorder are readily apparent, and suggests the hypothesis that the ACE D allele will function as a genetic modifier, accelerate disease progression, and worsen survival.

This role of the ACE D/I polymorphism as a genetic modifier has been confirmed in three independent clinical investigations that documented an adverse impact of the ACE D allele on heart failure survival. The first investigation was in a population of 193 subjects with idiopathic dilated cardiomyopathy and demonstrated poorer survival for subjects homozygous for the D allele [10]. This heart failure impact is independent of etiology, as more recently the adverse impact of the ACE D allele was demonstrated in 978 subjects post-myocardial infarction [11]. The impact in the cohort post-infarction was primarily evident in subjects with lower left ventricular ejections fraction (LVEF) or higher brain natriuretic peptide (BNP) levels. Neither study addressed the potential pharmacogenetic interactions of the ACE D/I polymorphism with the medical therapy of heart failure. Forty five percent of the subjects in the post-myocardial infarction study were on ACE inhibitor therapy, compared to only 25% of subjects in the earlier study of idiopathic dilated cardiomyopathy.

## Pharmacogenetics of the ACE D/I polymorphism: GRACE

The pharmacogenetic interactions of the ACE D/I polymorphism and heart failure therapy have been most extensively examined in the GRACE study, a single center study at the University of Pittsburgh of Genetic Risk Assessment of Cardiac Events. Four hundred and seventy-nine subjects with systolic dysfunction (mean LVEF $0.25 \pm 0.08$) from both ischemic and nonischemic etiologies were followed for a median of 3 years until death or cardiac transplantation. The D allele was associated with poorer outcome in transplant free survival, and demonstrated the same "gene ordered" effect shown

earlier for ACE activity: II homozygotes demonstrated the best survival, DD homozygotes the poorest, with heterozygotes displayed the predicted "intermediate" survival between the homozygotes. The adverse impact of the D allele on survival for this cohort was first reported on an analysis of the first 328 subjects [12], and remained evident during analysis for the entire cohort [13] (Figure 16.1a).

## β-blocker therapy

The GRACE study was the first to demonstrate that the impact of the ACE D/I polymorphism on heart failure outcomes may be altered by the pharmacological milieu. Ninety-five percent of subjects in GRACE were on ACE inhibitors or angiotensin receptor antagonists (ARBs), while only 42% were on beta-blockers reflecting the evolution of care at the time of the initiation of the study. Analysis by treatment subset demonstrated the effects of ACE D on outcomes were primarily in subjects not treated with β-blockers [12,13] (Figure 16.1b) and that impact of the polymorphism is virtually eliminated by β-blocker therapy (Figure 16.1c). The elimination of the effect of the D allele by beta-blocker therapy likely reflects their role as inhibitors of renin activation. Sympathetic activation is an important stimulus for renin release and beta-blockers markedly reduce angiotensin-2 levels [14]. For subjects not on beta-blockers, the 2-year event-free survival for DD subjects was only 51%, versus 80% for the II homozygotes. In contrast, for subjects on beta-blockers no effect of the D-allele on outcomes was apparent.

The potential role for the ACE D/I polymorphism in individualized treatment decisions is evident when examining the impact of β-blocker therapy *within ACE D/I genetic subsets* (Figure 16.2). While beta-blockers overall improved survival in the GRACE cohort the benefit for the entire cohort is driven by a marked treatment effect for the DD homozygotes. In contrast to the benefits in the ACE DD subjects the impact of therapy is diminished in the heterozygotes, and in this small cohort is no longer evident for subjects who are II homozygotes. These results suggest the ACE D/I polymorphism delineates genetic subsets of heart failure patients in whom the therapeutic impact of beta-blockade on heart failure survival is distinctly different. This

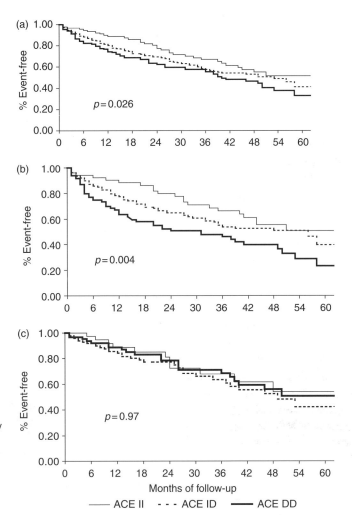

**Figure 16.1** Transplant-free survival by ACE D/I genotype, GRACE study, University of Pittsburgh [13]. (a) Overall cohort, ACE D allele associated with poorer event-free survival, $n = 479$, $p = 0.026$. (b) Subset with no beta-blocker therapy, $n = 277$, $p = 0.004$. (c) Subset treated with beta-blocker therapy, $n = 202$, $p = 0.97$.

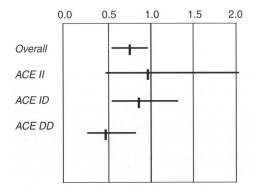

**Figure 16.2** Relative risk of event (death or transplantation) by beta-blocker use, GRACE study: overall cohort and by ACE D/I genotype, DD, DI, and II. (Adapted from table 4, [13]).

pharmacogenetic interaction will require further prospective validation prior to a determination of its clinical role. In contrast to the impact in GRACE, a recent study [15] of the effect of beta-blockers for 199 subjects with chronic heart failure demonstrated similar improvements in LVEF in all three genetic subsets, and suggests the ACE D/I polymorphism does not predict this particular endpoint of beta-blocker response.

## ACE-inhibitor therapy

The linkage of the ACE D allele to higher ACE activity should have significant impact on the therapeutic effects of ACE inhibitors. The widespread utilization of ACE inhibitors in heart failure treatment complicates the analysis of pharmacogenetic interactions due to the absence of an untreated "control" group. In GRACE, the pharmacogenetic interaction of ACE inhibitors with the ACE D/I polymorphism was investigated using a dose analysis, which compared higher-dose ACE therapy (>50% of target daily dose defined by national guidelines) to low-dose therapy (≤50%). This breakdown resulted in a roughly three-fold difference in the mean dose for the high-dose group compared to low-dose group. In contrast, the multicenter Assessment of Treatment with Lisinopril and Survival (ATLAS) trial [16] evaluated the impact of a 10-fold difference in the mean dose of ACE inhibitor. In a similar fashion to the effect seen with beta-blockers higher-dose ACE inhibitors markedly diminished the adverse impact of the ACE D allele on survival [13]. Analysis by treatment subset further suggests the effect of high-dose therapy was particularly evident in subjects not treated with beta-blockers (Figure 16.3).

In the analysis of relative risk the benefits of high-dose ACE inhibitors compared to low dose were modest with the risk of events on high-dose therapy of 0.88. This 12% reduction was not significant statistically, but was similar to the trend in survival benefit seen in ATLAS. The relative risk reduction with higher-dose therapy within ACE genotype class demonstrated a gene-ordered effect similar to that seen with $\beta$-blockers, with the greatest impact within the DD subset though this failed to reach significance (Figure 16.4). The increased impact of high-dose therapy in DD homozygotes may reflect greater resistance to ACE inhibition in this subset. Clinical studies of blood pressure response to captopril demonstrates minimal effects in DD subjects, an intermediate response in heterozygotes, and the greatest impact in II patients [17]. A similar interaction has been reported for chronic therapy with angiotensin receptor antagonists in hypertensive subjects [18], which studies suggest a diminished response to ACE inhibition or blockade with the ACE D allele.

## Aldosterone receptor antagonists: ACE D/I and aldosterone synthase promoter polymorphisms

The addition of aldosterone receptor antagonists to ACE inhibitor therapy has been demonstrated to improve survival in class IIIb to IV heart failure in the RALES trial [19], and in subjects post-myocardial infarction [20]; however, the impact of genetic background have not been fully investigated. The prevalence of "aldosterone escape" on ACE inhibitors is greatest in the ACE DD genotype [21]. The impact of the aldosterone-receptor antagonist spironolactone on left ventricular remodeling is also diminished in ACE DD subset compared to the ID and II subsets [22] in a manner that closely parallels the diminished clinical response to ACE inhibitors. The influence of the ACE D/I polymorphism on therapy with aldosterone receptor antagonists was not investigated in GRACE due to the small number of subjects on treatment. A promoter polymorphism of the aldosterone synthase gene exists in which the C allele is associated with higher aldosterone levels [23]. Analysis of gene–gene interactions in GRACE does suggests that coinheritance of the C promoter variant magnifies the impact of the ACE D allele [24]. The impact of this aldosterone synthase promoter variant on aldosterone-receptor antagonist therapy remains to be determined.

## The angiotensin-II type 1 receptor

The majority of intracellular effects of a-2 are mediated through interaction with the G-protein coupled receptor AT$_1$. A polymorphism (A1166C) of the AT$_1$ receptor gene (*ATRG*) has been described, in which there is a base substitution of adenosine for cytosine at position 1166 of the 3′ untranslated region of *AT1R* gene. The C allele has been associated with coronary vasoconstriction and stenosis [25], although its association with the development of hypertension and ischemic heart disease [26,27] remains more controversial. The A1166C polymorphism has been studied in patients with heart failure, yet the results are inconsistent. Anderson *et al.* demonstrated that for patients with heart failure the C allele as a single modifier did not appear to influence clinical outcomes; however, subjects who coinherited the C allele in addition to the ACE DD genotype did appear to have a poorer prognosis [28].

## Beta-adrenergic receptor variation

Sympathetic activation is a critical component of heart failure progression and variation at multiple

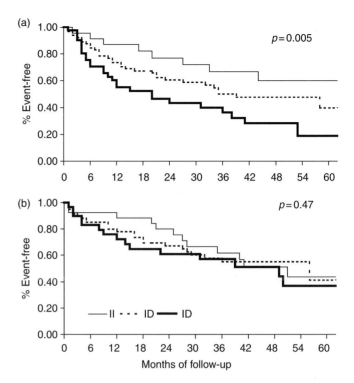

**Figure 16.3** Transplant-free survival by ACE D/I genotype, GRACE study, University of Pittsburgh [13]. (a) Subset on low-dose ACE inhibitors and no beta-blockers, ACE D allele associated with poorer event free survival, $n = 130$, $p = 0.005$. (b) Subset with high-dose ACE inhibitor therapy and no beta-blockers, $n = 117$, $p = 0.47$.

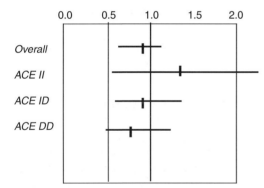

**Figure 16.4** Relative risk of event (death or transplantation) by ACE inhibitor dose use, GRACE study: Overall cohort and by ACE D/I genotype, DD, DI, and II (adapted from table 4, [13]).

loci will modulate its impact on heart failure progression and therapy. Beta-blockers may have beneficial effects on plasma renin; however, they also inhibit the deleterious effects of circulating catecholamines directly on the myocardium itself. This therapeutic aspect of beta-blocker therapy is mediated through $\beta_1$ and $\beta_2$ adrenergic receptors, and examination of the functional significance of their common genetic polymorphisms has been an area of intense research [29].

### Structure and function

Activation of both $\beta$ receptor subtypes is linked to increased cAMP formation through the interaction with the stimulatory guanine nucleotide binding protein ($G_s$). In the normal heart, $\beta_1$ receptors predominate over $\beta_2$ receptors at a ratio of roughly $4:1$ while in the failing myocardium sympathetic overactivation leads to selective downregulation of $\beta_1$ receptors to a much greater extent than $\beta_2$ and as a result the percentage of $\beta_2$ receptors may increase up to 40% [30]. In contrast, $\beta_2$ receptors do not decrease in receptor number, but become deactivated or less responsive to agonist stimulation.

The $\beta_1$ adrenergic receptor (Figure 16.5) is encoded for by an intronless gene and consists of a protein with 477 amino acid residues and 7 transmembrane domains (TMDs). The first 60 amino acids of the amino terminus comprise the extracellular surface of the receptor while the final 90 amino acids are located in the cytoplasmic domain. The $\beta_2$ receptor subtype (Figure 16.6) has a similar

$\beta_1$ adrenergic receptor

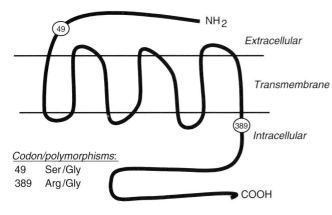

Codon/polymorphisms:
49    Ser/Gly
389    Arg/Gly

**Figure 16.5** Structure of the $\beta_1$ adrenergic receptor: Common polymorphisms: Ser = serine, Gly = glycine, Arg = arginine, $NH_2$ = aminoterminus, COOH = carboxyl terminus (Reproduced from [29]).

$\beta_2$ adrenergic receptor

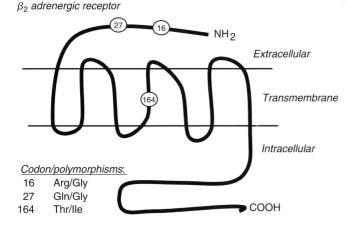

Codon/polymorphisms:
16    Arg/Gly
27    Gln/Gly
164    Thr/Ile

**Figure 16.6** Structure of the $\beta_2$ adrenergic receptor: Common polymorphisms: Arg = arginine, Gly = glycine, Gln = glutamine, Glu = glutamate, Thr = threonine, Ile = Isoleucine, $NH_2$ = aminoterminus, COOH = carboxylterminus. (Reproduced from [29]).

genomic and protein structure [31] with a coding region of 1239 nucleic acids encoding for 413 amino acids. Between $\beta_1AR$ and $\beta_2ARs$, the greatest amino acid identity (71%) is found in the TMDs, and the tertiary structure in the lipid bilayer takes on a ring or barrel shape that allows for multiple ligand contact points [32]. The cytoplasmic regions of the two receptor classes are more distinct, which allows for more diversity in their signaling interactions with other intracellular proteins [33].

## Functional variation and heart failure outcomes: $\beta_2$

Initial investigations focused on the clinical implications of $\beta_2$ receptor polymorphisms given their importance in the pharmacologic treatment of asthma and were led by Dr Stephen Liggett at the University of Cincinnati [34]. Three common polymorphisms exist in the coding region:

Arg16Gly, Glu27Gln, and Thr164Ile, which have demonstrated functional consequences in terms of receptor function or regulation *in vitro* [35]. The substitution of Ile for Thr occurs with allele frequency of approximately 3 to 5%, and the Ile164 receptor has significantly lower binding affinity for isoproterenol, epinephrine, and norepinephrine [36] (Table 16.1). Agonist stimulation of the Ile variant produces a lower level of adenylyl cyclase activity with the Thr wild type receptor. Transgenic mice that overexpress the Ile164 receptor in the heart have a decrease in resting and (agonist stimulated) contractile function *in vivo* when compared to transgenic controls overexpressing the wild type Thr164 receptor [37].

A clinical role of this polymorphism in modulating heart failure outcomes was demonstrated in a prospective study of 259 patients at the University of Cincinnati, which found that the presence of the

**Table 16.1** $\beta_1$ and $\beta_2$ polymorphisms: frequency and function.

| Codon | Region | Polymorphism | Allele frequency | Function in vitro |
|---|---|---|---|---|
| $\beta_1$ | | | | |
| 389 | Cytoplasmic | Arg/Gly | 0.70/0.30 | Arg = gain of function (↑cAMP) |
| 49 | Extracellular | Ser/Gly | 0.85/0.15 | No data |
| $\beta_2$ | | | | |
| 16 | Extracellular | Arg/Gly | 0.40/0.60 | Gly = enhanced downregulation |
| 27 | Extracellular | Gln/Glu | 0.55/0.45 | Glu = resistance to downregulation |
| 164 | Transmembrane Domain #4 | Thr/Ile | 0.95/0.05 | Ile = loss of function ↓agonist binding, ↓cAMP |

Gly = glycine, Arg = arginine, Ser = serine, Gln = glutamine, Glu = glutamate, Thr = threonine, Ile = Isoleucine (Reproduced from [29]).

Ile164 receptor polymorphism markedly decreased transplant-free survival with a relative risk of death or transplant of 4.8 compared to those homozygous for Thr164 [38]. Subjects with the Ile164 receptor in this population also demonstrated a marked reduction in functional capacity, as measured by metabolic-stress testing [39]. Consistent with these findings in heart failure subjects a study of normal Thr164Ile heterozygotes demonstrate blunted agonist responsiveness compared to subjects homozygous for Thr164 [40,41]. The effect of the Ile164 variant in these investigations support the importance of the $\beta_2$ receptor in heart failure progression, though the small number of subjects with the variant limits pharmacogenetic investigations. Several studies have linked the more common Arg16Gly or Glu27Gln polymorphisms to hypertension [42,43]; however, no influence on heart failure outcomes has been evident [38].

## Functional variation and heart failure outcomes: $\beta_1$

Two common polymorphisms exist in the coding region of the $\beta_1$ receptor: Ser49Gly and Arg389Gly [44], and both have been reported to modulate heart failure outcomes. The codon 49 polymorphism is located in the extracellular domain of the receptor (Figure 16.5), with relative allele frequencies of the Ser49 and Gly49 alleles of 0.85 and 0.15 respectively. The Gly49 variant demonstrated increased receptor downregulation in vitro compared to Ser49 receptors in two independent investigations [45,46]. The Arg389Gly polymorphism for codon 389 (allele frequency Arg389 = 0.70, Gly389 = 0.30) is located

near the carboxyl-terminus cytoplasmic tail and in vitro the Arg389 receptor demonstrates a higher basal adenylyl cyclase activity than the Gly389 variant. With agonist stimulation this distinction was greatly magnified suggesting the Arg389 variant results in a gain of function for G-protein coupling [47].

The Gly49 variant was associated with lower resting heart rates in an examination of more than 1000 normal individuals [48]. In an outcomes study of 184 subjects with heart failure due to systolic dysfunction the Gly49 variant was associated with improved survival [49]. An examination of the GRACE cohort suggests the Gly49 variant is linked to greater benefit from adrenergic-receptor blockade [50]. The Arg389 variant was linked to a greater risk of heart failure in an African American cohort, but only when coinherited with a deletion of the alpha 2C receptor [51]. The genetic substudy of the BEST trial of bucindilol suggests the presence of the 389Arg variant predicts a greater improvement of survival with beta-blocker therapy [52]; however, this linkage of 389Arg to beta-blocker benefit was not evident with metoprolol in the MERIT-HF substudy [53]. In a similar fashion, examination of the impact of 389Arg on blood pressure response in hypertensive subjects has led to conflicting results [54,55].

## Endothelial nitric oxide synthase (NOS3)

Nitric oxide (NO) plays an important protective role in heart failure [56–58] and endothelial nitric oxide synthase (NOS3) is the predominant source of vascular NO. A common polymorphism (G894T) exists on exon 7 (codon 298 : Glu298Asp) for which the wild type glutamate is replaced with aspartic acid [58]. The functional role of this apparently charge neutral amino acid change remains controversial; however, the Asp298 variant has a shorter half-life and therefore less NO activity in endothelial cell culture [59]. For subjects with heart failure functional assessment by metabolic-stress testing demonstrates significantly higher $VO_2$ max in subjects with the Glu298Glu phenotype compared to those with the Asp298 variant [60]. This modulation of functional capacity is consistent with the impact of this polymorphism on clinical outcomes as poorer transplant-free survival was evident for subjects with the Asp298 variant compared to individuals homozygous for Glu298 (Figure 16.7) [60].

## Pharmacogenetic interactions with NOS3 and ACE inhibitors

Nitric oxide synthase plays a central role in the therapeutic effects of ACE inhibitors. Murine models demonstrate that the post-infarction benefit of ACE inhibitors on remodeling is dependent on NOS3 [61]. In studies of vascular reactivity the effects of ACE inhibitors are diminished by pretreatment with NOS inhibitors. In GRACE, the examination of high-dose versus low-dose ACE inhibitor suggest a pharmacogenetic interaction with the NOS3 Glu298Asp polymorphism as the impact of Asp298 was primarily in subjects on low-dose ACE inhibitor, and was not evident in those receiving high-dose therapy [62]. Analysis of the impact of ACE-inhibitor dose by genetic

subset suggests the variable benefit of ACE inhibitors may be partially explained by variation at the NOS3 locus; however, this will need additional investigation in larger cohorts.

## Additional genetic modifiers of heart failure progression

Genetic variation in several additional mediators of heart failure progression has been demonstrated to influence clinical outcomes. While no clinical studies of specific pharmacogenetic interactions have yet been performed for these variants the ability to genetically delineate subjects at greater risk for poor outcomes has significant clinical implications for future targeting strategies.

### AMP deaminase-1

Adenosine monophosphate deaminase-1 (AMPD1) catalyzes the conversion of adenosine monophosphate to inosine monophosphate [63], the rate-limiting step for entry into the purine nucleotide cycle. A common polymorphism occurs, C to T transition at nucleotide 34, in exon 2 of the *AMPD1* gene. The T allele is a nonsense mutation that results in a truncated and inactive enzyme and increased levels of adenosine, and this variant is present in approximately 20–25% of Caucasians [64]. Adenosine has a cardioprotective effect, leading to vasodilatation, less platelet aggregation, reduced levels of oxidative stress and inflammatory markers, and facilitates myocardial ischemic preconditioning [65]. Consistent with the protective effects of adenosine the presence of the truncated variant of AMPD1 has been associated

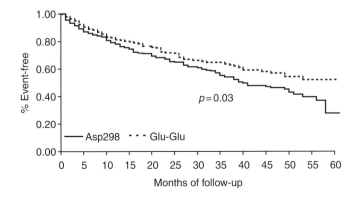

**Figure 16.7** Transplant-free survival by endothelial nitric oxide synthase (NOS3) codon 298 polymorphism, GRACE study, University of Pittsburgh: Overall cohort ($n = 469$): Asp$^{298}$ variant (solid line, $n = 266$), Glu$^{298}$ homozygotes (dashed line, $n = 203$). Event-free survival significantly poorer in subjects with the Asp$^{298}$ variant, $p = 0.03$. (Reproduced from [60]).

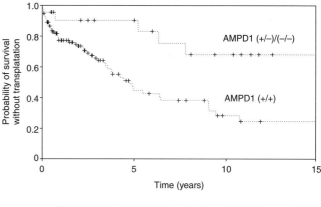

**Figure 16.8** Probability of transplant-free survival by adenosine monophosphate deaminase-1 (AMPD1) exon 2 genotype, retrospective analysis from the University of Pennsylvania (*n* = 132): Subjects heterozygous (−/+) or homozygous (−/−) for the T allele (truncated inactive enzyme) combined and had compared to subjects homozygous for the wild type (+/+) enzyme. Presence of the T allele was associated with significantly improved event-free survival (*p* = 0.002). (Reproduced from [67]).

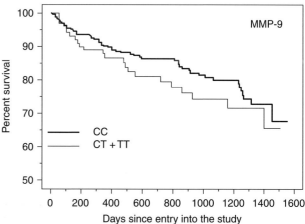

**Figure 16.9** Transplant-free survival by MMP-9 (−1562C > T) promoter genotypes for 444 subjects with heart failure due to systolic dysfunction. Subjects with the T allele (homzygotes T/T and heterozygotes T/C) combined and compared to subjects homozygous for the C allele (C/C). Event-free survival poorer for subjects with the T variant (*p* < 0.03). (Reproduced from [90]).

with improved clinical outcomes in patients with coronary artery disease [66].

Two studies have examined the impact of this polymorphism on clinical outcomes in patients with heart failure. Loh *et al.* [67] determined the AMPD1 genotype in 132 patients with advanced HF referred for cardiac transplantation. Investigators demonstrated that presence of the truncated variant (T allele) was associated with a prolonged probability of survival without transplantation (Figure 16.8). Yazaki *et al.* examined 390 subjects with HF, of whom 210 had ischemic cardiomyopathy [68]. The presence of the T allele in this study was an independent predictor of transplant-free cardiovascular survival in patients with ischemic cardiomyopathy, but not in nonischemics. A recent study [69] demonstrated that in the presence of the T allele subjects with heart failure had an improved exercise tolerance as measured by peak oxygen consumption during cardiopulmonary

testing. The impact of therapy on patients based on their AMPD1 genotype is yet to be explored.

## Tumor necrosis factor

Tumor necrosis factor (TNF) has been implicated in the development and progression of heart failure [70–73]. There is a biallelic polymorphism that has been identified at position 308 of the promoter region of the *TNFA* gene. A G to A substitution occurs at this nucleotide position leading to increased TNFA production (G = TNFA1 and A = TNFA2) [74,75]. The TNFA2 allele occurs at a higher frequency in patients with autoimmune diseases [76,77]. Only two studies have examined this polymorphism in patients with HF. Ito *et al.* [78] demonstrated that in a group of 48 Japanese patients with idiopathic cardiomyopathy the TNFA2 allele was more common than in a control group (13.5% versus 3.0%). In contrast, Kubota *et al.* [79] demonstrated that the frequency of the TNFA2 allele was similar in a group of patients with HF as compared to a control group. In addition, the TNFA2 allele did not correlate in these subjects with higher circulating levels of TNF alpha.

## Matrix metalloproteinases

A group of zinc-dependent proteolytic enzymes, known as matrix metalloproteinases (MMPs), are responsible for degradation of myocardial extracellular proteins. Their proteolytic activity is regulated by tissue inhibitors of metalloproteinases (TIMPs) [80,81]. The left ventricular remodeling process is a net result of the balance of MMP and TIMP activity in the myocardium. In patients with HF, elevated plasma levels of MMPs are associated with increased remodeling and worse clinical outcomes [82], and TNF activation may trigger MMP production [83].

Several MMP subtypes have associated polymorphisms that have been identified and for the most part affect the gene transcription process [84–86]. The two most frequently studied polymorphisms are those of MMP-3 (stromelysin) and MMP-9 (gelatinase-B). The MMP-3 polymorphism results from differing numbers of sequential adenosines in the promoter region (5 = 5A, 6 = 6A). The 5A allele is associated with increased MMP-3 promoter activity when compared to the 6A allele [84], and is reportedly associated with increased vascular remodeling, coronary restenosis, and aneurysmal coronary artery disease [87–89]. The MMP-9 polymorphism is also a common polymorphism involving a C-T substitution at position 1562 in the promoter region of the gene that leads to increased levels of MMP-9 with the T allele [86].

Several studies have examined the impact of these polymorphisms on outcomes in patients with HF, with variable results. Mizon-Gerard *et al.* [90] demonstrated that the MMP-9 T allele was an independent predictor of mortality (Figure 16.9). Shah *et al.* [91] have also demonstrated that the MMP-9 polymorphism influenced left ventricular dimensions in a group of patients with chronic heart failure, but showed no influence of the MMP-3 5A/6A polymorphism on clinical outcomes or phenotype [92]. Further studies are required to examine the influence of these polymorphisms on left ventricular remodeling and heart failure progression. In

addition, the impact of therapy on the remodeling process may be influenced by these functional genetic variants, and should be explored further.

## Future of pharmacogenetics: polygenic targeting

Clinical investigations have demonstrated that these neurohormonal polymorphisms influence HF outcomes and alter the effectiveness of drug therapy. Genetic variation of disease modifiers such as the ACE and $\beta$-adrenergic receptors ($\beta$AR) influences the effectiveness of ACE inhibitor and beta-blocker. Predictably, genetic influences on heart failure therapy are polygenic. Pharmacogenetic investigations to date have not integrated more than one genetic locus into a clinical outcomes model, and larger cohorts will be required for adequate statistical power to address polygenic "background" effects. Genetic background has become a potential clinical tool for predicting HF outcomes and targeting therapeutic intervention. Prospective validation of the predictive impact of genetic variants will be required prior to the routine implementation of genetically individualized treatments. Ultimately, functional genomics will allow pharmacologic therapeutics to be tailored to an individual's specific genetic background.

## References

1 Thomas Coar. *The Aphorisims of Hippocrates.* Longman and Co., London, 1822:26.
2 Osler W. *The Principles and Practice of Medicine.* D. Appleton and Co., New York, 1892:623.
3 Liggett SB. Pharmacogenetic applications of the human genome project. *Nat Med* 2001; **7**:281–283.
4 Rigat B, Hubert C, Alhenc-Gelas F, Cambien F, Corvol P, Soubrier F. An insertion/deletion polymorphism in the angiotensin I-converting enzyme gene accounting for half the variance of serum enzyme levels. *J Clin Invest* 1990; **86**:1343–1346.
5 Rigat B, Hubert C, Corvol P, Soubrier F. PCR detection of the insertion/deletion polymorphism of the human angiotensin converting enzyme gene (DCP) (dipeptidyl carboxypeptidase 1). *Nucleic Acids Res* 1992; **20**:1433.
6 Tiret L, Rigat B, Visvikis S *et al.* Evidence, from combined segregation and linkage analysis, that a variant of the angiotensin I-converting enzyme (ACE) gene controls plasma ACE levels. *Am J Hum Genet* 1992; **51**:197–205.

7  Danser AH, Derkx FH, Hense HW *et al.* Angiotensino-gen (M235T) and angiotensin-converting enzyme (I/D) polymorphisms in association with plasma renin and prorenin levels. *J Hypertens* 1998; **16**:1879–1883.

8  Cambien F, Poirier O, Lecerf L *et al.* Deletion polymorphism in the gene for angiotensin-converting enzyme is a potent risk factor for myocardial infarction. *Nature* 1992; **359**:641–644.

9  Ihnken R, Verho K, Gross M, Marz W. Deletion polymorphism of the angiotensin I-converting enzyme gene is associated with increased plasma angiotensin-converting enzyme activity but not with increased risk for myocardial infarction and coronary artery disease. *Ann of Intern Med* 1996; **125**: 19–25.

10  Andersson B, Sylven C. The DD genotype of the angiotensin-converting enzyme gene is associated with increased mortality in idiopathic heart failure. *J Am Coll Cardiol* 1996; **28**:162–167.

11  Palmer BR, Pilbrow AP, Yandle TG *et al.* Angiotensin-converting enzyme gene polymorphism interacts with left ventricular ejection fraction and brain natriuretic peptide levels to predict mortality after myocardial infarction. *J Am Coll Cardiol* 2003; **41**:729–736.

12  McNamara DM, Holubkov R, Janosko K *et al.* Pharmacogenetic interactions between $\beta$-blocker therapy and the angiotensin-converting enzyme deletion polymorphism in patients with congestive heart failure. *Circulation* 2001; **103**:1644–1648.

13  McNamara DM, Holubkov R, Postava L *et al.* Phamacogenetic interactions between ACE inhibitor therapy and the angiotensin-converting enzyme deletion polymorphism in patients with congestive heart failure. *J Amer Coll Cardiol* 2004; **44**:2019–2026.

14  Campbell D. Aggrarwal A, Esler M *et al.* Beta blockers, angiotensin II, and ACE inhibitors in patients with heart failure. *Lancet* 2001; **358**:1609–1610.

15  de Groote P, Helbecque N, Lamblin N *et al.* Beta-adrenergic receptor blockade and the angiotensin-converting enzyme deletion polymorphism in patients with chronic heart failure. *Eur J Heart Fail* 2004; **6**:17–21.

16  Packer M, Poole-Wilson PA, Armstrong PW *et al.* Comparative effects of low and high doses of the angiotensin-converting enzyme inhibitor, lisinopril, on morbidity and mortality in chronic heart failure. *Circulation* 1999; **100**:2312–2318.

17  O'Toole L, Stewart M, Padfield P, Channer K. Effect of the insertion/deletion polymorphism of the angiotensin-converting enzyme gene on the response to angiotensin-converting inhibitors in patients with heart failure. *J Cardiovasc Pharmacol* 1998; **32**:988–994.

18  Kurland L, Melhus H, Karlsson J *et al.* Angiotensin-converting enzyme gene polymorphism predicts blood pressure response to angiotensin II receptor type 1 antagonist treatment in hypertensive patients. *J Hypertens* 2001; **19**:1783–1787.

19  Pitt B, Zannad F, Remme WJ *et al.* for the Randomized Aldactone Evaluation Study Investigators. The effect of spironolactone on morbidity and mortality in patients with severe heart failure. *N Engl J Med* 1999; **341**: 709–717.

20  Pitt B, Remme W, Zannad F *et al.* Eplerenone, a selective aldosterone blocker, in patients with left ventricular dysfunction after myocardial infarction. *N Engl J Med* 2003; **348**:1309–1321.

21  Cicoira M, Zanolla L, Rossi A *et al.* Failure of Aldosterone suppression despite angiotensin-converting enzyme (ACE) inhibitor administration in chronic heart failure associated with the ACE DD genotype. *J Am Coll Cardiol* 2001; **37**:1808–1812.

22  Ciocoira M, Rossi A, Bonapace S *et al.* Effects of ACE gene insertion/deletion polymorphism on response to sprironolactone in patients with chronic heart failure. *Am J Med* 2004; **116**:657–661.

23  Postava LA, Holubkov R, Janosko KM *et al.* The aldosterone synthase promoter polymorphism modulates the effect of the ACE D-allele on heart failure survival. *Circulation* 2001; **104**:9.

24  Pojoga L, Gautier L, Blanc H *et al.* Genetic determination of plasma aldosterone levels in essential hypertension. *Am J Hypertens* 1998; **11**:856–860.

25  Van Geel PP, Pinto YM, Voors AA *et al.* Angiotensin II Type I receptor A1166C gene polymorphism is associated with an increased response to angiotensin II in human arteries. *Hypertension* 2000; **35**: 717–721.

26  Liyou N, James K, Simons L *et al.* The A1166C mutation in the angiotensin II type I receptor and hypertension in the elderly. *Clin Exp Pharmacol Physiol* 1999; **26**: 525–526.

27  Berge KE, Bakken A, Bohn M, Erikssen J, Berg K. A DNA polymorphism at the angiotensin type I receptor (AT1R) locus and myocardial infarction. *Clin Genet* 1997; **52**:71–76.

28  Anderson B, Blange I, Sylven C. Angiotensin-II type 1 receptor gene polymorphism and long-term survival in patients with idiopathic congestive heart failure. *Eur J Heart Fail* 1999; **1**:363–369.

29  McNamara DM, MacGowan GA, London B. Clinical importance of beta adrenoceptor polymorphisms in cardiovascular disease. *Am J Pharmacogenomics* 2002; **2**:73–78.

30  Bristow MR. Beta adrenergic receptor blockade in the failing heart. *Circulation* 2000; **101**:558–569.

31  Buscher R, Herrmann V, Insel PA. Human adrenoceptor polymorphisms: Evolving recognition of clinical importance. *Trends Pharmacol Sci* 1999; **20**:94–99.

32 Steinberg SF. The molecular basis for distinct beta adrenergic receptor subtype action in cardiomyocytes. *Circ Res* 1999; **85**:1101–1111.

33 Lefkowitz RF, Rockman HA, Koch WJ. Catecholamines, cardiac beta adrenergic receptors and heart failure. *Circulation* 2000; **101**:1634–1637.

34 Liggett SB. Pharmacogenetics of relevant targets in asthma. *Clin Exp Allergy* 1998; **28**:77–79.

35 Liggett SB. $\beta_2$ adrenergic receptor pharmacogenetics. *Am J Respir Cirt Care Med* 2000; **161**:S197–S201.

36 Green SA, Cole G, Jacinro M *et al.* A polymorphism of the beta 2-adrenergic receptor within the fourth membrane domain alters ligand binding and functional properties of the receptor. *J Biol Chem* 1993; **268**:32166–32121.

37 Turki J, Lorenz JN, Green SA *et al.* Myocardial signaling defects and impaired cardiac function of human beta 2-adrenergic receptor polymorphism expressed in transgenic mice. *Proc Natl Acad Sci* 1996; **93**:10483–10488.

38 Liggett SB, Wagoner LE, Craft LL *et al.* The Ile164 $\beta_2$ adrenergic receptor polymorphism adversely affects the outcome of congestive heart failure. *J Clin Invest* 1998; **102**:1534–1539.

39 Wagoner LE, Craft LL, Singh B *et al.* Polymorphisms of the $\beta_2$ adrenergic receptor determine exercise capacity in patients with heart failure. *Circ Res* 2000; **86**:834–840.

40 Brodde OE, Busher R, Tellkamp R, Radke J, Dhein S, Insel PA. Blunted cardiac responses to receptor activation in subjects with Thr164Ile $\beta_2$ adrenoceptors. *Circulation* 2001; **103**:1048–1050.

41 Feldman RD. Adrenergic receptor polymorphisms in cardiac function (and dysfunction): A failure to communicate? *Circulation* 2001; **103**:1042–1043.

42 Timmermann B, Mo R, Luft FC *et al.* $\beta_2$ adrenoceptor genetic variation is associated with genetic predisposition to essential hypertension: The Bergen blood pressure study. *Kidney Int* 1998; **53**:1455–1460.

43 Busjahn A, Li GH, Faulhaber HD *et al.* $\beta_2$ adrenergic receptor gene variations, blood pressure, and heart size in normal twins. *Hypertension* 2000; **35**:555–562.

44 Maqbool A, Hall AS, Paul SG, Balmforth AJ. Common polymorphisms of $\beta_1$ adrenoceptor: Identification and rapid screening assay. *Lancet* 1999; **353**:897–899.

45 Levin MC, Marullo S, Muntaner O *et al.* The myocardium protective variant of the Gly-49 variant of the beta 1 adrenergic receptor exhibits constitutive activity and increased desensitization and down-regulation. *J Biol Chem* 2002; **34**:30429–30435.

46 Rathz DA, Brown KM, Kramer LA, Liggett SB. Amino acid 49 polymorphisms of the human beta 1 adrenergic receptor affect agonist promoted trafficking. *J Cardiovasc Pharmacol* 2002; **39**:155–160.

47 Mason DA, Moore JD, Green SA, Liggett SB. A gain of function polymorphism in a g-protein coupling domain of the human $\beta_1$ adrenergic receptor. *J Biol Chem* 1999; **274**:12670–12474.

48 Ranade K, Jorgenson E, Sheu WH *et al.* A polymorphism in the beta 1 receptor is associated with resting heart rate. *Am J Hum Genet* 2002; **70**:935–942.

49 Borjesson M, Magnusson Y, Hjalmarson A, Andersson B. A novel polymorphism in the gene coding for the $\beta_1$ adrenergic receptor associated with survival in patients with heart failure. *Eur Heart J* 2000; **21**:1810–1812.

50 Postava L, Mahlab D, Holubkov R *et al.* $\beta_1$ and $\beta_2$ Adrenergic receptor Polymorphisms and heart failure survival: interaction with beta blockade (Abstract). *Circulation* 2002; **19**:II–611.

51 Liggett SB, Wagoner LE, Levin AM *et al.* Synergistic polymorphisms of Beta 1 and alpha 2c adrenergic receptors and the risk of congestive heart failure. *N Engl J Med* 2002; **347**:1135–1142.

52 Liggett SB. Presentation at the Heart Failure Society of America, Late Breaking Clinical Trials, (with permission), Toronto, September, 2004.

53 White HL, de Boar RA, Maqbool A *et al.* An evaluation of the beta-1 adrenergic receptor Arg389Gly polymorphism in individuals with heart failure: a MERIT-HF substudy. *Eur J Heart Fail* 2003; **5**:463–468.

54 Johnson JA, Zineh I, Puckett BJ *et al.* Beta-1 adrenergic receptor polymorphisms and antihypertensive response to metoprolol. *Clin Pharmacol Ther* 2003; **74**:44–52.

55 Brodde OR, Stein CM. The Gly389Arg beta 1 adrenergic receptor polymorphism: a predictor of response to beta-blocker treatment? *Clin Pharmacol Ther* 2003; **74**:299–302.

56 Kelly RA, Balligand JL, Smith TW. Nitric oxide and cardiac function. *Circ Res* 1996; **79**:363–380.

57 Drexler H. Nitric oxide synthases in the failing human heart: A double-edged sword? *Circulation* 1999; **99**:2972–2975.

58 Philip I, Plantefeve G, Vuillaumier-Barrot S *et al.* G894T polymorphism in the endothelial nitric oxide synthase gene is associated with an enhanced vascular responsiveness to phenylephrine. *Circulation* 1999; **99**:3096–3098.

59 Tesauro M, Thompson WC, Rogliani P *et al.* Intracellular processing of endothelial nitric oxide synthase isoforms associated with differences in severity of cardiopulmonary diseases: Cleavage of proteins with aspartate vs. glutamate at position 298. *Proc Natl Acad Sci USA* 2000; **97**:2832–2835.

60 McNamara DM, Holubkov R, Postava L *et al.* The Asp[298] variant of endothelial nitric oxide synthase: Effect on Survival for patients with congestive heart failure. *Circulation* 2003; **107**:1598–1602.

61 Yang XP, Liu YH, Sheseley EG *et al.* Endothelial nitric oxide gene knockout mice cardiac phenotypes and the effect of angiotensin-converting enzyme inhibitor on

myocardial ischemia/reperfusion injury. *Hypertension* 1999; **34**:24–30.

62 Bedi M, Murali S, MacGowan G *et al*. High dose ACE inhibitors reduces the impact of the NOS3 Asp298 variant on heart failure survival (Abstract). *Circulation* 2003; **1085**:IV–444.

63 Morisaki T, Gross M, Morisaki H *et al*. Molecular basis of AMP deaminase deficiency in skeletal muscle. *Proc Natl Acad Sci USA* 1992; **89**:6457–6461.

64 Sinkeler SP, Joosten EM, Weavers RA *et al*. Myoadenylate Deaminase deficiency: a clinical, genetic, and biochemical study in nine families. *Muscle Nerve* 1988; **11**: 312–317.

65 Dubey RK, Gillespie DG, Mi Z, Jackson EK. Exogenous and endogenous adenosine inhibits fetal calf serum-induced growth of rat cardiac fibroblasts: role of A2B receptors. *Circulation* 1997; **96**:2656–2666.

66 Anderson JL, Habashi J, Carlquist JF *et al*. A common variant of the AMPD1 gene predicts improved cardiovascular survival in patients with coronary artery disease. *J Am Coll Cardiol* 2000; **36**:1248–1252.

67 Loh E, Rebbeck TR, Mahoney PD *et al*. Common variant in AMPD1 gene predicts improved clinical outcome in patients with heart failure. *Circulation* 1999; **99**: 1422–1425.

68 Yazaki Y, Muhlestein JB, Carlquist JF *et al*. A common variant of the AMPD1 gene predicts improved survival in patients with ischemic left ventricular dysfunction. *J Card Fail* 2004; **10**:316–320.

69 Auseon AJ, Ferguson JP, Cooke GE, Binkley PF. Association of a common variant in the AMPD1 gene with exercise capacity in patients with heart failure: prelude to a positive prognosis? *J Card Fail* 2004; **10**:S58.

70 Levine B, Kalman J, Mayer L *et al*. Elevated circulating levels of tumor necrosis factor in severe chronic heart failure. *N Engl J Med* 1990; **223**:236–241.

71 Ferrari R, Bachetti T, Confortini R *et al*. Tumor necrosis factor soluble receptors in patients with various degrees of congestive heart failure. *Circulation* 1995; **92**: 1479–1486.

72 Torre-Amione G, Kapadia S *et al*. Proinflammatory cytokine levels in patients with depressed left ventricular ejection fraction: a report from the studies of left ventricular dysfunction (SOLVD). *J Am Coll Cardiol* 1996; **27**:1201–1206.

73 Nozaki N, Yamaguchi S, Shirakabe M *et al*. Soluble tumor necrosis factor receptors are elevated in relation to severity of congestive heart failure. *Jpn Circ J* 1997; **61**:657–664.

74 Wilson AG, di Giovine FS, Blakemore AIF, Duff GW. Single base polymorphism in the human tumor necrosis factor alpha (TNF-$\alpha$) gene detected by Nco1 restriction of the PCR product. *Hum Mol Genet* 1992; **1**:353.

75 Wilson AG, Symons JA, McDowell TL *et al*. Effects of a tumor necrosis factor (TNF-$\alpha$) promoter base transition on transcriptional activity. *Br J of Rheumatol* 1994; **33**:89.

76 Wilson AG, Giovine FS, Duff GW. Genetics of tumor necrosis factor in autoimmune, infectious and neoplastic diseases. *J Inflamm* 1995; **45**:1–12.

77 Danis V, Millington M, Hyland V *et al*. Increased frequency of the uncommon allele of a tumor necrosis factor $\alpha$ gene polymorphism in Rheumatoid Arthritis and Systemic Lupus Erythematosus. *Dis Markers* 1994; **12**:127–133.

78 Ito M, Takahashi H, Fuse K *et al*. Polymorphisms of tumor necrosis factor-alpha and interleukin-10 genes in Japanese patients with idiopathic dilated cardiomyopathy. *Jpn Heart J* 2000; **41**:183–191.

79 Kubota T, McNamara DM *et al*. Effect of tumor necrosis factor gene polymorphisms on patients with congestive heart failure. *Circulation* 1998; **97**:2499–2501.

80 Spinale FG. Matrix metalloproteinases: regulation and dysregulation in the failing heart. *Circ Res* 2002; **90**:520–530.

81 Spinale FG, Gunasinghe H, Sprunger PD *et al*. Extracellular degradative pathways in myocardial remodeling and progression to heart failure. *Card Fail* 2002; **8**: S332–S338.

82 Wilson EM, Gunasinghe HR, Coker ML *et al*. Plasma matrix metalloproteinase and inhibitor profiles in patients with heart failure. *J Card Fail* 2002; **8**:390–398.

83 Bradham WS, Moe G, Wendt KA *et al*. TNF-alpha and myocardial matrix metalloproteinases in heart failure: relationship to LV remodeling. *Am J Physiol Heart Circ Physiol* 2002; **282**:H1288–1295.

84 Medley TL, Kingwell BA, Gatzka CD *et al*. Matrix metalloproteinase-3 genotype contributes to age-related aortic stiffening through modulation of gene and protein expression. *Circ Res* 2003; **92**:1254–1261.

85 Blankenberg S, Rupprecht HJ, Poirier O *et al*. AtheroGene Investigators, Plasma concentrations and genetic variation of matrix metalloproteinase 9 and prognosis of patients with cardiovascular disease. *Circulation* 2003; **107**:1579–1578.

86 Zhang B, Ye S, Herrmann SM *et al*. Functional polymorphism in the regulatory region of gelatinase B gene in relation to severity of coronary atherosclerosis. *Circulation* 1999; **99**:1788–1794.

87 Lamblin N, Bauters C, Hermant X *et al*. Polymorphisms in the promoter regions of MMP-2, MMP-3, MMP-9 and MMP-12 genes as determinants of aneurysmal coronary artery disease. *J Am Coll Cardiol* 2002; **40**:43–48.

88 Beyzade S, Zhang S, Wong YK *et al*. Influences of matrix metalloproteinase-3 gene variation on extent of coronary atherosclerosis and risk of myocardial infarction. *J Am Coll Cardiol* 2003; **41**:2130–2137.

89  Cho HJ, Chae IH, Park KW *et al.* Functional polymorph-
    ism in the promoter region of the gelatinase B gene in
    relation to coronary artery disease and restenosis after
    percutaneous coronary intervention. *J Hum Genet* 2002;
    **47**:88–91.

90  Mizon-Gerard F, de Groote P *et al.* Prognostic impact
    of matrix metalloproteinase gene polymorphisms in
    patients with heart failure according to the aetiology of
    left ventricular systolic dysfunction. *Eur Heart J* 2004;
    **25**:688–693.

91  Shah AN, Tobelmann P, Afari-Armah N *et al.*
    Genetic variation in MMP-3 (stromelysin), pheno-
    type and clinical outcomes in patients with congest-
    ive heart failure (Abstract). *Circulation* 2004; **110**:
    III–555.

92  Shah AN, Tobelmann P, Sheppard R *et al.* Genetic
    Variation in MMP-9 (Gelatinase-B) LV Remodeling
    and Clinical Outcomes in Patients with Congest-
    ive Heart Failure (Abstract). *Circulation* 2004; **110**:
    III–445.

**CHAPTER 17**

# Management of diastolic dysfunction

*Arthur M. Feldman,* MD, PHD *& Bonita Falkner,* MD

## Introduction

Patients with 'heart failure' present with a classic triad of symptoms including shortness of breath, overwhelming fatigue, and edema and have physical findings that include signs of diminished cardiac output and/or volume overload. Historically, the pattern of signs and symptoms attributable to 'heart failure' were thought to reflect abnormalities in the systolic performance of the ventricular myocardium. However, it is being increasingly recognized that a significant proportion of patients with signs and symptoms of 'heart failure' have normal or near normal ejection fractions. Indeed, studies demonstrate that between 30% and 55% of patients with clinical heart failure have an ejection fraction of ≥45% [1–4]. These patients with normal ejection fractions have symptoms secondary to marked impairment in diastolic function [5]. While systolic dysfunction represents an inability of the myofibrils to shorten against a load diastolic dysfunction occurs when the myofibrils do not rapidly or completely return to their resting length thereby resulting in a slowing of ventricular filling [6]. These changes in diastolic function appear to be more common in women, the elderly, and those with a history of hypertension [1,7–9]. In addition, recent studies have also demonstrated an important relationship between diabetes and the development of diastolic dysfunction [2,10].

Overall annual mortality rates in patients with diastolic heart failure have been reported between 5% and 8% [11–15]. While less than the annual mortality rates reported for patients with systolic heart failure (10–15%) the presence of diastolic dysfunction is not without serious consequences even in the absence of symptoms. For example, in the Cardiovascular Health Study of the elderly, Aurigemma *et al.* obtained echocardiographic data from 2671 subjects without known coronary artery disease, heart failure, or atrial fibrillation. After a mean follow-up of 5.2 years, 6.4% of the cohort developed heart failure – 57% had a normal or borderline ejection fraction at the time of development of heart failure [16]. Similarly, in the Strong Heart Study, a population-based assessment of 3008 middle-aged and elderly American Indians, abnormal diastolic function was associated with a marked increase in the risk of death [17]. Furthermore, although survival appears to be somewhat better in heart failure patients with normal ejection fractions, the hospitalization rates for both populations appear to be very similar [4,18,19].

Because of the growing recognition that a large proportion of patients presenting with symptomatic 'heart failure' have a normal or only slightly reduced ejection fraction, there has been an increasing interest in developing strategies for the treatment of this challenging group of patients. Unfortunately, historically, patients with heart failure and normal ejection fractions have been systematically excluded from large multicenter heart failure trials and therefore there is no proven treatment for this group of patients. However, recent gains in our understanding of the biology of cardiac function and remodeling, new investigator-initiated clinical trials, and several recent multicenter industry-sponsored clinical trials have begun to

**Table 17.1** Management principles for patients with diastolic heart failure.

| Goal | Treatment |
|---|---|
| Reduce the congestive state | Salt restriction |
| | Diuretics |
| | ACE inhibitors |
| | Angiotensin II – receptor blockers |
| Maintain atrial contraction and prevent tachycardia | Cardioversion of atrial fibrillation |
| | Sequential atrioventricular pacing |
| | Beta blockers |
| | Calcium channel blockers |
| | Radiofrequency ablation modification of atrioventricular node and pacing |
| Treat and prevent myocardial ischemia | Nitrates |
| | Beta blockers |
| | Calcium channel blockers |
| | Coronary-artery bypass surgery, percutaneous coronary intervention |
| Control hypertension | Antihypertensive agents |
| Measures with theoretical benefit in diastolic heart failure | |
| Promote regression of hypertrophy and prevent myocardial fibrosis | ACE inhibitors |
| | ARBs |
| | Spironolactone |

*Source*: Adapted from [21].

allow us to formulate a more rational and effective treatment strategy for this complex group of patients (Table 17.1).

## Pathophysiology of diastolic dysfunction

Diastolic dysfunction has been defined as a group of abnormalities in the mechanical properties of the heart that include decreased left ventricular (LV) diastolic distensibility, impaired ventricular filling, and a slowing or delay in myocardial relaxation [6]. These changes can be associated with heart failure symptoms or can be found by non-invasive (echocardiography) or invasive (cardiac catheterization) assessment of an otherwise asymptomatic individual. Cardiac diastole is biphasic and begins with the energy-dependent relaxation of the ventricular myocardium as individual myofibrils return to their resting length. This relaxation of the ventricular myocardium facilitates rapid ventricular filling as blood moves from an area of higher pressure in the atria to the area of lower pressure in the ventricle.

During the second phase of diastole, the atria contract and further facilitate ventricular filling with the amount of late filling being determined by the force of the atrial contraction, the pressure of the left atria and the stiffness of the ventricle [20]. Thus, diastolic function is determined by the efficiency with which the ventricle actively relaxes during isovolumic relaxation and the passive elastic properties of the left ventricle [21].

When ventricular filling is impaired during the rapid filling phase, the shape of the diastolic pressure–volume relationship changes and higher left atrial pressures are required to provide optimal filling volumes especially at rapid heart rates [22]. This leads to an elevated left ventricular end-diastolic pressure. Similarly, diastolic dysfunction during the late filling phase of diastole due to ventricular stiffness can also lead to an increased left ventricular end-diastolic pressure. Thus, even a small increase in central blood volume, an increase in venous tone, or an increase in arterial stiffness or in peripheral vascular resistance can result in a profound increase in left atrial and pulmonary venous pressures resulting in a marked diminution in exercise tolerance or in the development of acute pulmonary edema [23].

Energy-dependent ventricular diastolic relaxation can be decreased by a number of biologic changes in the heart including decreased energy availability and changes in calcium homeostasis [24]. Relaxation can be delayed by anything that interferes with cross-bridge detachment or with preceding calcium removal from the cytosol including prolongation of the calcium transient because of reduced resequestration into the sarcoplasmic reticulum, abnormal extrusion by the sodium/calcium exchanger, interference with cross-bridge uncoupling by abnormal high-energy phosphate metabolism, and abnormalities of the contractile proteins themselves that affect their interaction or calcium sensitivity [25]. Indeed, alterations in the expression of the calcium handling proteins including calcium-ATPase and phospholamban and by proteins that modify their function through phosphorylation including protein kinase A and protein kinase C have been identified in failing human heart [26–29]. Relaxation can also be delayed by alterations in the contractile proteins [30]. Since most of these processes are energy dependent, conditions that are associated with decreased ATP availability including ischemia, increased diastolic calcium concentration, or a delay in the decline of diastolic calcium concentration may also significantly impair relaxation [31]. Recent interest has also focused on titin a macromolecule located within the sarcomere that appears to alter passive stiffness in heart through expression of alternative isoforms but which can also be post-translationally modified by calcium and by phosphorylation [32–36].

Diastolic function can also be altered by changes in the passive properties of the ventricle. For example, ventricular hypertrophy can increase ventricular stiffness and thereby impair diastolic function when wall thickness increases disproportionately to changes in chamber size – a phenomenon seen commonly in patients with long standing hypertension or with aortic stenosis [20]. This pathologic hypertrophy must be distinguished from hypertrophy secondary to exercise training in which the growth of muscular and nonmuscular elements is proportional and diastolic dysfunction

does not occur [37]. Another potentially important, though controversial, contributor to myocardial stiffness in patients with cardiac disease is intracellular fibrosis and changes in collagen isoforms [38]. Individual myocytes are surrounded by a collagen network that is composed of filamentous struts, perimysial fibers, and epimysial fibers. These fibers form an intricate latticework that supports both contractile and vascular cells and allows the movement of individual myocytes to be translated into a unified contraction by the entire muscle mass. The homeostasis of this collagen network is modulated over time by the balanced activity of a group of matrix metalloproteinases (MMPs) and inhibitors of matrix metalloproteinases (TIMPs) that are found in the ventricular myocardium [39,40]. Studies suggest that alterations in the amount and isoform structure of these collagen fibers can contribute to changes in diastolic function and that alterations in the expression of MMPs and TIMPs can be correlated with the functional integrity of the heart in patients with both hypertrophy and failure [41,42]. Furthermore, collagen turnover and deposition in the heart appears to be regulated by neurohormones including angiotensin II and aldosterone that are elevated in patients with both heart failure and hypertension and are associated with increased myocardial fibrosis and stiffness while inhibition of the renin–angiotensin–aldosterone system has been associated with reduced myocardial stiffness and fibrosis [43,44]. However, recent studies have questioned whether MMP activity is associated with increased myocardial stiffness because of direct changes in collagen turnover or due to non-collagen related pathways [45,46]. Regardless, the MMPs and TIMPs are being pursued as potential therapeutic targets in the treatment of patients with both systolic and diastolic cardiac dysfunction.

## Diagnosing diastolic heart failure

According to guidelines provided by the American College of Cardiology/American Heart Association, the diagnosis of diastolic heart failure is 'based on the finding of typical symptoms and signs of heart failure in a patient who is shown to have a normal left ventricular ejection fraction and no

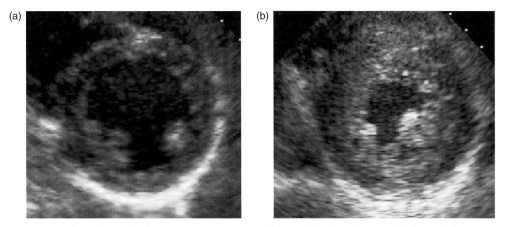

**Figure 17.1** 2D echocardiographic short axis images of a normal left ventricle (a) and concentric left ventricular hypertrophy (b).

valvular abnormalities on echocardiogram' [47]. The echocardiogram also allows the clinician to rule out other diagnosis that might also cause heart failure or heart failure symptoms in the setting of a normal ejection fraction including acute mitral or aortic regurgitation or myocardial constriction (Figure 17.1). The addition of Doppler imaging may be helpful in assessing the presence of diastolic dysfunction by measuring the height and timing of the E and A waves that reflect early diastolic filling and late diastolic filling respectively (Figure 17.2). An E/A ratio less than 0.75 or greater than 1.5 is consistent with diastolic dysfunction. However, diastolic dysfunction may also be present with an E/A ratio between 0.75 and 1.5 if other parameters, such as the deceleration time, are abnormal [48,49]. Furthermore, a recent study suggests that the diagnosis of diastolic dysfunction should not be based on a single echo-Doppler parameter but rather multiple parameters should be examined in concert and should be related to the clinical observation [21]. The recent development of tissue Doppler echocardiography, which uses pulsed wave Doppler to measure the velocity of myocardial motion rather than blood flow, has provided another method to measure diastolic performance that is less influenced by preload [50]. Cardiac catheterization using conductance catheters and measurement of pressure–volume relationships remains the gold standard for the evaluation of left ventricular filling pressures and left ventricular diastolic function; however, an invasive

assessment is usually performed only when there is a suspicion that myocardial ischemia is playing an important role in the rapid onset of heart failure [21].

## Pharmacolgic treatment of diastolic dysfunction

### Initial management of a patient with new onset heart failure

The initial management of patients with diastolic heart failure is aimed at reducing pulmonary venous pressure and thereby reducing symptoms of congestion. Diuretics play a key role in lowering total systemic volume and in relieving the symptoms of pulmonary congestion. In addition, patients may benefit from supplemental oxygen, morphine, and nitroglycerin. Diuresis is a double-edged sword in patients with diastolic dysfunction because of their steep curve for left ventricular diastolic pressure in relation to volume [21]. These patients often require higher filling pressures in order to insure that atrial pressures exceed ventricular pressures during the early ventricular filling period. Attention must also be given to precipitating causes of worsening heart failure symptoms including severe hypertension, ischemia, sinus tachycardia, or loss of sinus rhythm. In the acute setting, in the presence of severe hypertension, patients may respond most effectively to the parenteral administration of sodium nitroprusside which can allow for careful titration of the blood

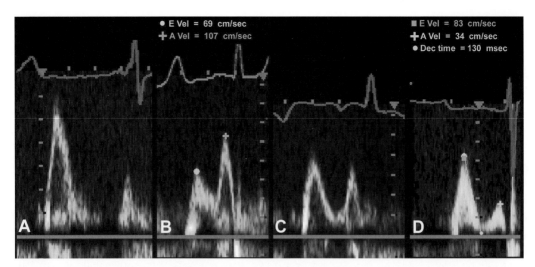

**Figure 17.2** Transmitral Doppler flow demonstrating the stages of diastolic dysfunction. Panel A represents a young normal, with brisk early filling after the opening of the mitral valve (E wave), and a smaller atrial component (A wave), with a ratio of greater than 1.5 : 1. With early diastolic dysfunction (stage 1), impaired early relaxation leads to a lower gradient between the left atrium and left ventricle after mitral opening, and the E wave component lessens in velocity and increases in duration (Panel B). The ratio of E to A lessens to the 0.75 : 1, and deceleration time increases, usually between 150–270 ms. Panel C demonstrates the phenomenon of 'pseudonormalization', known as stage 2 diastolic dysfunction. As left atrial pressure rises, the pressure gradient between the left atrium and left ventricle increases, and the E wave velocity increases relative to the A wave. This 1 : 1 ratio is seen in older normals, and is therefore called pseudonormalization. The underlying relaxation abnormality can be elicited by Valsalva maneuver which decreases left atrial pressure and unmasks the underlying E to A reversal. Stage 3 diastolic dysfunction is shown in Panel D. Further decrease in left ventricular compliance, elevation of left atrial pressure and loss of atrial function lead to a restrictive pattern, with shortened early filling (deceleration time less than 140 ms) and diminished A wave (E to A ratio >1.5 : 1), as the atrium fails to generate pressure. Note the similarity between end stage restrictive physiology and the young normal.

pressure to appropriate levels. Nitroglycerin may be useful when ischemia complicates the clinical setting; however, appropriate actions must be taken consistent with published guidelines in the setting of an acute coronary syndrome. Even in the absence of obstructive coronary artery disease, tachycardia can have important consequences in patients with diastolic dysfunction because it shortens relaxation time in an already compromised ventricle thereby increasing end-diastolic pressure and further compromising ventricular filling. When tachycardia is secondary to atrial fibrillation with a rapid ventricular response and is accompanied by pulmonary edema and/or hypertension urgent cardioversion is often indicated [21]. In patients who have a less urgent need for rate control beta blockers or nondihyrdropyridine calcium channel blockers may be useful [47,51]. Although many clinicians begin neurohormonal modulators in the acute setting, neither an intravenous beta blocker nor a calcium channel blocker acutely alters left

ventricular compliance in patients with ventricular hypertrophy and normal resting systolic function. Thus, at least in the acute sense, chamber compliance is principally determined by passive structural elements rather than by active processes in the heart and immediate measures must be utilized that alter ventricular filling pressures by modulating pre-load and after-load.

## Chronic management of patients with diastolic dysfunction

Unlike the wealth of information regarding the efficacy of pharmacologic therapy in patients with heart failure secondary to systolic dysfunction, there have been virtually no large randomized and placebo-controlled clinical trials that have evaluated the role of selective pharmacologic strategies in patients with diastolic dysfunction. None-the-less, investigators have pursued smaller, investigator-initiated trials for nearly two decades. While these trials have often involved short term follow-up and have often measured surrogate endpoints they have influenced physician perspectives. However, they illustrate the limitations of our knowledge base regarding the therapy of diastolic dysfunction as they represent the only fundamental knowledge base that is available. Therefore, we will review a representative number of these trials – and in particular those that may have influenced both clinicians and investigators in their approach to this disease.

## Angiotensin converting enzyme inhibitors and angiotensin receptor antagonists

Because angiotensin II mediates myocyte hypertrophy, extracellular collagen matrix formation, peripheral vasoconstriction, and release of aldosterone, investigators hypothesized that an Angiotensin converting enzyme (ACE) inhibitor might diminish left ventricular hypertrophy and left ventricular mass in patients with cardiovascular disease. Indeed, ACE inhibitors reduce both left ventricular mass and regress left ventricular hypertrophy in animal models and reduce left ventricular volumes and improve left ventricular systolic function in patients with coronary disease when administered early after a myocardial infarction or in patients with left ventricular systolic dysfunction [52–54]. Initial studies focused on patients with systemic hypertension – a group of patients who develop diastolic dysfunction earlier and in parallel to an increase in blood pressure and left ventricular mass [55]. For example, reductions in left ventricular hypertrophy were seen in the Prospective Randomized Enalapril Study Evaluating Regression of Ventricular Enlargement (PRESERVE) that was designed to assess whether the calcium channel blocker nifedipine or the ACE inhibitor enalapril was more effective in reducing left ventricular mass in a group of patients with essential hypertension [56]. Although a significant difference could not be shown between enalapril and long-acting nifedipine both effected a moderately beneficial and statistically significant regression in left ventricular hypertrophy.

In a recent substudy of the Heart Outcomes Prevention Evaluation (HOPE) trial, investigators assessed the effects of the ACE inhibitor ramipril in a subset of patients with controlled blood pressure and preserved left ventricular ejection fraction. When compared with placebo, ramipril (10 mg/day) significantly decreased left ventricular mass, left ventricular end-diastolic volume, and left ventricular end-systolic volumes [57]. In the Valsartan in Acute Myocardial Infarction (VALIANT) Echo substudy, either the ACE inhibitor captopril, the angiotensin receptor blocker (ARB) valsartan, or the combination of captopril plus valsartan effectively reduced ventricular volumes to an equal degree in patients who had left ventricular enlargement and systolic dysfunction [58]. While these studies were consistent with studies demonstrating the ability of both ACE inhibitors and ARBs to reduce left ventricular mass [59–63], they assessed a surrogate endpoint, that is, left ventricular hypertrophy, and did not address the question of whether either ACE inhibitors or ARBs could improve survival and decrease morbidity in patients with heart failure and preserved systolic function.

Recently, the Candesartan in Heart Failure – Assessment of Reduction in Mortality and Morbidity (CHARM) study attempted to address the role of angiotensin receptor blockade in patients with symptomatic diastolic dysfunction [64]. The CHARM study consisted of three investigational arms: CHARM-alternative examined the efficacy of candesartan in patients with systolic heart failure (EF ≤40%) who were intolerant of ACE inhibitors, CHARM-added assessed the efficacy of candesartan in patients who remained symptomatic despite therapy with an ACE inhibitor, while CHARM-preserved assessed the efficacy of candesartan in patients with an ejection fraction ≥40% [65]. In over 3000 patients in the CHARM-preserved arm who were followed for a mean of 36.6 months, candesartan did not effect a significant benefit when assessing the primary endpoint of cardiovascular death or heart failure hospitalizations as cardiovascular deaths were not different in the two groups. However, fewer patients in the candesartan group were hospitalized for worsening heart failure. Although disappointing, the results of CHARM-preserved may not accurately have represented outcomes in patients who have symptomatic heart failure secondary to diastolic dysfunction because the demographics of the population was somewhat different than would be expected in a population with pure diastolic dysfunction: the mean age was younger (67 years), only 40% of the subjects were women, coronary disease was far more frequent than expected, and patients had mild systolic dysfunction as evidenced by a mean ejection fraction <50%. Thus, the population in CHARM might have represented a group of patients with predominantly systolic dysfunction who improved their ejection fraction as a result of earlier aggressive therapy with beta blockers [66]. However, the importance of CHARM is that it demonstrates clearly that large randomized and placebo-controlled clinical trials can be carried out in a large population of patients with heart failure and normal systolic function.

Definitive information regarding the role of ACE inhibitors and angiotensin receptor antagonists in the therapy of patients with preserved ejection fraction and heart failure symptoms will hopefully be forthcoming from the results of the ongoing Irbesartan in Heart Failure with preserved EF (I-PRESERVE) trial that is presently enrolling patients [66]. In contrast with CHARM, the I-PRESERVE trial will enroll only patients who are ≥60 years of age and have an EF >45%. Importantly, patients with a history of moderate or severe systolic dysfunction are excluded. Follow-up is expected to be completed in early 2007.

## Calcium channel blockers

The calcium channel blockers nifedipine and verapamil have been used extensively in the treatment of hypertension [67] and have been demonstrated to decrease left ventricular mass after sustained therapy [68,69]. The Prospective Randomized Enalpril Study Evaluating Reversal of Ventricular Enlargement (PRESERVE) study was planned to test the hypothesis that the ACE inhibitor enalpril was more effective than the calcium channel blocker mifedipine in reversing left ventricular hypertrophy and improving diastolic left ventricular filling [70]. However, in an ethnically diverse population of 303 men and women with essential hypertension and increased left ventricular mass at screening echocardiography, the investigators could not demonstrate a difference in diastolic filling when comparing the two treatment options; although both left ventricular mass and diastolic filling improved in both

groups during the course of the trial. These results differed from an early meta-analysis that had suggested that ACE inhibitors reduced left ventricular mass more than calcium channel blockers or other treatments when the degree of reduction in blood pressure and the baseline left ventricular mass were factored into the analysis [59] and also differed from an earlier study that had failed to demonstrate an effect of the dihydropyridine calcium channel blockers on left ventricular hypertrophy [71]. However, the investigators suggested that the salutary benefits with dihydropyridine calcium channel blockers reported in the PRESERVE trial might have been due to the use of longer-acting preparations with a lower profile of sympathetic activation and edema [56]. This hypothesis is supported by the recent finding that diltiazem significantly improved diastolic properties in patients with hypertrophic cardiomyopathy [72].

## Beta-blocker therapy

Several early reports in small populations suggested that beta-blocker therapy improved diastolic function [73–76]. However, these studies were limited by their relatively small size, the inclusion of relatively younger subjects with dilated cardiomyopathy and systolic dysfunction, and the lack of long-term follow-up. However, interesting information comes from the echocardiographic substudy of the Metoprolol CR/XL Randomized Intervention Trial in Heart Failure (MERIT-HF) trial [77]. A total of 66 patients were examined three times during a 12-month period by physicians who were blinded to their treatment group. In those patients receiving metoprolol CR/XL, there was a significant increase in ejection fraction. In addition, there were changes in the deceleration time of the early mitral filling wave, the time velocity integral of the E-wave, and the duration of the late mitral filling wave that were significant and were reflective of an improvement in diastolic performance. Interestingly, the improvement in systolic function did not predict the changes in diastolic function, thus suggesting that improved diastolic function was not due solely to the improvement in systolic function. These salutary benefits of beta blockade were not metoprolol-specific as similar results were seen in a substudy of the CHRISTMAS trial (carvedilol hibernation reversible ischaemia trial;

marker of success) [78,79]. The substudy analysis of both the MERIT-HF and CHRISTMAS trials were limited by the fact that these studies included patients who had both systolic and diastolic dysfunction. Important information regarding the efficacy of beta-blocker therapy in patients with diastolic dysfunction also comes from the recent Swedish Doppler-echocardiographic study (SWEDIC) [80]. In this trial, 113 patients with diastolic heart failure who were symptomatic with normal systolic left ventricular function and abnormal diastolic function were randomized to receive either carvedilol or placebo. After uptitartion, treatment was continued for 6 months. Although a composite endpoint of four integrated quantitative assessments was not statistically significant, there was a statistically significant improvement in E:A ratio in patients treated with carvedilol when compared with those receiving placebo. This effect was particularly robust in those patients with a higher heart rate at baseline. Thus, taken together, these studies suggest that beta blockers might have salutary benefits in patients with heart failure and normal systolic performance. However, larger, placebo-controlled randomized trials will be necessary to definitively test this hypothesis.

The Study of Effects of Nebivolol Intervention on Outcomes and Rehospitalizations in Seniors with Heart Failure (SENIORS) recently assessed the effectiveness of a $\beta$1-selective antagonist in a large cohort of patients over the age of 70 [81,82]. Nebivolol effected a significant reduction in the primary endpoint of death or cardiovascular hospitalization and there was a modest trend towards an improvement in mortality. Approximately 20% of the treatment group had an ejection fraction $\geq$45% – similar to that group of patients in CHARM-preserved. Although the results in this select group of patients was not presented, subgroup analysis suggested no apparent difference between those with an EF of less than or greater than 35%. However, this data is somewhat difficult to interpret because of the enrollment of patients with systolic heart failure who may simply have improved their ejection fractions secondary to optimal pharmacologic therapy. Regardless of the lack of clarity in this group of studies, many clinicians view beta blockers as being a key therapeutic intervention in patients with heart failure.

## Aldosterone antagonists

Aldosterone has been implicated in the development of myocardial fibrosis, hypertrophy, and dysfunction. Improved outcome in patients with systolic heart failure who have received the aldosterone antagonist spironolactone have been associated with an antifibrotic effect of the drug [83–85]. Thus, investigators hypothesized that aldosterone antagonism might decrease left ventricular remodeling in patients with diastolic dysfunction secondary hypertensive heart disease and normal left ventricular function. To test this hypothesis, Mottram et al. randomized 30 medically treated ambulatory hypertensive patients with exertional dyspnea, echocardiographically verified diastolic dysfunction, and an ejection fraction of >50% to receive either 25 mg/day spironolactone or placebo for 6 months [86]. Patients who received spironlactone demonstrated an increase in long-axis strain rate, peak systolic strain, and cyclic variation of integrated backscatter at 6 months when compared with patients receiving placebo. These changes were consistent with a change in systolic performance. However, spironolactone-treated patients also exhibited a reduction in posterior wall thickness, and a trend to a reduced left atrial area, changes consistent with a reduction in LV stiffness, and/or end-diastolic pressure. Thus, in this albeit small study, the investigators provided the first suggestion that an aldosterone antagonist could improve function in patients with diastolic dysfunction. However, additional studies are required.

## Digoxin

An interesting therapeutic conundrum has been the role of digoxin in the therapy of patients with diastolic dysfunction. The DIG ancillary trial enrolled nearly 1000 patients who were in sinus rhythm and had a left ventricular ejection fraction >45%. Although the results of this trial have not been published, the results in the total population did not show a benefit of digoxin when assessing the primary outcome of mortality [66,87]. However, digoxin effected a significant benefit in reducing heart failure hospitalizations and a trend towards a decrease in the risk of either death or a hospitalization for worsening heart failure. Although these results have led investigators to suggest that digoxin might benefit patients with both systolic and diastolic dysfunction, the inotropic properties of digoxin are intuitively counterproductive in patients who have a normal or near normal ejection fraction. Indeed, inotropic agent are considered contraindicated in patients with hypertrophic obstructive cardiomyopathy – and should probably not be considered in the treatment of patients with normal left ventricular ejection fractions and diastolic dysfunction.

## Control of hypertension

Perhaps the most fundamental therapy for the treatment of diastolic dysfunction is control of systemic blood pressure. In many patients, blood pressure control can be obtained simply with a single agent. However, in other patients, blood pressure control is more challenging and requires poly-pharmacy. Therefore, it is relevant to at least review in brief the current recommendations for blood pressure control in the adult population (Table 17.2).

Of the several risk factors for heart failure, hypertension is the most common risk factor in the general population [88]. The benefits of antihypertensive therapy in reducing cardiovascular events and improving outcome have been firmly established [89]. Heart failure is considered a compelling indication in management of hypertension, indicating that the heart failure is managed in parallel with the blood pressure reduction [90]. In parallel with selecting drugs to control blood pressure, the choice of antihypertensive medication should also extend benefit by attenuating the deterioration in cardiac structure and function. The clinical trial data discussed above reinforce the importance of achieving optimal blood pressure control in the management of patients with diastolic heart failure.

Rigorous control of blood pressure and cholesterol are important preventive measures for patients at risk for heart failure as well as those in an early stage of heart failure [91]. The oral antihypertensive drugs and the usual dose range, as described in the most recent national guidelines on management of hypertension [90], are provided in Table 17.2. Thiazide type diuretics should, in general, be used in initial therapy for most patients with hypertension, and provide some benefit in reduction of volume overload in patients with heart failure.

However, combinations of medications from several classes of antihypertensive medications will be necessary to achieve optimal management of heart failure patients (Table 17.3). For patients who are asymptomatic, but who have evidence of ventricular dysfunction, it is recommended that the ACE inhibitors and the beta blockers be used to lower blood pressure to an optimal range (<140/90 mmHg) of blood pressure control [92,93]. For patients with a more advanced stage of heart failure or end-stage heart disease, ACE inhibitors, beta blockers, ARBs, and also aldosterone blockers are recommended, along with a loop diuretic [90]. The preceding discussion in this chapter describes the parallel benefits of these classes of drugs on hemodynamic function and vascular remodeling. Because there is now evidence that aldosterone contributes to myocardial fibrosis and diastolic stiffness the aldosterone blocking agents have an important therapeutic role in heart failure, in addition to a blood pressure lowering effect [94]. When a patient is receiving drugs from these classes and the blood pressure control is still not optimal a long-acting calcium channel blocker could be added for further blood pressure reduction.

Lifestyle modifications have added benefit for reduction of blood pressure and enhancing antihypertensive drug efficacy [90]. The lifestyle changes that should be encouraged include weight reduction in patients who are overweight or obese, dietary sodium reduction, moderation of alcohol consumption, and physical activity.

## Summary: pharmacologic management of patients with diastolic heart failure

In contrast with patients with systolic dysfunction and heart failure, there are far fewer clinical guidelines that can help the practitioner to care for this often challenging group of patients. However, Table 17.1 provides some of the general goals that can serve as a focus for pharmacologic intervention. First, the clinician must strive to reduce blood volume and in turn reduce both pre-load and after-load. This can be accomplished by a variety of medications that have already been discussed including diuretics, ACE inhibitors, and angiotensin II-receptor blockers.

**Table 17.2** Oral antihypertensive drugs*.

| Class | Drug (Trade name) | Usual dose range (mg/day) | Usual daily frequency* |
|---|---|---|---|
| Thiazide diuretics | | | |
| | Chlorothiazide (Diuril) | 125–500 | 1–2 |
| | Chlorthalidone (generic) | 12.5–25 | 1 |
| | Hydrochlorothiazide (Microzide, HydroDIURIL*) | 12.5–50 | 1 |
| | Polythiazide (Renese) | 2–4 | 1 |
| | Indapamide (Lozol*) | 1.25–2.5 | 1 |
| | Metolazone (Mykrox) | 0.5–1.0 | 1 |
| | Metolazone (Zaroxolyn) | 2.5–5 | 1 |
| Loop diuretics | | | |
| | Bumetanide (Bumex[†]) | 0.5–2 | 2 |
| | Furosemide (Lasix[†]) | 20–80 | 2 |
| | Torsemide (Demadex[†]) | 2.5–10 | 1 |
| Potassium-sparing diuretics | | | |
| | Amiloride (Midamor[†]) | 5–10 | 1–2 |
| | Triamterene (Dyrenium) | 50–100 | 1–2 |
| Aldosterone receptor blockers | | | |
| | Eplerenone (Inspra) | 50–100 | 1 |
| | Spironolactone (Aldactone[†]) | 25–50 | 1 |
| BBs | | | |
| | Atenolol (Tenormin[†]) | 25–100 | 1 |
| | Betaxolol (Kerlone[†]) | 5–20 | 1 |
| | Bisoprolol (Zebeta[†]) | 2.5–10 | 1 |
| | Metoprolol (Lopressor[†]) | 50–100 | 1–2 |
| | Metoprolol extended release (Toprol XL) | 50–100 | 1 |
| | Nadolol (Corgard[†]) | 40–120 | 1 |
| | Propranolol (Inderal[†]) | 40–160 | 2 |
| | Propranolol long-acting (Inderal LA[†]) | 60–180 | 1 |
| | Timolol (Blocadren[†]) | 20–40 | 2 |
| BBs with intrinsic sympathomimetic activity | | | |
| | Acebutolol (Sectral[†]) | 200–800 | 2 |
| | Penbutolol (Levatol) | 10–40 | 1 |
| | Pindolol (generic) | 10–40 | 2 |
| Combined alpha- and BBs | | | |
| | Carvedilol (Coreg) | 12.5–50 | 2 |
| | Labetalol (Normodyne, Trandate[†]) | 200–800 | 2 |
| ACEIs | | | |
| | Benazepril (Lotensin[†]) | 10–40 | 1 |
| | Captopril (Capoten[†]) | 25–100 | 2 |
| | Enalapril (Vasotec[†]) | 5–40 | 1–2 |
| | Fosinopril (Monopril) | 10–40 | 1 |
| | Lisinopril (Prinivil, Zestril[†]) | 10–40 | 1 |
| | Moexipril (Univasc) | 7.5–30 | 1 |
| | Perindopril (Aceon) | 4–8 | 1 |
| | Quinapril (Accupril) | 10–80 | 1 |
| | Ramipril (Altace) | 2.5–20 | 1 |
| | Trandolapril (Mavik) | 1–4 | 1 |

*Continued*

**Table 17.2** Continued.

| Class | Drug (Trade name) | Usual dose range (mg/day) | Usual daily frequency* |
|---|---|---|---|
| Angiotensin II antagonists | | | |
| | Candesartan (Atacand) | 8–32 | 1 |
| | Eprosartan (Teveten) | 400–800 | 1–2 |
| | Irbesartan (Avapro) | 150–300 | 1 |
| | Losartan (Cozaar) | 25–100 | 1–2 |
| | Olmesartan (Benicar) | 20–40 | 1 |
| | Telmisartan (Micardis) | 20–80 | 1 |
| | Valsartan (Diovan) | 80–320 | 1–2 |
| CCBs – nondihydropyridines | | | |
| | Diltiazem extended release (Cardizem CD, Dilacor XR, Tiazac[†]) | 180–420 | 1 |
| | Diltiazem extended release (Cardizem LA) | 120–540 | 1 |
| | Verapamil immediate release (Calan, Isoptin[†]) | 80–320 | 2 |
| | Verapamil long acting (Calan SR, Isoptin SR[†]) | 120–480 | 1–2 |
| | Verapamil (Coer, Covera HS, Verelan PM) | 120–360 | 1 |
| CCBs – dihydropyridines | | | |
| | Amlodipine (Norvasc) | 2.5–10 | 1 |
| | Felodipine (Plendil) | 2.5–20 | 1 |
| | Isradipine (Dynacirc CR) | 2.5–10 | 2 |
| | Nicardipine sustained release (Cardene SR) | 60–120 | 2 |
| | Nifedipine long-acting (Adalat CC, Procardia XL) | 30–60 | 1 |
| | Nisoldipine (Sular) | 10–40 | 1 |
| Alpha-1 blockers | | | |
| | Doxazosin (Cardura) | 1–16 | 1 |
| | Prazosin (Minipress[†]) | 2–20 | 2–3 |
| | Terazosin (Hytrin) | 1–20 | 1–2 |
| Central alpha-2 agonists and other centrally acting drugs | | | |
| | Clonidine (Catapres[†]) | 0.1–0.8 | 2 |
| | Clonidine patch (Catapres-TTS) | 0.1–0.3 | 1-weekly |
| | Methyldopa (Aldomet[†]) | 250–1000 | 2 |
| | Reserpine (generic) | 0.1–0.25 | 1 |
| | Guanfacine (Tenex[†]) | 0.5–2 | 1 |
| Direct vasodilators | | | |
| | Hydralazine (Apresoline[†]) | 25–100 | 2 |
| | Minoxidil (Loniten[†]) | 2.5–80 | 1–2 |

ACEIs, angiotensin converting enzyme inhibitors; BBs, beta blockers; CCBs, calcium channel blockers.
* In some patients treated once daily, the antihypertensive effect may diminish toward the end of the dosing interval (trough effect). BP should be measured just prior to dosing to determine if satisfactory BP control is obtained. Accordingly, an increase in dosage or frequency may need to be considered. These dosages may vary from those listed in the *Physicians Desk Reference* (57th edn).
[†] Available now or becoming available soon in generic preparations.
*Source: Physicians' Desk Reference*. 57th edn, Thompson PDR, Montvale, NJ, 2003.

The ACE inhibitors may have ancillary benefits including regression of hypertrophy and attenuation of maladaptive remodeling and fibrosis. Second, the clinician should strive to maintain sinus rhythm and to prevent tachycardia in order to assure the most effective myocardial hemodynamics. These goals can be achieved pharmacologically through the use of beta blockers and calcium channel blockers; however, invasive procedures to maintain sinus rhythm may be required

**Table 17.3** Combination drugs for hypertension.

| Combination type* | Fixed-dose combination, mg[†] | Trade name |
|---|---|---|
| ACEIs and CCBs | | |
| | Amlodipine-benazepril hydrochloride (2.5/10, 5/10, 5/20, 10/20) | Lotrel |
| | Enalapril-felodipine (5/5) | Lexxel |
| | Trandolapril-verapamil (2/180, 1/240, 2/240, 4/240) | Tarka |
| ACEIs and diuretics | | |
| | Benazepril-hydrochlorothiazide (5/6.25, 10/12.5, 20/12.5, 20/25) | Lotensin HCT |
| | Captopril-hydrochlorothiazide (25/15, 25/25, 50/15, 50/25) | Capozide |
| | Enalapril-hydrochlorothiazide (5/12.5, 10/25) | Vaseretic |
| | Fosinopril-hydrochlorothiazide (10/12.5, 20/12.5) | Monopril/HCT |
| | Lisinopril-hydrochlorothiazide (10/12.5, 20/12.5, 20/25) | Prinzide, Zestoretic |
| | Moexipril-hydrochlorothiazide (7.5/12.5, 15/25) | Uniretic |
| | Quinapril-hydrochlorothiazide (10/12.5, 20/12.5, 20/25) | Accuretic |
| ARBs and diuretics | | |
| | Candesartan-hydrochlorothiazide (16/12.5, 32/12.5) | Atacand HCT |
| | Eprosartan-hydrochlorothiazide (600/12.5, 600/25) | Teveten-HCT |
| | Irbesartan-hydrochlorothiazide (150/12.5, 300/12.5) | Avalide |
| | Losartan-hydrochlorothiazide (50/12.5, 100/25) | Hyzaar |
| | Olmesartan medoxomil-hydrochlorothiazide (20/12.5,40/12.5,40/25) | Benicar HCT |
| | Telmisartan-hydrochlorothiazide (40/12.5, 80/12.5) | Micardis-HCT |
| | Valsartan-hydrochlorothiazide (80/12.5, 160/12.5, 160/25) | Diovan-HCT |
| BBs and diuretics | | |
| | Atenolol-chlorthalidone (50/25, 100/25) | Tenoretic |
| | Bisoprolol-hydrochlorothiazide (2.5/6.25, 5/6.25, 10/6.25) | Ziac |
| | Metoprolol-hydrochlorothiazide (50/25, 100/25) | Lopressor HCT |
| | Nadolol-bendroflumethiazide (40/5, 80/5) | Corzide |
| | Propranolol LA-hydrochlorothiazide (40/25, 80/25) | Inderide LA |
| | Timolol-hydrochlorothiazide (10/25) | Timolide |
| Centrally acting drug and diuretic | | |
| | Methyldopa-hydrochlorothiazide (250/15, 250/25, 500/30, 500/50) | Aldoril |
| | Reserpine-chlorthalidone (0.125/25, 0.25/50) | Demi-Regroton, Regroton |
| | Reserpine-chlorothiazide (0.125/250, 0.25/500) | Diupres |
| | Reserpine-hydrochlorothiazide (0.125/25, 0.125/50) | Hydropres |
| Diuretic and diuretic | | |
| | Amiloride-hydrochlorothiazide (5/50) | Moduretic |
| | Spironolactone-hydrochlorothiazide (25/25, 50/50) | Aldactazide |
| | Triamterene-hydrochlorothiazide (37.5/25, 75/50) | Dyazide, Maxzide |

ACEIs, angiotensin converting enzyme inhibitors; ARBs, angiotensin receptor blockers; BBs, beta blockers; CCBs, calcium channel blockers.
[†] Some drug combinations are available in multiple fixed doses. Each drug dose is reported in milligrams.

including cardioversion, sequential atrioventricular pacing, or radiofrequency ablation. Third, it is imperative that myocardial ischemia be prevented and/or treated when present as ischemia worsens diastolic relaxation through a variety of mechanisms. Interestingly, the same pharmacologic agents that reduce pulmonary congestion and/or prevent tachycardia can provide salutary benefits in the treatment of ischemia, that is, beta blockers and calcium channel blockers. However, nitrates might also play a role. Finally, the most important pharmacologic intervention in patients with diastolic dysfunction is one that controls hypertension. While attaining these goals is an important key to management of patients with diastolic dysfunction, it is also of critical importance that measures be undertaken that can potentially improve diastolic performance and/or regress myocardial hypertrophy. Four groups of agents have been shown to benefit patients with both systolic and diastolic dysfunction including the ACE inhibitors, ARBs, spironolactone, and beta blockers. However, virtually no objective data is available as to which drug to add first, the optimal doses in patients with diastolic dysfunction, or the most reliable combinations. Thus, the clinician must individualize their therapy to each individual patient based on an assessment of their symptoms and their overall risk profile. Furthermore, it must be recognized that regression of hypertrophy is a time-dependent process and therefore agents targeting cardiac remodeling should be evaluated for at least 3 to 6 months in any given patient. Hopefully, both the scientific community and the pharmaceutical industry will undertake trials in the future that are focused on developing a data-driven algorithm for the treatment of this increasing population of patients.

# References

1 Senni M, Tribouilloy CM, Rodeheffer RJ et al. Congestive heart failure in the community: a study of all incident cases in Olmsted County, Minnesota, in 1991. *Circulation* 1998;**98**:2282–2289.

2 Kitzman DW, Gardin JM, Gottdiener JS et al. Importance of heart failure with preserved systolic function in patients ≥65 years of age. CHS Research Group. Cardiovascular Health Study. *Am J Cardiol* 2001;**87**:413–419.

3 MacCarthy PA, Kearney MT, Nolan J et al. Prognosis in heart failure with preserved left ventricular systolic function: prospective cohort study. *BMJ* 2003;**327**: 78–79.

4 Vasan RS, Larson MG, Benjamin EJ, Evans JC, Reiss CK, Levy D. Congestive heart failure in subjects with normal versus reduced left ventricular ejection fraction: prevalence and mortality in a population-based cohort. *J Am Coll Cardiol* 1999;**33**:1948–1955.

5 Zile MR, Gaasch WH, Carroll JD et al. Heart failure with a normal ejection fraction: is measurement of diastolic function necessary to make the diagnosis of diastolic heart failure? *Circulation* 2001;**104**:779–782.

6 Gaasch WH, Zile MR. Left ventricular diastolic dysfunction and diastolic heart failure. *Annu Rev Med* 2004;**55**:373–394.

7 Gaasch WH. Diagnosis and treatment of heart failure based on left ventricular systolic or diastolic dysfunction. *JAMA* 1994;**271**:1276–1280.

8 Vasan RS, Benjamin EJ, Levy D. Prevalence, clinical features and prognosis of diastolic heart failure: an epidemiologic perspective. *J Am Coll Cardiol* 1995;**26**: 1565–1574.

9 Banerjee P, Clark AL, Cleland JG. Diastolic heart failure: a difficult problem in the elderly. *Am J Geriatr Cardiol* 2004;**13**:16–21.

10 Piccini JP, Klein L, Gheorghiade M, Bonow RO. New insights into diastolic heart failure: role of diabetes mellitus. *Am J Med* 2004;**116**:64S–75S.

11 Dauterman KW, Massie BM, Gheorghiade M. Heart failure associated with preserved systolic function: a common and costly clinical entity. *Am Heart J* 1998;**135**: S310–319.

12 O'Connor CM, Gattis WA, Shaw L, Cuffe MS, Califf RM. Clinical characteristics and long-term outcomes of patients with heart failure and preserved systolic function. *Am J Cardiol* 2000;**86**:863–867.

13 Setaro JF, Soufer R, Remetz MS, Perlmutter RA, Zaret BL. Long-term outcome in patients with congestive heart failure and intact systolic left ventricular performance. *Am J Cardiol* 1992;**69**:1212–1216.

14 Judge KW, Pawitan Y, Caldwell J, Gersh BJ, Kennedy JW. Congestive heart failure symptoms in patients with preserved left ventricular systolic function: analysis of the CASS registry. *J Am Coll Cardiol* 1991;**18**: 377–382.

15 Brogan WC, 3rd, Hillis LD, Flores ED, Lange RA. The natural history of isolated left ventricular diastolic dysfunction. *Am J Med* 1992;**92**:627–630.

16 Aurigemma GP, Gottdiener JS, Shemanski L, Gardin J, Kitzman D. Predictive value of systolic and diastolic function for incident congestive heart failure in the elderly: the cardiovascular health study. *J Am Coll Cardiol* 2001;**37**:1042–1048.

17 Bella JN, Palmieri V, Roman MJ et al. Mitral ratio of peak early to late diastolic filling velocity as a predictor of mortality in middle-aged and elderly adults: the Strong Heart Study. *Circulation* 2002;**105**:1928–1933.

18 Gottdiener JS, McClelland RL, Marshall R et al. Outcome of congestive heart failure in elderly persons: influence of left ventricular systolic function. The Cardiovascular Health Study. *Ann Intern Med* 2002;**137**:631–639.

19 Elesber AA, Redfield MM. Approach to patients with heart failure and normal ejection fraction. *Mayo Clin Proc* 2001;**76**:1047–1052.

20 Litwin SE, Grossman W. Diastolic dysfunction as a cause of heart failure. *J Am Coll Cardiol* 1993;**22**:49A–55A.

21 Aurigemma GP, Gaasch WH. Clinical practice. Diastolic heart failure. *N Engl J Med* 2004;**351**:1097–1105.

22 Hay I, Rich J, Ferber P, Burkhoff D, Maurer MS. Role of impaired myocardial relaxation in the production of elevated left ventricular filling pressure. *Am J Physiol Heart Circ Physiol* 2005;**288**:H1203–1208.

23 Zile MR, Baicu CF, Gaasch WH. Diastolic heart failure – abnormalities in active relaxation and passive stiffness of the left ventricle. *N Engl J Med* 2004;**350**:1953–1959.

24 Zile MR, Brutsaert DL. New concepts in diastolic dysfunction and diastolic heart failure: Part II: causal mechanisms and treatment. *Circulation* 2002;**105**:1503–1508.

25 Kass DA, Bronzwaer JG, Paulus WJ. What mechanisms underlie diastolic dysfunction in heart failure? *Circ Res* 2004;**94**:1533–1542.

26 Hasenfuss G, Pieske B. Calcium cycling in congestive heart failure. *J Mol Cell Cardiol* 2002;**34**:951–969.

27 Schwinger RH, Munch G, Bolck B, Karczewski P, Krause EG, Erdmann E. Reduced Ca(2+)-sensitivity of SERCA 2a in failing human myocardium due to reduced serin-16 phospholamban phosphorylation. *J Mol Cell Cardiol* 1999;**31**:479–491.

28 MacLennan DH, Kranias EG. Phospholamban: a crucial regulator of cardiac contractility. *Nat Rev Mol Cell Biol* 2003;**4**:566–577.

29 Frank KF, Bolck B, Brixius K, Kranias EG, Schwinger RH. Modulation of SERCA: implications for the failing human heart. *Basic Res Cardiol* 2002;**97**:172–78.

30 Fitzsimons DP, Patel JR, Moss RL. Role of myosin heavy chain composition in kinetics of force development and relaxation in rat myocardium. *J Physiol* 1998;**513**: 171–183.

31 Apstein CS MJ. Cellular Mechanism underlying left ventricular diastolic failure. In: Gaasch WH, LeWinter, MM, ed. *Left Ventricular Diastolic Dysfunction and Heart Failure*. Lea & Febriger, Philadelphia, 1994: 3–24.

32 Linke WA, Popov VI, Pollack GH. Passive and active tension in single cardiac myofibrils. *Biophys J* 1994;**67**: 782–792.

33 Wu Y, Cazorla O, Labeit D, Labeit S, Granzier H. Changes in titin and collagen underlie diastolic stiffness diversity of cardiac muscle. *J Mol Cell Cardiol* 2000;**32**: 2151–2162.

34 Neagoe C, Kulke M, del Monte F *et al.* Titin isoform switch in ischemic human heart disease. *Circulation* 2002;**106**:1333–1341.

35 Yamasaki R, Wu Y, McNabb M, Greaser M, Labeit S, Granzier H. Protein kinase A phosphorylates titin's cardiac-specific N2B domain and reduces passive tension in rat cardiac myocytes. *Circ Res* 2002;**90**:1181–1188.

36 Warren CM, Jordan MC, Roos KP, Krzesinski PR, Greaser ML. Titin isoform expression in normal and hypertensive myocardium. *Cardiovasc Res* 2003;**59**:86–94.

37 Lewis JF, Spirito P, Pelliccia A, Maron BJ. Usefulness of Doppler echocardiographic assessment of diastolic filling in distinguishing 'thlete's heart' from hypertrophic cardiomyopathy. *Br Heart J* 1992;**68**:296–300.

38 Kato S, Spinale FG, Tanaka R, Johnson W, Cooper Gt, Zile MR. Inhibition of collagen cross-linking: effects on fibrillar collagen and ventricular diastolic function. *Am J Physiol* 1995;**269**:H863–868.

39 Li YY, McTiernan CF, Feldman AM. Interplay of matrix metalloproteinases, tissue inhibitors of metalloproteinases and their regulators in cardiac matrix remodeling. *Cardiovasc Res* 2000;**46**:214–224.

40 Dollery CM, McEwan JR, Henney AM. Matrix metalloproteinases and cardiovascular disease. *Circ Res* 1995;**77**:863–868.

41 King MK, Coker ML, Goldberg A *et al.* Selective matrix metalloproteinase inhibition with developing heart failure: effects on left ventricular function and structure. *Circ Res* 2003;**92**:177–185.

42 Gunasinghe SK, Ikonomidis J, Spinale FG. Contributory role of matrix metalloproteinases in cardiovascular remodeling. *Curr Drug Targets Cardiovasc Haematol Disord* 2001;**1**:75–91.

43 Zannad F, Dousset B, Alla F. Treatment of congestive heart failure: interfering the aldosterone-cardiac extracellular matrix relationship. *Hypertension* 2001;**38**:1227–1232.

44 Brilla CG, Funck RC, Rupp H. Lisinopril–mediated regression of myocardial fibrosis in patients with hypertensive heart disease. *Circulation* 2000;**102**:1388–1393.

45 Senzaki H, Paolocci N, Gluzband YA, *et al.* beta-blockade prevents sustained metalloproteinase activation and diastolic stiffening induced by angiotensin II combined with evolving cardiac dysfunction. *Circ Res* 2000;**86**: 807–815.

46 Deschamps AM, Spinale FG. Disruptions and detours in the myocardial matrix highway and heart failure. *Curr Heart Fail Rep* 2005;**2**:10–17.

47 Hunt SA, Baker DW, Chin MH *et al.* ACC/AHA guidelines for the evaluation and management of chronic heart failure in the adult: executive summary. A report of the American College of Cardiology/American Heart Association Task Force on Practice Guidelines (Committee to revise the 1995 Guidelines for the Evaluation and Management of Heart Failure). *J Am Coll Cardiol* 2001;**38**:2101–2113.

48 Haney S, Sur D, Xu Z. Diastolic heart failure: a review and primary care perspective. *J Am Board Fam Pract* 2005;**18**:189–198.

49 Whalley GA, Wasywich CA, Walsh H, Doughty RN. Role of echocardiography in the contemporary management of chronic heart failure. *Expert Rev Cardiovasc Ther* 2005;**3**:51–70.

50 Ommen SR, Nishimura RA, Appleton CP *et al.* Clinical utility of Doppler echocardiography and tissue Doppler imaging in the estimation of left ventricular

filling pressures: a comparative simultaneous Doppler-catheterization study. *Circulation* 2000;**102**:1788–1794.

51 Fuster V, Ryden LE, Asinger RW *et al.* ACC/AHA/ESC guidelines for the management of patients with atrial fibrillation: executive summary. A Report of the American College of Cardiology/American Heart Association Task Force on Practice Guidelines and the European Society of Cardiology Committee for Practice Guidelines and Policy Conferences (Committee to Develop Guidelines for the Management of Patients With Atrial Fibrillation): developed in Collaboration With the North American Society of Pacing and Electrophysiology. *J Am Coll Cardiol* 2001;**38**:1231–1266.

52 Nagano M, Higaki J, Mikami H *et al.* Converting enzyme inhibitors regressed cardiac hypertrophy and reduced tissue angiotensin II in spontaneously hypertensive rats. *J Hypertens* 1991;**9**:595–599.

53 Greenberg B, Quinones MA, Koilpillai C *et al.* Effects of long-term enalapril therapy on cardiac structure and function in patients with left ventricular dysfunction. Results of the SOLVD echocardiography substudy. *Circulation* 1995;**91**:2573–2581.

54 Lonn EM, Yusuf S, Jha P *et al.* Emerging role of angiotensin–converting enzyme inhibitors in cardiac and vascular protection. *Circulation* 1994;**90**:2056–2069.

55 Mattioli AV, Zennaro M, Bonatti S, Bonetti L, Mattioli G. Regression of left ventricular hypertrophy and improvement of diastolic function in hypertensive patients treated with telmisartan. *Int J Cardiol* 2004;**97**:383–388.

56 Devereux RB, Palmieri V, Sharpe N *et al.* Effects of once-daily angiotensin-converting enzyme inhibition and calcium channel blockade-based antihypertensive treatment regimens on left ventricular hypertrophy and diastolic filling in hypertension: the prospective randomized enalapril study evaluating regression of ventricular enlargement (preserve) trial. *Circulation* 2001;**104**: 1248–1254.

57 Lonn E, Shaikholeslami R, Yi Q *et al.* Effects of ramipril on left ventricular mass and function in cardiovascular patients with controlled blood pressure and with preserved left ventricular ejection fraction: a substudy of the Heart Outcomes Prevention Evaluation (HOPE) Trial. *J Am Coll Cardiol* 2004;**43**:2200–2206.

58 Solomon SD, Skali H, Anavekar NS *et al.* Changes in ventricular size and function in patients treated with valsartan, captopril, or both after myocardial infarction. *Circulation* 2005;**111**:3411–3419.

59 Dahlof B, Pennert K, Hansson L. Reversal of left ventricular hypertrophy in hypertensive patients. A meta-analysis of 109 treatment studies. *Am J Hypertens* 1992;**5**: 95–110.

60 Dahlof B. Left ventricular hypertrophy and angiotensin II antagonists. *Am J Hypertens* 2001;**14**:174–182.

61 Malmqvist K, Kahan T, Edner M *et al.* Regression of left ventricular hypertrophy in human hypertension with irbesartan. *J Hypertens* 2001;**19**:1167–1176.

62 Isobe N, Taniguchi K, Oshima S *et al.* Candesartan cilexetil improves left ventricular function, left ventricular hypertrophy, and endothelial function in patients with hypertensive heart disease. *Circ J* 2002;**66**:993–999.

63 Thurmann PA, Kenedi P, Schmidt A, Harder S, Rietbrock N. Influence of the angiotensin II antagonist valsartan on left ventricular hypertrophy in patients with essential hypertension. *Circulation* 1998;**98**:2037–2042.

64 Yusuf S, Pfeffer MA, Swedberg K, *et al.* Effects of candesartan in patients with chronic heart failure and preserved left-ventricular ejection fraction: the CHARM-Preserved Trial. *Lancet* 2003;**362**:777–781.

65 Swedberg K, Pfeffer M, Granger C *et al.* Candesartan in heart failure – assessment of reduction in mortality and morbidity (CHARM): rationale and design. Charm-Programme Investigators. *J Card Fail* 1999;**5**:276–282.

66 Massie BM, Fabi MR. Clinical trials in diastolic heart failure. *Prog Cardiovasc Dis* 2005;**47**:389–395.

67 Kaplan NM. Calcium entry blockers in the treatment of hypertension. Current status and future prospects. *JAMA* 1989;**262**:817–823.

68 Phillips RA, Ardeljan M, Shimabukuro S *et al.* Normalization of left ventricular mass and associated changes in neurohormones and atrial natriuretic peptide after 1 year of sustained nifedipine therapy for severe hypertension. *J Am Coll Cardiol* 1991;**17**:1595–1602.

69 Diamond JA KL, Martin K, Wallenstein S, Phillips RA. Comparison of ambulatory blood pressure and amounts of left ventricular hypertrophy in men versus women with similar levels of hypertensive clinic blood pressures. *Am J Cardiol* 1997;**79**:505–508.

70 Devereux RB, Dahlof B, Levy D, Pfeffer MA. Comparison of enalapril versus nifedipine to decrease left ventricular hypertrophy in systemic hypertension (the PRESERVE trial). *Am J Cardiol* 1996;**78**:61–65.

71 Cruickshank JM, Lewis J, Moore V, Dodd C. Reversibility of left ventricular hypertrophy by differing types of antihypertensive therapy. *J Hum Hypertens* 1992;**6**: 85–90.

72 Ito T, Suwa M, Imai M, Hozumi T, Tonari S, Kitaura Y. Acute effects of diltiazem on regional left ventricular diastolic filling dynamics in patients with hypertrophic cardiomyopathy as assessed by color kinesis. *Circ J* 2004;**68**:1035–1040.

73 Eichhorn EJ, Grayburn PA. beta-blocker improvement in diastolic performance: the yin and yang of ventricular function changes. *Am Heart J* 2000;**139**:584–586.

74 Eichhorn EJ, Bedotto JB, Malloy CR *et al.* Effect of beta-adrenergic blockade on myocardial function and energetics in congestive heart failure. Improvements in

hemodynamic, contractile, and diastolic performance with bucindolol. *Circulation* 1990;**82**:473–483.

75 Kim MH, Devlin WH, Das SK, Petrusha J, Montgomery D, Starling MR. Effects of beta-adrenergic blocking therapy on left ventricular diastolic relaxation properties in patients with dilated cardiomyopathy. *Circulation* 1999;**100**:729–735.

76 Capomolla S, Febo O, Gnemmi M *et al*. Beta-blockade therapy in chronic heart failure: diastolic function and mitral regurgitation improvement by carvedilol. *Am Heart J* 2000;**139**:596–608.

77 Effect of metoprolol CR/XL in chronic heart failure: Metoprolol CR/XL Randomised Intervention Trial in Congestive Heart Failure (MERIT-HF). *Lancet* 1999;**353**:2001–2007.

78 Cleland JG, Pennell DJ, Ray SG *et al*. Myocardial viability as a determinant of the ejection fraction response to carvedilol in patients with heart failure (CHRISTMAS trial): randomised controlled trial. *Lancet* 2003;**362**:14–21.

79 Bellenger NG, Rajappan K, Rahman SL *et al*. Effects of carvedilol on left ventricular remodelling in chronic stable heart failure: a cardiovascular magnetic resonance study. *Heart* 2004;**90**:760–764.

80 Bergstrom A, Andersson B, Edner M, Nylander E, Persson H, Dahlstrom U. Effect of carvedilol on diastolic function in patients with diastolic heart failure and preserved systolic function. Results of the Swedish Doppler-echocardiographic study (SWEDIC). *Eur J Heart Fail* 2004;**6**:453–461.

81 Shibata MC, Flather MD, Bohm M *et al*. Study of the Effects of Nebivolol Intervention on Outcomes and Rehospitalisation in Seniors with Heart Failure (SENIORS). Rationale and design. *Int J Cardiol* 2002;**86**: 77–85.

82 Flather MD, Shibata MC, Coats AJ, *et al*. Randomized trial to determine the effect of nebivolol on mortality and cardiovascular hospital admission in elderly patients with heart failure (SENIORS). *Eur Heart J* 2005;**26**:215–225.

83 Weber KT, Brilla CG. Pathological hypertrophy and cardiac interstitium. Fibrosis and renin-angiotensin-aldosterone system. *Circulation* 1991;**83**:1849–1865.

84 Lacolley P, Safar ME, Lucet B, Ledudal K, Labat C, Benetos A. Prevention of aortic and cardiac fibrosis by spironolactone in old normotensive rats. *J Am Coll Cardiol* 2001;**37**:662–667.

85 Zannad F, Alla F, Dousset B, Perez A, Pitt B. Limitation of excessive extracellular matrix turnover may contribute to survival benefit of spironolactone therapy in patients with congestive heart failure: insights from the randomized aldactone evaluation study (RALES). Rales Investigators. *Circulation* 2000;**102**:2700–2706.

86 Mottram PM, Haluska B, Leano R, Cowley D, Stowasser M, Marwick TH. Effect of aldosterone antagonism on myocardial dysfunction in hypertensive patients with diastolic heart failure. *Circulation* 2004;**110**:558–565.

87 The Digitalis Investigation Group. The effect of digoxin on mortality and morbidity in patients with heart failure. *N Engl J Med* 1997;**336**:525–533.

88 Levy D, Larson MG, Vasan RS, Kannel WB, HO KKL. The progression from hypertension to congestive heart failure. *JAMA* 1996;**275**:1557–1562.

89 Neal B, MacMahon S, Chapman N. Effects of ACE inhibitors, calcium anagonists, and other blood-pressure-lowering drugs: Results of prospectively designed overviews of randomized trials. Blood Pressure Lowering Treatment Trialists' Collaboration. *Lancet* 2000;**356**:1955–1964.

90 Chobanian AV, Bakris GL, Black HR *et al*. The Seventh Report of the Joint National Committee on Prevention, Detection, Evaluation, and Treatment of High Blood Pressure. *Hypertension* 2003;**42**:1206–1252.

91 Hunt SA, Baker DW, Chin MH *et al*. ACC/AHA guidelines for the evaluation and management of chronic heart failure in the adult: Executive summary. A repot of the American College of Cardiology/American Heart Association Task Force on Practice Guidelines (Committee to revise the 1995 Guidelines for the Evaluation and Management of Heart Failure. *J Am Coll Cardiol* 2001;**38**:2101– 2113.

92 Pfeffer MA, Braunwald E, Moye LA *et al*. Effect of captopril on mortality and morbidity in patients with left ventricular dysfunction after myocardial infarction. Results of the Survival and Ventricular Enlargement trial. The SAVE Investigators. *N Engl J Med* 1992;327:669–677.

93 The Capricorn Investigators. Effect of carvedilol on outcome after myocardial infarction in patients with left-ventricular dysfunction. The CAPRICORN randomized trial. *Lancet* 2001;**357**:1385–1390.

94 Pitt B, Zannad F, Remme WJ *et al*. The effect of spironolacctone on morbidity and mortality in patients with severe heart failure. Randomized Aldactone Evaluation Study Investigators. *N Engl J Med* 1999;**341**:709–717.

## CHAPTER 18

# Multidrug pharmacy for treatment of heart failure: an algorithm for the clinician

*Mariell Jessup,* MD

## Introduction

Knowing that the many therapies detailed in previous chapters of this book are available for the management of heart failure is comforting and wondrous to contemplate. Confronted with a new patient experiencing severe orthopnea, significant ascites, and massive leg edema, who presents with a barely palpable blood pressure and cool extremities, a busy clinician may be bewildered as to where to start in the use of these miraculous new treatments. This chapter is designed to provide an algorithm or roadmap of drugs with which to approach the patient with heart failure (Figure 18.1). However, to use a roadmap effectively while driving a car other skills have to be mastered. Likewise, it is important to define the skills that must be mastered to effectively use the roadmap in heart failure.

## Establishing a foundation of heart failure skills

### Identify the risk factors for the development of heart failure and the patients at risk

The lifetime risk of developing heart failure is 20% in both men and women; this risk changes with age and time [1,2]. The ACC/AHA Guidelines for the Evaluation and Management of Chronic Heart Failure in the Adult have been instrumental in more clearly articulating the early stages of heart failure [3], or the preclinical phase of the disease, and the patterns of disease associated with subsequent progression to clinical symptoms (Figure 18.2).

Those risk factors include hypertension, diabetes, hyperlipidemia, coronary artery disease, or any of these factors in combination. (Obviously, there are less readily identifiable risks as well, such as inherited forms of cardiomyopathy, that will one day be easily recognized through gene profiling, but that are currently unclear and therefore unhelpful to a busy clinician.) It is extremely important to notice that there are well-established practice guidelines for the management of the very same diseases that confer a risk for heart failure [4–11]. Moreover, effective treatment of hypertension and coronary artery disease, for example, often incorporates the same classes of drugs that are suggested for the management of heart failure [12,13]. Indeed, it can be argued that quality care of the heart failure patient flows naturally when a clinician renders optimal care of the comorbid conditions associated with heart failure. This may be particularly true when a patient has heart failure with a preserved ejection fraction (EF) [14,15]. Thus, an awareness of the risk factors associated with heart failure arms the clinician with a great deal of the knowledge necessary to manage heart failure.

### Develop a standard physical exam to perform serial assessments of patients with heart failure

A great many of the symptoms experienced by patients with heart failure are a result of fluid retention and volume expansion. Breathlessness, abdominal bloating, peripheral edema, orthopnea, and dyspnea on exertion are often quickly relieved

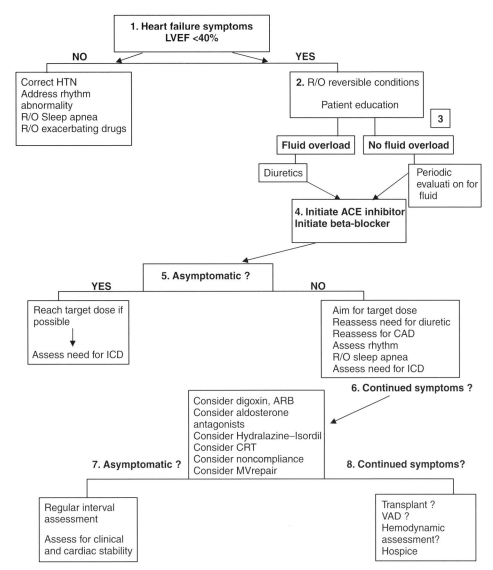

**Figure 18.1** A multidrug algorithm for the clinical management of patients with heart failure symptoms.
ARB = angiotensin receptor antagonists; CAD = coronary artery disease; CRT = cardiac resynchronization therapy;
HTN = hypertension; ICD = implantable cardiodefibrillator; LVEF = left ventricular ejection fraction; MV = mitral valve;
R/O = rule out; VAD = ventricular assist device.

with judicious use of diuretic agents. Clinicians need to develop an office system that allows for the routine record of body weight of each patient, and a periodic assessment of height so that BMI (body mass index) can be calculated. Other measurements that should be undertaken at each office visit include blood pressure recordings in supine and standing positions with corresponding heart rate, so that orthostasis or undue bradycardia may

be documented. Clinicians likewise need to look for evidence of jugular venous distension, hepatic congestion, or edema at each visit [16–20]. These simple items from a more extensive physical exam can be extremely helpful in the determination of fluid overload in an individual patient, and be the first indication that drug therapy may need to be altered or added. When cardiac palpation and auscultation of the heart and lungs are added to this

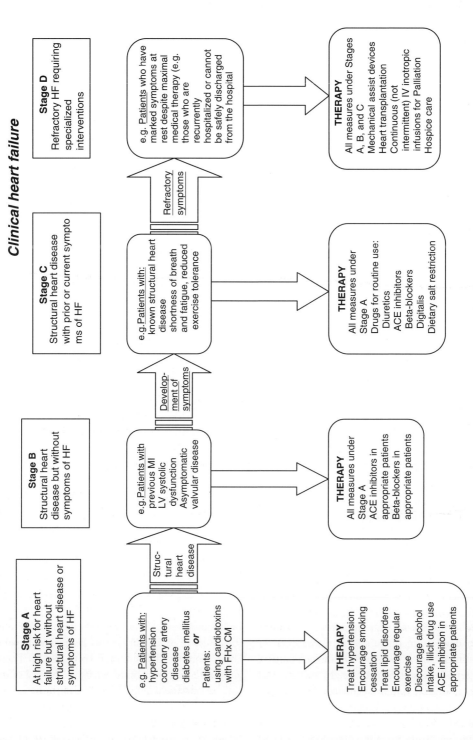

**Figure 18.2** Stages in the evolution of heart failure and recommended therapy by stage. Proposed by the ACC/AHA Guidelines for the Evaluation and Management of Chronic Heart Failure in Adults of 2001. FHx CM = family history of cardiomyopathy; IV = intravenous; LV = left ventricular; MI: myocardial infarction. (Reproduced with permission from Hunt *et al.* [3].)

list the clinician has many of the tools necessary to supplement an interval history of a regular patient.

The above items observed during an interval office visit seem rudimentary and easy to accomplish. Yet it is important to recognize that most of these measurements are not routinely done in a busy office practice, and many clinicians examine patients fully clothed! Incorporating these simple measures will ensure that additional drugs used to treat heart failure will result in the stabilization of symptoms while the disease is stabilized as well.

### Develop a standard set of measures to serially assess the symptomatic status of heart failure patients

It is important to assess a patient in a routine manner at each visit to accurately determine their symptomatic status. Patients with heart failure often begin to decrease their attempts at physical activity, usually subconsciously, so that over time their subjective complaints may diminish despite progressive cardiac deterioration. Ask about one or two items that a patient must do on a regular basis, such as making a bed or showering and dressing without stopping, as a routine at each visit. Always ask about social outings, or visits with family members, as patients with severe heart failure or profound fatigue will stop undertaking even pleasurable encounters but may not volunteer this information. Think about incorporating some simple assessment of submaximal exercise into an office visit periodically. This may involve watching the patient walk in a place, a measured walk in a hall, or a more formal treadmill test [21]. The amount of information gained, including the possibility of noting marked increases in blood pressure, failure of heart rate to augment, or the aggravation of arrhythmias can often justify the time and expense of the test. There are also some standardized questionnaires that assess quality of life in patients with heart failure that can be self-administered in the office and maintained in the office file [22,23].

Additional information that must be acquired and documented at each visit includes any emergency room visits or hospitalizations the patient may have experienced. A review must be made of each medication the patient is taking, including over-the- counter medications that could be exacerbating the heart failure syndrome. Certain arthritis or pain formulations are common culprits, as are some drugs used for diabetic management [24–26]. Other important historical information includes the possibility of dizziness, syncope, chest pain, or severe sleep disturbances; all of these symptoms may be amenable to treatment or may require intervention.

## Establishing goals of treatment in heart failure

Having established a foundation of clinical skills necessary for the management of the patient with heart failure it is critical to outline the goals of treatment for these patients. Using the skills detailed above a clinician may quickly determine how well the goals are being met at each office visit.

### Improve quality of life

A number of studies have clearly documented that patients with heart failure, especially severe heart failure, value the absence of discomfort and breathlessness as much or more than the actual duration of their lives [27]. Improving quality of life may mean different things to different patients and may include the absence of hospitalizations, the ability to go shopping with family, or the capacity to continue gainful employment. It is a useful exercise to ask each patient what aspect of his or her illness is most troubling, and then follow the impact of disease management on this perceived disability. Certainly, an improvement of score on a formalized questionnaire used in heart failure to assess quality of life is an indication of enhanced function. Likewise, an increasing ability to perform during exercise testing is another way to document that this goal is being achieved. Irrespective of the method used to chart functional capacity clinicians need to periodically assess whether their patients with heart failure are maintaining or improving quality of life. This is an important goal of therapy and one in which individual patients can be monitored.

### Enhance survival

Obviously, there has been a deserved emphasis on the high-mortality rate of patients with heart failure, and as public health advocates we want to impact favorably on survival [28–30]. However, as practicing clinicians our patients' care cannot be dictated by our predictions of their demise. To date, there have been very few reliable methods to accurately calculate an individuals' prognosis after heart failure becomes evident [31]. Rather, clinicians must use those treatments that have been shown in well-designed trials to improve survival, and hope that the broad results are applicable to the single patient at hand. This, then, is the art of medicine. Clinicians must forge ahead with the prescription of drugs that have been shown to be life saving in large studies for an individual patient who may not resemble the study population [32,33].

Having emphasized the importance of practicing evidenced-based medicine it is also useful now to refer back to the roadmap. Clinicians in a busy office-practice have lots more to do than worry about the nuances of multiple practice guidelines. An overall strategy of care can be reasonably uniform for most patients with heart failure, and is outlined below in eight broad categories.

## A strategy for care of the heart failure patient

### In the patient with symptoms of heart failure is the left ventricular ejection fraction normal or depressed, that is, less than 40%?

The overwhelming numbers of studies performed in a heart failure population have been in those patients with dilated left ventricles that are poorly contracting, a syndrome often referred to as systolic dysfunction. Although there is a growing recognition that as many as 30 to 50% of all hospitalized patients with heart failure have normal cardiac contractility, or a preserved EF, there remains a paucity of evidence-based recommendations for this group. (This syndrome has been called a variety of names including diastolic heart failure or nondilated heart failure.) Most reviews stress the importance of excluding significant coronary ischemia as an exacerbating cause of heart failure symptoms, and all agree that meticulous control of hypertension is critical [14,15,34]. Many of these patients with heart failure and a normal EF present

with atrial arrhythmias, usually atrial fibrillation, and control of heart rate in this situation can be very useful. Obesity, diabetes, arthritis, and renal insufficiency are typical comorbid conditions in this group of patients, so a search for exacerbating drugs used to treat these conditions may be fruitful. Sleep apnea is common and a screening interview for sleep disturbances is appropriate [35,36]. There have been a number of excellent reviews of this nondilated heart failure syndrome that cover additional therapeutic principals.

### In the patient with heart failure and a low LVEF look for correctable causes of the cardiac dysfunction

If the patient has heart failure in the setting of a dilated left ventricle and has a low LVEF as determined by an echocardiogram, nuclear ventriculography, or angiography then the next phase is to pursue, by means of a complete history and physical examination and a few simple diagnostic tests, a search for reversible or correctable causes of the low systolic function. In the United States, the most common cause of dilated cardiomyopathy is chronic ischemia related to coronary artery obstruction [37–43]. A complete list of potentially correctable etiologies is beyond this review, but may include illicit drug use or alcohol abuse, thyroid disorders, or uncontrolled hypertension.

Fundamental to our algorithm is the initiation of patient (and family) education [44]. There are some key principals to cover with the patient including, the potential seriousness of the diagnosis; recommendations about diet, that is, whether the patient needs to restrict fluid or sodium; recommendations about exercise; develop a routine for the patient to self-monitor his or her volume status at home, usually done by daily weights; counsel about alcohol and/or nicotine use; an action plan for the patient who may develop increasing symptoms; and finally discuss end-of-life wishes. Although these instructions do take time initially they will serve both the office staff and the patient well in the future. Moreover, there are an increasing number of electronic educational sites available on the internet that will reinforce the instructions and teaching done in the office.

## Determine whether the patient has symptoms and signs of volume expansion

Diuretics produce symptomatic benefits more rapidly than any other drug used for heart failure; they can relieve peripheral or pulmonary edema with hours or days [45–50]. Diuretics are the only drugs used in the outpatient management of heart failure that can adequately control fluid retention. Nevertheless, they should never be the sole treatment for patients with stage C or D heart failure, even if the patient becomes asymptomatic after the initiation of a diuresis. Using the skills outlined earlier a clinician needs to determine whether a patient has signs or symptoms of fluid retention, and then begin a maintenance diuretic regimen. Although some patients with dilated cardiomyopathy who have been stabilized on a standard regimen of neurohormonal antagonists may be effectively managed without diuretics, the large majority of patients will need a regular dose of diuretic, usually daily.

Diuretic dosage may need to be adjusted as time and other circumstances change. Periodic physical exams coupled with home weight monitoring and laboratory testing should be done to avoid azotemia or electrolyte imbalances. A key reason for follow-up office visits of the heart failure patient is to assess the need for diuretic dose adjustment.

## Initiate ACE-inhibitor and beta-blocker therapy

All patients with a low EF (in the absence of aortic outflow obstruction) should be initiated and maintained on both an ACE inhibitor and a beta-blocker [3]. For historical reasons, clinicians commonly start an ACE inhibitor first and add a beta-blocker as a second agent, but recent data suggests that starting a beta-blocker as initial therapy has some advantages [51]. Clinicians need to keep in focus that their ultimate task is to maintain patients on both drugs at the highest-tolerated dosages. Thus, it is reasonable to start both drugs at very low doses and then up-titrate each drug alternately until target doses are reached or patients become intolerant. If hypotension or azotemia develops reducing diuretics or staggering the dosing time of the drugs may alleviate symptoms.

Clinicians, in their eagerness, may simultaneously start a patient with newly diagnosed dilated cardiomyopathy and heart failure on diuretics, ACE inhibitors and beta-blockers, all within a 12-h period. The result is often hypotension, azotemia or both, and the clinician may wrongly conclude that the patient is intolerant of these life-saving drugs. Once a patient is euvolemic there is no specific time course that necessitates rushing to get a patient on both drugs. A slow steady approach over several weeks is usually more successful. Many times this can be done without an office visit, but rather through a nurse-administered titration protocol supervised by phone calls.

Patients with an intractable cough secondary to an ACE inhibitor should be placed on an angiotensin-receptor antagonist (ARB). Patients, on the other hand, with a rapid increase in creatinine, BUN, or potassium after an ACE inhibitor is initiated will not likely tolerate an ARB either [52,53]. Every effort should be made to maintain patients with dilated cardiomyopathy on beta-blockers even the majority of patients with some degree of lung disease and most certainly diabetic patients. ARBs are appropriate substitutes for the patient intolerant of ACE inhibitors, but the available data suggests there are no good substitutes for the benefits accrued by beta-blockade in these patients.

## Reassess the functional status of the patient after neurohormonal therapy has been initiated and maintained

It takes time for the beneficial effects of the ACE inhibitor and beta-blocker combination to be quantifiable, especially when observing for evidence of reverse LV remodeling. After target dosages of the two neurohormonal antagonists have been maintained for approximately 3 or 4 months it is appropriate to reassess the functional status of the patient. If the patient is able to perform an acceptable level of daily living activities and is free from fluid retention [equivalent to a New York Heart Association (NYHA) functional class I or II] the only remaining task is to assess whether the patient should be considered for an implantable cardiodefibrillator (ICD) [54–57]. These patients should then be followed at intervals often enough to detect any worsening of symptoms or the addition of comorbid conditions.

However, if the patient continues to complain of fatigue, breathlessness, and fluid retention, there are some steps to consider before additional drug classes are initiated. These considerations include the following. Is it possible to try again to reach target doses of the ACE inhibitor and beta-blocker? Perhaps the patient will benefit from an increased dose or frequency of diuretics, or a combination of loop and distal tubule diuretics. Is there evidence of new or exacerbated ischemia that accounts for the patient's symptoms, and a reevaluation for coronary artery disease should be undertaken. Is the rhythm appropriate for the patient, and both undue bradycardia and tachycardia have been excluded. Is the patient's fatigue and nocturnal restlessness a manifestation of sleep apnea rather than worsening heart failure with orthopnea? Is the patient's depression mimicking heart failure symptoms [58,59]? These patients also must be considered for their risk of sudden death, and the timing of an ICD procedure.

## The patient with continued symptoms of heart failure

If a patient with dilated cardiomyopathy continues to have symptomatic heart failure despite all of the measures outlined earlier, they fall into unchartered territory as to the proper sequence of pharmacotherapy. There are a number of drugs that can be added to baseline ACE inhibitor and beta-blocker but the relative value of one additional drug over another cannot be compared. Currently, there are three possible therapeutic alternatives that have been explored in randomized, clinical trials: the addition of an ARB, the addition of an aldosterone antagonist [60–62], or the addition of the drug combination hydralazine–isosorbide dinitrate [63,64]. All have been shown to have a meaningful and beneficial impact on outcome. Less well-studied in a population already on ACE inhibitor and beta-blocker therapy is the addition of digoxin, but this drug has historically been a mainstay of heart failure treatment [65–67]. Nevertheless, clinicians should make every effort to add one of the above therapies to a patient with ongoing symptoms with a preference to the use of one

of the first three regimens, as they have been shown to significantly reduce morbidity and mortality.

Another approach that should be explored for this persistently symptomatic population includes consideration of cardiac resynchronization therapy (CRT), which may be identified by a prolonged QRS on the surface electrocardiogram or by more sensitive methods of detecting cardiac dysynchrony [68–70]. Patients with severe mitral regurgitation could be considered for mitral valve repair, which has not been investigated in a controlled clinical trial [71–73]. Finally, an effort should be made to ensure that the patient is indeed taking their prescribed medications. Noncompliance to a medical regimen is a frequent cause for heart failure decompensation.

## Has the stage C, NYHA class III patient become less symptomatic or free of symptoms?

Gratifying as it may be to have made the right choice and instituted the appropriate drug combination for the persistently symptomatic patient it should be emphasized that this patient continues to have a very limited prognosis. Patients who have stabilized only after they are on an ACE inhibitor, beta-blocker, and either an ARB or aldosterone antagonist have a high 5-year mortality rate, and need to be followed quite carefully. Clinical and cardiac stability may deteriorate surreptitiously and these unfortunate patients must be seen at regular intervals.

## The patient has progressed to stage D, with persistent symptoms despite optimal medical therapy

Despite great advances in our management strategies for heart failure there will always be patients who do not respond to our best efforts or our most efficacious drugs. Cardiac transplantation is an option for only a very select few of this group [74]. Permanent ventricular assist devices (VAD) may improve survival and quality of life in an additional group of patients [75–78]. These devices may become technologically improved in the future and may provide a solution for a larger and more meaningful group of patients. Other, perhaps investigational approaches might begin with a thorough hemodynamic assessment or a repeat left heart catheterization. Most importantly, a repeat discussion about end-of-life decisions and wishes must be undertaken. Hospice is an appropriate alternative for many patients, as compared to an endless cycle of increasingly longer hospital admissions [79].

## Summary

It may be useful to view the above algorithm as a finite set of building blocks. The base or foundation of this structure begins with a clinician who interviews the patient with the aim of determining symptomatic status, and examines the patient to search for fluid retention. Diuretics are part of this foundation. The next block to be added, for the patient with heart failure and a low LVEF, is the floor of our structure: ACE inhibition and beta-blockade. For patients who continue to have many symptoms or ongoing evidence of fluid overload, a number of maneuvers may be done to reaffirm the solidity of the foundation and floor. Both groups of patients, however, those who are asymptomatic and those who are persistently in failure, need a discussion about ICD implantation; the analogy might be for some electrical wiring for our building. Finally, a series of blocks representing additional drugs may be added in an attempt to improve quality of life while prolonging survival. Increasingly, a firm structure of pharmacotherapy can be maintained for a majority of patients with heart failure out of these individual building blocks of drugs.

## References

1 Levy D, Kenchaiah S, Larson MG et al. Long-term trends in the incidence of and survival with heart failure (Comment). N Engl J Med 2002;**347**:1397–1402.

2 Lloyd-Jones DM, Larson MG, Leip EP et al. Lifetime risk for developing congestive heart failure: the Framingham Heart Study (Comment). Circulation 2002;**106**: 3068–3072.

3 Hunt HA, Baker DW, Chin MH et al. ACC/AHA Guidelines for the Evaluation and Management of Chronic Heart Failure in the Adult: Executive Summary A Report of the American College of Cardiology/American Heart Association Task Force on Practice Guidelines (Committee to Revise the 1995 Guidelines for the Evaluation and Management of Heart Failure): Developed in Collaboration With the International Society for Heart and Lung Transplantation; Endorsed by the Heart Failure Society of America. Circulation 2001;**104**:2996–3007.

4 Klein L, Gheorghiade M. Coronary artery disease and prevention of heart failure. Med Clin North Am 2004;**88**:1209–1235.

5 Kaplan NM. New JNC-6 guidelines. Joint National Committee. Am J Kidney Dis 1998;**31**:864–865.

6 Harris SB, Lank CN. Recommendations from the Canadian Diabetes Association. 2003 guidelines for prevention and management of diabetes and related cardiovascular risk factors (See comment). Can Fam Physician 2004;**50**:425–433.

7 Grundy SM. United States Cholesterol Guidelines 2001: expanded scope of intensive low-density lipoprotein-lowering therapy. Am J Cardiol 2001;**88**:23J–27J.

8 Flack JM, Peters R, Shafi T, Alrefai H, Nasser SA, Crook E. Prevention of hypertension and its complications: theoretical basis and guidelines for treatment. J Am Soc Nephrol 2003;**14**:592–598.

9 Fihn SD, Williams SV, Daley J et al. Guidelines for the management of patients with chronic stable angina: treatment (See comment). Ann Intern Med 2001;**135**:616–632.

10 Eagle KA, Guyton RA, Davidoff R et al. ACC/AHA guidelines for coronary artery bypass graft surgery: executive summary and recommendations : A report of the American College of Cardiology/American Heart Association Task Force on Practice Guidelines (Committee to revise the 1991 guidelines for coronary artery bypass graft surgery). Circulation 1999;**100**:1464–1480.

11 Chobanian AV, Bakris GL, Black HR et al. The Seventh Report of the Joint National Committee on Prevention, Detection, Evaluation, and Treatment of High Blood Pressure: the JNC 7 report (Comment) (erratum appears in JAMA 2003;**290**:197). JAMA 2003;**289**:2560–2572.

12 Bristow MR. Mechanisms of development of heart failure in the hypertensive patient. Cardiology 1999;**92**:3–6; discussion 7–9, 20–21.

13 Cleland JG. Progression from hypertension to heart failure. Mechanisms and management. Cardiology 1999;**92**:10–19; discussion 20–21.

14 Zile MR, Brutsaert DL. New concepts in diastolic dysfunction and diastolic heart failure: Part I: diagnosis, prognosis, and measurements of diastolic function. Circulation 2002;**105**:1387–1393.

15 Zile MR, Brutsaert DL. New concepts in diastolic dysfunction and diastolic heart failure: Part II: causal mechanisms and treatment. Circulation 2002;**105**: 1503–1508.

16 Konstam M, Dracup K, Baker D et al. Heart Failure: Evaluation and care of patients with left-ventricular systolic dysfunction. Clinical Practice Guideline No. 11. Rockville, MD: Agency for Health Care Policy and

Research Public Health Service US Department of Health and Human Services, 1994.

17 Candlish P, Watts P, Redman S, Whyte P, Lowe J. Elderly patients with heart failure: a study of satisfaction with care and quality of life. *Int J Qual Health Care* 1998;**10**: 141–146.

18 Doba N, Tomiyama N, Nakayama T. Drugs, heart failure and quality of life: what are we achieving? What should we be trying to achieve? *Drugs Aging* 1999;**14**:153–163.

19 Friedman MM. Gender differences in the health related quality of life of older adults with heart failure. *Heart Lung* 2003;**32**:320–327.

20 Hawthorne MH, Hixon ME. Functional status, mood disturbance and quality of life in patients with heart failure. *Prog Cardiovasc Nurs* 1994;**9**:22–32.

21 Demers C, McKelvie RS, Negassa A, Yusuf S, Investigators RPS. Reliability, validity, and responsiveness of the six-minute walk test in patients with heart failure. *Am Heart J* 2001;**142**:698–703.

22 Rector T, Cohn J. Assessment of patient outcome with the Minnesota Living with Heart Failure questionnaire: Reliability and validity during a randomized, double-blind, placebo-controlled trial of pimobendan. *Am Heart J* 1992;**124**:1017.

23 Alla F, Briancon S, Guillemin F *et al.* Self-rating of quality of life provides additional prognostic information in heart failure. Insights into the EPICAL study. *Eur J Heart Fail* 2002;**4**:337–343.

24 Tang WH, Francis GS, Hoogwerf BJ, Young JB. Fluid retention after initiation of thiazolidinedione therapy in diabetic patients with established chronic heart failure (See comment). *J Am Coll Cardiol* 2003;**41**:1394–1398.

25 Page J, Henry D. Consumption of NSAIDs and the development of congestive heart failure in elderly patients: an underrecognized public health problem. *Arch Intern Med* 2000;**160**:777–784.

26 Feenstra J, Heerdink ER, Grobbee DE, Stricker BH. Association of nonsteroidal anti-inflammatory drugs with first occurrence of heart failure and with relapsing heart failure: the Rotterdam Study. *Arch Intern Med* 2002;**162**:265–270.

27 Lewis EF, Johnson PA, Johnson W, Collins C, Griffin L, Stevenson LW. Preferences for quality of life or survival expressed by patients with heart failure. *J Heart Lung Transplant* 2001;**20**:1016–1024.

28 Baker DW, Einstadter D, Thomas C, Cebul RD. Mortality trends for 23,505 Medicare patients hospitalized with heart failure in Northeast Ohio, 1991 to 1997. *Am Heart J* 2003;**146**:258–264.

29 Cicoira M, Davos CH, Florea V *et al.* Chronic heart failure in the very elderly: clinical status, survival, and prognostic factors in 188 patients more than 70 years old. *Am Heart J* 2001;**142**:174–180.

30 Cowie MR, Wood DA, Coats AJ *et al.* Survival of patients with a new diagnosis of heart failure: a population based study. *Heart* (British Cardiac Society). 2000;**83**: 505–510.

31 Cowie MR. Estimating prognosis in heart failure: time for a better approach (Comment). *Heart* (British Cardiac Society). 2003;**89**:587–588.

32 Khand A, Gemmel I, Clark A, Cleland J. Is the prognosis of heart failure improving? *J Am Coll Cardiol* 2000;**36**: 2284–2286.

33 Konstam MA. Progress in heart failure management? Lessons from the real world. *Circulation* 2000;**102**: 1076–1078.

34 Gaasch WH, Zile MR. Left ventricular diastolic dysfunction and diastolic heart failure. *Annu Rev Med* 2004;**55**:373–394.

35 Bradley TD, Floras JS. Sleep apnea and heart failure: Part I: obstructive sleep apnea. *Circulation* 2003;**107**: 1671–1678.

36 Bradley TD, Floras jS. Sleep apnea and heart failure: Part II: central sleep apnea. *Circulation* 2003;**107**: 1822–1826.

37 Adams KF, Jr. New epidemiologic perspectives concerning mild-to-moderate heart failure. *Am J Med* 2001;**110**:6S–13S.

38 Adams KF, Jr., Dunlap SH, Sueta CA *et al.* Relation between gender, etiology and survival in patients with symptomatic heart failure. *J Am Coll Cardiol* 1996;**28**:1781–1788.

39 Cowie MR, Wood DA, Coats AJ *et al.* Incidence and aetiology of heart failure; a population-based study. *Eur Heart J* 1999;**20**:421–428.

40 Dunlap SH, Sueta CA, Tomasko L, Adams KF, Jr. Association of body mass, gender and race with heart failure primarily due to hypertension. *J Am Coll Cardiol* 1999;**34**:1602–1608.

41 Guertl B, Noehammer C, Hoefler G. Metabolic cardiomyopathies. *Int J Exp Pathol* 2000;**81**:349–372.

42 Haas GJ. Etiology, evaluation, and management of acute myocarditis. *Cardiol Rev* 2001;**9**:88–95.

43 Mair FS, Crowley TS, Bundred PE. Prevalence, aetiology and management of heart failure in general practice. *Br J Gen Pract* 1996;**46**:77–79.

44 Colonna P, Sorino M, D'Agostino C *et al.* Nonpharmacologic care of heart failure: counseling, dietary restriction, rehabilitation, treatment of sleep apnea, and ultrafiltration. *Am J Cardiol* 2003;**91**:41F–50F.

45 Brater DC. Drug therapy: diuretic therapy. *N Eng J Med* 1998;**339**:387–395.

46 Gheorghiade M, Cody RJ, Francis GS, McKenna WJ, Young JB, Bonow RO. Current medical therapy for advanced heart failure. *Am Heart J* 1998;**135**: S231–S248.

47 Haller H. Diuretics in congestive heart failure: new evidence for old problems. *Nephrol Dial Transplant* 1999;**14**:1358–1360.

48 Kramer EK, Schweda F, Riegger GAJ. Diuretic treatment and diuretic resistance in heart failure. *Am J Med* 1999;**106**:90–96.

49 Neuberg GW, Miller AB, O'Connor CM *et al.* Diuretic resistance predicts mortality in patients with advanced heart failure. *Am Heart J* 2002;**144**: 31–38.

50 Sica DA. Diuretic-related side effects: development and treatment. *J Clin Hypertens* 2004;**6**:532–540.

51 Sliwa K, Norton GR, Kone N *et al.* Impact of initiating carvedilol before angiotensin-converting enzyme inhibitor therapy on cardiac function in newly diagnosed heart failure.[see comment]. *J Am Coll Cardiol* 2004;**44**: 1825–1830.

52 Jong P, Demers C, McKelvie RS, Liu PP. Angiotensin receptor blockers in heart failure: meta-analysis of randomized controlled trials. *J Am Coll Cardiol* 2002;**39**: 463–470.

53 Gring CN, Francis GS. A hard look at angiotensin receptor blockers in heart failure. *J Am Coll Cardiol* 2004;**44**: 1841–1846.

54 Boehmer JP. Device therapy for heart failure. *Am J Cardiol* 2003;**91**:53D–59D.

55 Bansch D, Antz M, Boczor S *et al.* Primary prevention of sudden cardiac death in idiopathic dilated cardiomyopathy: the Cardiomyopathy Trial (CAT). *Circulation* 2002;**105**:1453–1458.

56 Moss AJ, Zareba W, Hall WJ *et al.* Prophylactic implantation of a defibrillator in patients with myocardial infarction and reduced ejection fraction. *N Eng J Med* 2002;**346**:877–883.

57 Stevenson WG, Stevenson LW. Prevention of sudden death in heart failure. *J Cardiovasc Electrophysiol* 2001;**12**:112–114.

58 MacMahon KM, Lip GY. Psychological factors in heart failure: a review of the literature. *Arc Intern Med* 2002;**162**:509–516.

59 Vaccarino V, Kasl SV, Abramson J, Krumholz HM. Depressive symptoms and risk of functional decline and death in patients with heart failure. *J Am Coll Cardiol* 2001;**38**:199–205.

60 Pitt B, Zannad F, Remme W *et al.* The effect of spironolactone on morbidity and mortality in patients with severe heart failure. *N Eng J Med* 1999;**341**:709–717.

61 Pitt B, Remme W, Zannad F *et al.* Eplerenone, an aldosterone-receptor blocker, in patients with left ventricular dysfunction after myocardial infarction. *N Eng J Med* 2003;**348**;1309–1321.

62 Jessup M. Aldosterone blockade and heart failure (Comment). *N Eng J Med* 2003;**348**:1380–1382.

63 Steimle AE, Stevenson LW, Chelimsky-Fallick C *et al.* Sustained hemodynamic efficacy of therapy tailored to reduce filling pressures in survivors with advanced heart failure. *Circulation* 1997;**96**:1165–1172.

64 Gomberg-Maitland M, Baran DA, Fuster V. Treatment of congestive heart failure: guidelines for the primary care physician and the heart failure specialist. *Arc Intern Med* 2001;**161**:342–352.

65 Eichhorn EJ, Gheorghiade M. Digoxin – new perspective on an old drug. *N Eng J Med* 2002;**347**:1394–1395.

66 Rahimtoola SH. Digitalis therapy for patients in clinical heart failure. *Circulation* 2004;**109**:2942–2946.

67 The Digitalis Investigators Group. The effect of digoxin on mortality and morbidity in patients with heart failure. *N Eng J Med* 1997;**336**:525–533.

68 Abraham WT. Cardiac resynchronization therapy: a review of clinical trials and criteria for identifying the appropriate patient. *Rev Cardiovasc Med* 2003;**4**:S30–37.

69 Abraham WT, Fisher WG, Smith AL *et al.* Cardiac resynchronization in chronic heart failure. *N Eng J Med* 2002;**346**:1845–1853.

70 Bradley D, Bradley E, Baughman KL *et al.* Cardiac resynchronization and death from progressive heart failure: a meta-analysis of randomized controlled trials. *JAMA* 2003;**289**:730–740.

71 Bitran D, Merin O, Klutstein MW, Od-Allah S, Shapira N, Silberman S. Mitral valve repair in severe ischemic cardiomyopathy. *J Card Surg* 2001;**16**:79–82.

72 Bolling SF, Smolens IA, Pagani FD. Surgical alternatives for heart failure. *J Heart Lung Transplant* 2001;**20**: 729–733.

73 Gummert JF, Rahmel A, Bucerius J *et al.* Mitral valve repair in patients with end stage cardiomyopathy: who benefits? *Eur J Cardiothorac Surg* 2003;**23**:1017–1022; discussion 1022.

74 Hunt SA. Current status of cardiac transplantation. *JAMA* 1998;**280**:1692–1698.

75 Frazier OH, Rose EA, Oz MC *et al.* Multicenter clinical evaluation of the HeartMate vented electric left ventricular assist system in patients awaiting heart transplantation. *J Thorac Cardiovasc Surg* 2001;**122**:1186–1195.

76 Goldstein D, Oz MC, Rose EA. Implantable left ventricular assist devices. *N Eng J Med* 1998;**339**:1522–1533.

77 Holman WL, Davies JE, Rayburn BK *et al.* Treatment of end-stage heart disease with outpatient ventricular assist devices. *Ann Thorac Surg* 2002;**73**:1489–1493; discussion 1493–1494.

78 Mancini D, Oz M, Beniaminovitz A. Current experience with left ventricular assist devices in patients with congestive heart failure. *Curr Cardiol Rep* 1999;**1**:33–37.

79 Albert NM, Davis M, Young J. Improving the care of patients dying of heart failure. *Cleve Clinic J Med* 2002;**69**:321–328.

# Index

Note: page numbers in *italics* refer to figures, those in **bold** refer to tables.